SAFER SURGERY

Safer Surgery
Analysing Behaviour in the Operating Theatre

RHONA FLIN
University of Aberdeen, UK

&

LUCY MITCHELL
University of Aberdeen, UK

ASHGATE

Published by
Ashgate Publishing Limited
Wey Court East
Union Road
Farnham
Surrey, GU9 7PT
England

Ashgate Publishing Company
Suite 420
101 Cherry Street
Burlington
VT 05401-4405
USA

www.ashgate.com

British Library Cataloguing in Publication Data
Safer surgery : analysing behaviour in the operating
    theatre.
    1. Surgical errors--Prevention. 2. Operating room
    personnel--Psychology. 3. Operating room
    personnel--Evaluation. 4. Teams in the workplace.
    5. Surgical errors.
    I. Flin, Rhona H. II. Mitchell, Lucy.
    617.9-dc22

ISBN: 978-0-7546-7536-5 (hbk); 978-0-7546-9577-6 (ebk)

Library of Congress Cataloging-in-Publication Data
Safer surgery : analysing behaviour in the operating theatre / [edited] by Rhona Flin and
Lucy Mitchell.
    p. cm.
    Includes bibliographical references and index.
    ISBN 978-0-7546-7536-5
    1. Surgical errors--Prevention. 2. Surgery. 3. Operating rooms. I. Flin, Rhona H. II.
Mitchell, Lucy.
    [DNLM: 1. Medical Errors--prevention & control. 2. Surgical Procedures, Operative-
-methods. 3. Accident Prevention. 4. Interprofessional Relations. 5. Operating Rooms.
WO 500 S128 2009]
    RD27.85.S24 2009
    617--dc22

                                                                                    2009004030

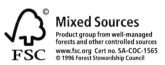

Mixed Sources
Product group from well-managed
forests and other controlled sources
www.fsc.org Cert no. SA-COC-1565
© 1996 Forest Stewardship Council

Printed and bound in Great Britain by
MPG Books Group, UK

Contents

List of Figures

List of Tables

Notes on Contributors

Sonal Arora is a doctor of medicine and a trainee in general surgery, with a further degree in psychology. Her research interests include surgical education and training for patient safety, with a focus upon simulation and non-technical skills training. She is currently completing her PhD, entitled 'Stress, Safety and Surgical Performance.' sonal.arora06@imperial.ac.uk

Bianca Balvert is an OR-nurse specialized in endoscopic surgery in Sint Lucas Andreas Hospital in Amsterdam. She graduated having studied the improvement of OR patient tracking efficiency. She is involved in a patient safety project in collaboration with Erasmus MC. b.balvert@slaz.nl

Jonathan Beard is a consultant vascular surgeon at the Sheffield Vascular Institute, Professor of Surgical Education at the University of Sheffield and Education Tutor at the Royal College of Surgeons of England. He has published widely on surgical skill assessment and helped to develop the Intercollegiate Surgical Curriculum Project. Jonathan.D.Beard@sth.nhs.uk

Doug Bonacum is vice president – safety management for Kaiser Permanente. He leads the development, implementation and monitoring of programme-wide safety management strategies and plans with specific responsibilities for environmental, health and safety, patient safety and clinical risk management. He was formerly responsible for weapons and ships safety as well as nuclear power plant operations in the US Submarine Force. doug.bonacum@kp.org

Benno Bonke is an associate professor of medical psychology at Erasmus University Centre, Rotterdam and was trained as a clinical psychologist and psychotherapist. He is the coordinator of medical education in communication skills and professional behaviour in the core curriculum in Rotterdam. B.Bonke@Erasmusmc.nl

John Brookey is assistant medical director of quality for Southern California Permanente Medical Group, a large multi-specialty group that provides care for over three million Kaiser Permanente health-plan members. He is a paediatrician and practises at the Kaiser Permanente Pasadena Medical Office. john.brookey@kp.org

Cornelius Buerschaper is a management consultant and human factors psychologist specializing in crisis management. He is a team trainer for medical and managerial teams using computer simulated games for safety training and is co-author of *Crisis Management in Acute Care Settings: Human Factors and Team Psychology in a High Stakes Environment* (2007). cornelius.buerschaper@t-online.de

J. Forrest Calland is an assistant professor of surgery in the University of Virginia School of Medicine. His research focuses on outcomes, safety and human factors in high risk environments.calland@viginia.edu

Ken Catchpole is a human factors practitioner in the QRSTU, Nuffield Department of Surgery, University of Oxford. Taking a semi-ethnographic approach to understanding the complex nature of error in healthcare, he seeks to evaluate and improve the safety of surgical systems. Ken.Catchpole@nds.ox.ac.uk

Jim Crossley is senior fellow in the Academic Unit of Medical Education at the University of Sheffield and a consultant paediatrician in Chesterfield. He advises and publishes widely on workplace-based assessment and psychometrics.

Trevor Dale is a human factors training specialist and retired airline training captain. With Guy Hirst he is working with the NHS Institute, The Royal College of Surgeons of England and Oxford University Nuffield Department of Surgery.

Connie Dekker-van Doorn is an RN with a degree in HRD. She is now working on her PhD in collaboration with Delft University of Technology focusing on patient safety and human factors. c.dekker-vandoorn@erasmusmc.nl

Peter Dieckmann is a work and organizational psychologist working with the Danish Institute for Medical Simulation (DIMS) at the Copenhagen University Hospital in Herlev, Denmark. Peter studies the use of simulations for training and research focusing on human factors studies and training of simulation instructors. mail@peter-dieckmann.de.

John Duncan is a consultant general and vascular surgeon at Raigmore Hospital, Inverness. He is Clinical Tutor and member of the Specialist Advisory Board in General Surgery for the Royal College of Surgeons of Edinburgh. john.duncan@haht.scot.nhs.uk

Christoph Eich is consultant paediatric anaesthetist and co-director of the Centre for Education and Simulation in Anaesthesiology, Emergency and Intensive Care Medicine at University Medical Centre Göttingen (Germany). ceich@med.uni-goettingen.de

Li Felländer-Tsai is a professor and senior consultant in orthopaedic surgery. She is the chairperson of the Department of Clinical Science, Intervention and

Technology (CLINTEC) at Karolinska Institutet and the director of the Centre for Advanced Medical Simulation at Karolinska in Stockholm, Sweden. li.tsai@ki.se

Rhona Flin is professor of applied psychology, University of Aberdeen (www.iprc.ac.uk), and she leads the Scottish Patient Safety Research Network (www.spsrn.ac.uk). Her research on safety examines leadership, culture, team skills and decision-making in healthcare and high risk industry.

Kenneth T. Fong is a senior managerial consultant in the Pricing Underwriting Department for Kaiser Permanente's Northern and Southern California regions. Kenneth.t.fong@kp.org

David Gaba is a medical doctor (anaesthesiology), Professor of Anaesthesia and Associate Dean for Immersive and Simulation-based Learning at Stanford University School of Medicine. He is also a Staff Anaesthesiologist at VA Palo Alto Health Care System. gaba@stanford.edu

Fauzia Gardezi is a clinical research project manager at SickKids Learning Institute in Toronto and a research consultant with expertise in qualitative methodology and critical sociology. fauzia.gardezi@utoronto.ca

Emma Giles is a specialist anaesthetist at Sir Charles Gairdner Hospital in Perth, Western Australia. She has a strong interest in teaching and assessing anaesthesia registrars and in patient safety, and is an examiner for ANZCA. emma.k8@gmail. com

Ronnie Glavin is a consultant anaesthetist at the Victoria Infirmary in Glasgow. He also carries out various roles for NHS for Education in Scotland (NES). ronnie. glavin@ggc.scot.nhsuk

Dawn Goodwin is a social science lecturer in medical education. She teaches courses on various aspects of science, technology and medicine to both medical and social science students.

Jodi Graham is a specialist anaesthetist at Sir Charles Gairdner Hospital in Perth, Western Australia. She is a supervisor of anaesthesia training, and her main interests are in education and simulation. jgraham@meddent.uwa.edu.au

Suzanne Graham is director of patient safety for Kaiser Permanente. Suzanne has served in multiple roles within Kaiser Permanente at the medical centre, regional and national levels. She has a BSN in nursing as well as Masters degrees in school health and developmental disabilities from San Francisco State University. Her doctoral degree is from a combined programme at Baylor, University of Texas, and University of Houston. Suzanne.Graham@kp.org

Gudela Grote is professor of work and organizational psychology at the ETH Zurich, Switzerland. She is Associate Editor of the journal *Safety Science* and has consulted on safety management for companies like Swiss Re, Deutsche Bahn AG and the Swiss Nuclear Inspectorate. ggrote@ethz.ch

Stephanie Guerlain is associate professor of systems and information engineering at the University of Virginia, USA. Her research focuses on human–computer interaction, particularly information visualization, training system design and the design of decision support systems. guerlain@virginia.edu

Leif Hedman is a licensed psychologist and associate professor at the Department of Psychology, Umeå University, expert in medical human factors. He is also an affiliated researcher at the Department of Clinical Science, Intervention and Technology (CLINTEC) and the Centre for Advanced Medical Simulation at Karolinska in Stockholm, Sweden. Leif.Hedman@psy.umu.se

Guy Hirst founded Atrainability Limited with Trevor Dale in 2002. He recently retired as a training standards captain from British Airways. Since 2001 he has been involved in several research projects training multidisciplinary teams in various healthcare environments. guy.hirst@atrainability.co.uk

Graham Hocking is a specialist anaesthetist at Sir Charles Gairdner Hospital, Perth, Western Australia. His main interests are research, education and regional anaesthesia.

Gesine Hofinger is a human factors psychologist specializing in patient safety and management of critical incidents. She is a member of the advisory board of the German Coalition for Patient Safety and co-author of *Crisis Management in Acute Care Settings: Human Factors and Team Psychology in a High Stakes Environment* (2007). gesine.hofinger@t-online.de

Steve Howard is an associate professor of anaesthesia at Stanford University School of Medicine and a staff anaesthesiologist at the VA Palo Alto Health Care System. showard@stanford.edu

Robbert Huijsman is part-time professor of management of integrate care at the department of Health Policy and Management of Erasmus University Rotterdam. He combines his scientific work with a partnership in a healthcare consultancy firm (Zorg Consult Nederland).

Rosamond Jacklin is a specialist registrar in general surgery. After graduating from medical school in 2000, Ros undertook basic surgical training and the MRCS, then completed a PhD at Imperial College (2004–2008) entitled 'Judgment and Decision Making in Surgery'. r.jacklin03@imperial.ac.uk

Shelly Jeffcott is a senior research fellow at the NHMRC Centre of Research Excellence in Patient Safety and has a background in psychology and the examination of risk and safety in high hazard industries. Shelly.Jeffcott@med. monash.edu.au

Geert Kazemier is hepatobiliary and transplant surgeon at Erasmus Medical Centre. He is also responsible for the Operating Room Department at that institution. G.kazemier@erasmusmc.nl

Jan Klein is professor of anaesthesiology at the Erasmus University Medical Centre. He developed a special interest in peri-operative patient safety and is the President of the Netherlands Society of Anaesthesiology. j.klein@erasmusmc.nl

Michaela Kolbe is work and organizational psychologist and research assistant at the Organization, Work and Technology Group at ETH Zurich, Switzerland. mkolbe@ethz.ch

Barbara Künzle is work and organizational psychologist and research assistant at the Organization, Work and Technology Group at ETH Zurich, Switzerland. bkuenzle@ethz.ch

Johan Lange is professor of surgery in the department of surgery of the Erasmus University Medical Centre in Rotterdam, the Netherlands. He is Associate Dean of the Faculty of Medicine of the Erasmus University and President of the Committee of Patient Safety of the Dutch Society of Surgery. J.lange@erasmusmc.nl

Robert Lasky is a professor of paediatrics and the director of the Design and Analysis Support Services for the Centre of Clinical Research and Evidence Based Medicine at the University of Texas Medical School at Houston. Robert.E.Lasky@ uth.tmc.edu

Lorelei Lingard is senior scientist in the SickKids Research Institute and the Wilson Centre for Research in Education, University Health Network and University of Toronto. She is the inaugural holder of the BMO Financial Group Professorship in Health Professions Education Research. lorelei.lingard@utoronto.ca

Colin Mackenzie is professor of anaesthesiology and associate professor of physiology at the University of Maryland School of Medicine. His research interests include human factors in emergencies, and trauma resuscitation. He has been continuously funded by Federal grants for the past 18 years. cmack003@ umaryland.edu

Marlene Dyrløv Madsen works at the Danish Institute for Medical Simulation (DIMS) as a researcher in patient safety and safety culture. She has a PhD in patient safety and ethics of patient safety, and holds a Masters in philosophy and communication. mdyrloev@ruc.dk

Tanja Manser is a senior lecturer at the Centre for Organizational and Occupational Sciences, ETH Zurich, where she is heading a research group on human performance and safety in complex systems. tmanser@ethz.ch

Nikki Maran is a consultant anaesthetist in The Royal Infirmary of Edinburgh and Director of the Scottish Clinical Simulation Centre in Stirling. Her interests are in anaesthesia for emergency surgery, education for patient safety and non-technical skills training and assessment.

Joy Marriott is a specialty registrar in obstetrics and gynaecology, currently working towards an MD in surgical education and a Masters of Education at the University of Sheffield. Her research interests include workplace assessment and competency-based selection. Joy.Marriott@sth.nhs.uk

Karen R. Mazzocco is a nurse-attorney with 20 years of experience as a surgical director, primarily at the University of Cincinnati where she achieved her BSN and Juris Doctor. She practised law in hospitals in New York and New Mexico. Since 2001, she worked in research in surgical and perinatal patient safety during affiliations at Kaiser Permanente in California. Currently, she is affiliated with Sharp Healthcare in San Diego, CA, in the evolving field of patient service and satisfaction. karen.mazzocco@sharp.com

Peter McCulloch is clinical reader at the Nuffield Department of Surgery in Oxford. He founded the Quality, Reliability, Safety and Teamwork Unit (QRSTU) in 2005, which focuses on evaluating interventions to improve the functionality of modern healthcare systems. peter.mcculloch@nds.ox.ac.uk

Lisbet Meurling is specialist in anaesthesia and intensive care medicine and participant of the Scandinavian Society of Anaesthesiology training programme in intensive care medicine. She is a PhD student at CLINTEC, Karolinska Institutet. lisbet.meurling@karolinska.se

Ami Mishra is a surgical registrar on the Oxford rotation, whose MD project examined the value of an aviation-style team training approach to improving safety in the operating theatre. He hopes to maintain his research throughout and beyond his training. ami.mishra@nds.ox.ac.uk

Lucy Mitchell is a research assistant in the Industrial Psychology Research Centre, University of Aberdeen, investigating non-technical skills of nurses/scrub practitioners. She previously studied police firearms officers' decision-making skills and was formerly a police officer. l.mitchell@abdn.ac.uk

Maggie Mort is reader in the sociology of science, technology and medicine and co-director of the Centre for Science Studies at Lancaster University, UK. An ethnographer, her research interests include new medical technologies, telehealthcare and disaster recovery. m.mort@lancaster.ac.uk

Michael Müller is consultant anaesthetist at the Hospital of Technical University and Director of Interdisciplinary Medical Simulation Centre, Dresden, Germany. mp-mueller@web.de

David Musson is an assistant professor and Director of the Centre for Simulation-Based Learning at McMaster University in Hamilton, Canada. He received his MD from the University of Western Ontario, and PhD in psychology from the University of Texas at Austin. musson@mcmaster.ca

Andrea Nickut is a research student at the Centre for Education and Simulation in Anaesthesiology, Emergency and Intensive Care Medicine at University Medical Centre Göttingen (Germany). andreanickut@web.de

Simon Paterson-Brown is a consultant general and upper gastro-intestinal surgeon at the Royal Infirmary Edinburgh and an honorary senior lecturer at the University of Edinburgh. Simon.Paterson-Brown@luht.scot.nhs.uk

Rona Patey is a consultant anaesthetist at Aberdeen Royal Infirmary. She is also the Director of the Clinical Skills Centre at Foresterhill and Deputy Head of the University of Aberdeen Division of Medical and Dental Education. r.patey@abdn.ac.uk

Diana Petitti is a physician (preventive medicine) and medical doctor (MD) She is Professor in the Department of Biomedical Informatics in the Fulton School of Engineering at Arizona State University. diana.petitti@asu.edu

David Pitts is a psychologist with a background in management development. He is Project Coordinator of the UK orthopaedic curriculum (OCAP), Associate Director of Leadership and Educational Development at the Royal College of Surgeons of Edinburgh and Education Advisor to the British Orthopaedic Association. d.pitts@rcsed.ac.uk

Catherine Pope is reader in the school of health sciences, University of Southampton. Her research includes evaluations of organizational change and studies of surgical practice. She is currently researching the use of computer decision support in urgent and emergency care, and ambulance handovers.cjp@soton.ac.uk

Helen Purdie is a senior research sister at the Clinical Research Facility in Sheffield. She has also gained surgical experience as a surgical care practitioner (SCP) within the specialties of cardiac and vascular. helen.purdie@sth.nhs.uk

Marcus Rall is an anaesthetist and the director of the Centre for Patient Safety and Simulation (TüPASS) at the University of Tuebingen, Germany. Marcus is leading the two incident reporting systems and PaSOS. Marcus.rall@med.uni-tuebingen. de

Silke Reddersen is anaesthetist at Tuebingen University Hospital, Germany. She works for the Tuebingen Centre for Patient Safety and Simulation with an emphasis on in-situ trainings, instructor training and the German Incident Reporting systems PaSIS and PaSOS. silke.reddersen@freenet.de

Glenn Regehr is Richard and Elizabeth Currie Chair in Health Professions Education Research, Professor and Senior Scientist at the Wilson Centre for Research in Education, University Health Network and University of Toronto. g.regehr@utoronto.ca

David Rowley is an orthopaedic surgeon. He is Director of Education at the Royal College of Surgeons of Edinburgh as well as Visiting Professor of Surgery at Edinburgh University, and Emeritus Professor at Dundee University. d.i.rowley@ dundee.ac.uk

Nick Sevdalis is an experimental psychologist. Initially a post-doctoral researcher in the Imperial Department of Surgery (2004–2006), Nick was appointed Lecturer in Patient Safety (2006 to the present) – with two years spent jointly in Imperial and the National Patient Safety Agency (2006–2008). Nick investigates non-technical skills/teamwork in surgery. n.sevdalis@imperial.ac.uk

J. Bryan Sexton is a psychologist by training and is the Director of Safety Culture Research and Practice at the Johns Hopkins Quality and Safety Research Group. He has collected culture data in over 2000 hospitals, in 15 countries.

Andrew Smith is a consultant anaesthetist at the Royal Lancaster Infirmary and Honorary Professor of Clinical Anaesthesia at Lancaster University, UK. He has a strong interest in risk, safety and professional expertise in anaesthesia. andrew. f.smith@mbht.nhs.uk

Arnd Timmermann is consultant anaesthetist and co-director of the Centre for Education and Simulation in Anaesthesiology, Emergency and Intensive Care Medicine at University Medical Centre Göttingen (Germany). atimmer@med. uni-goettingen.de

Eric Thomas is a professor of medicine at the University of Texas – Houston Medical School and Director of the UT-Houston Memorial Hermann Center for Healthcare Quality and Safety. He studies several aspects of patient safety including diagnostic errors, teamwork and safety culture. Eric.Thomas@uth.tmc. edu

Paul Uhlig is a cardiothoracic surgeon and associate professor in the Department of Preventive Medicine and Public Health at the University of Kansas, School of Medicine – Wichita in Wichita, Kansas. His area of special expertise is social architecture in healthcare and methods for transformation of healthcare practice culture.

Shabnam Undre is a doctor of medicine and is a trainee in urology. She recently completed her PhD, 'Teamwork in the Operating Theatre', at Imperial College and is involved in various research projects for assessing and improving teamwork in surgery.

Charles Vincent trained as a clinical psychologist and has conducted research on risk management, medical error and patient safety in a number of settings. He is currently Director of the Centre for Patient Safety and Service Quality at Imperial College Academic Health Sciences Centre. c.vincent@imperial.ac.uk

Bart Vrouenraets is a surgeon working at the Department of Surgery at Sint Lucas Andreas Hospital in Amsterdam. His specialities are surgical oncology and general surgery. bc.vrouenraets@slaz.nl

Johannes Wacker is a board-certified specialist in anaesthesiology FMH and is working as a consultant anaesthetist at the Department of Anaesthesia, University Hospital Zurich, Zurich, Switzerland. johannes.wacker@usz.ch; http://www. anaesthesie.usz.ch

Carl-Johan Wallin is senior consultant in anaesthesia and intensive care medicine, Diplomate of the European Academy of Anaesthesiology (DEAA) and PhD in medical sciences. He is Director of Training at the Department of Anaesthesiology and Intensive Care at Karolinska University Hospital Huddinge, and the manager of the Division of Advanced Patient Simulation, Centre for Advanced Medical Simulation at Karolinska in Stockholm, Sweden. carl-johan. wallin@ki.se

Linda Wauben is an engineer working on her PhD in a collaborative project with the Erasmus MC and Delft University of Technology focusing on human factors. l.s.g.l.wauben@tudelft.nl

Theo Wehner is a professor and holds the Chair of Work and Organizational Psychology at the ETH Zurich's Department of Management, Technology and Economics. He specializes in human error, experiences and knowledge management. twehner@ethz.ch

Sarah Whyte worked for five years as a research coordinator in the operating room. She is currently a doctoral candidate in English Language and Literature at the University of Waterloo and a doctoral fellow at the Wilson Centre in Toronto, Canada. sarah.whyte@utoronto.ca

Yan Xiao is associate professor of anaesthesiology and director for research in patient safety at University of Maryland. He authored over 60 journal articles in the areas of patient safety including coordination, team performance, and technology enhanced performance. yxiao@maryland.edu

George Youngson is professor of paediatric surgery at Royal Aberdeen Children's Hospital. His other interests are surgical education and advising government on healthcare strategy. He is chairman of the Patient Safety Board at the Royal College of Surgeons of Edinburgh. ggyrach@abdn.ac.uk

Steven Yule is a lecturer in psychology at the University of Aberdeen with background training in human factors. His research is on psychological aspects of behaviour and safety in high-risk organizations, especially leadership and non-technical skills in surgery. www.abdn.ac.uk/~psy296/dept

Enikö Zala-Mezö is work and organizational psychologist, lecturer and researcher at Zurich University of Applied Sciences, Zurich, Switzerland. enikoe.zala@phzh.ch

Foreword

Charles Vincent

What could a background in psychology, medical error and safety bring to surgery and what would surgeons, anaesthetists and nurses make of patient safety? These were the questions that faced me when I moved, in 2002, from a department of psychology to a department of surgery. Initially I read the surgical literature to see how safety was approached. The journals were full of descriptions of the complex technicalities of operative procedure and of the influence of co-morbidities and risk factors on patient outcome. From the safety point of view, there was pioneering work on human factors and crisis training in anaesthesia and some impressive work on surgical skills. However, very little had been written on topics that would appear fundamental to safe surgery such as the nature of error and systems, teamwork, decision-making, the working environment, culture and all the other staples of the safety world. It was puzzling, and rather worrying, that the safety point of view and the surgical literature seemed so divergent.

Even more puzzling however was that the surgical literature did not seem to accord with the daily experience of clinicians. My colleagues were generous in explaining the challenges of their work; I watched and listened. Technical issues, risk factors and so on were certainly critical. However, their stories of the operating theatre revolved around difficult decisions, equipment problems, teams that just failed to gel, the difficulty of bringing a team together during a crisis, the way the wider hospital impacted on the operating theatre and so on … in fact a litany of classic safety issues. None of this appeared to be reflected in the surgical journals or in surgical research.

The chapters in this book mark the huge progress that has been made over the last five years in broadening the scope of research on the factors that create safety in the operating theatre and beyond. The issues that nurses, anaesthetists and surgeons have always dealt with, talked about and suffered are now regarded as worthy of serious study and recognized as being critical to safe care. The chapters are, both individually and collectively, extraordinarily rich and it would be pointless to anticipate the detailed arguments in a foreword. However, it is perhaps worth reflecting on some of the major themes of these studies which, to my mind, underpin the progress that has been made.

First, it is worth recalling that studies of clinical work, particularly on error and safety, can arouse considerable suspicion and even hostility between clinicians and researchers. In contrast, as the Edinburgh meeting made clear, these research teams are grounded in trust, mutual respect and the desire to work together for safer healthcare. This collaborative and optimistic spirit infuses the studies described and also, I believe, accounts for the richness and depth of understanding achieved across disciplines.

Second, these studies show a considerable sophistication in the development of measures. There is of course due attention to methodology and technical issues, but also recognition of the subtleties of teamwork and that communication does not only have to be recorded but also understood. Even silence may have multiple meanings, which will not be apparent to the casual observer. A researcher might take years to fully understand this environment and the meaning of such communications, but a team of researchers and clinicians can together reveal the nuances and subtleties.

Third, the studies almost all concern safety and yet are not dominated by the issue of error. These researchers are concerned to understand how safety is created and eroded in the fluid interplay of clinical work. Certainly, both clinicians and researchers need to understand failure and the many hazards of the operating theatre; but the study of failure is in a sense only a necessary step in the more general quest to understand how success is achieved and how safety can be gained or lost in a moment.

Finally, these studies carry lessons beyond their immediate focus. Although this book is apparently confined to the operating theatre, it points to much wider themes of relevance to safety in healthcare. Many authors speak, directly or indirectly, of the wider influences on teamwork in the operating theatre and the need to address these issues if theatre teams are to reach their full potential. These issues include staffing levels, organizational constraints and trade-offs, failure to train in teams, inter-professional rivalries, and the difficulties of engaging staff in safety procedures. In this sense the operating theatre, and the mirror these studies hold to it, is a microcosm of the healthcare system. If you read this book you will learn a great deal about the operating theatre, but also a great deal about the progress and challenges of patient safety across the whole of healthcare.

Preface

George Youngson

Since the primitive beginnings of operative surgery, surgeons have had a need to work with assistance, even if it was, in those early times, merely for the purposes of physical restraint. As surgical and anaesthetic practice became more sophisticated, so were the tasks becoming more complex and the demand on the surgical team ever increasing. It is only recently, however, with surgery becoming an ever more complex and technology-based clinical science that the dynamic and interaction between all members of the surgical team has become more important and seen as an element that contributes to a successful outcome or not as the case may be. As the severity of illness being treated increases and potency of the therapeutic surgical tools becoming ever greater, so does the risk of the treatment and the potential for harm. The safety of patients and their continued well-being while under operative care is therefore not a recent nor novel concern – but there is a new and increasing recognition of the need for a standardized approach to communication, leadership and teamworking in the operating theatre, if the team is to work at maximum efficiency and if error of understanding and performance between individual team members is to be avoided.

The Royal College of Surgeons of Edinburgh (RCSEd) has a long tradition of trying to build upon surgical standards of care and to further promote safe surgical practice; it has created a specific forum around which both technical but also nontechnical aspects of operative performance can be researched, discussed and developed. The Patient Safety Board of the College has formed out of developmental research on non-technical skills utilized by surgeons during their operative performance. Working in concert with the University of Aberdeen and surgeons in Edinburgh, Dundee, Aberdeen and Inverness a more scholastic approach to the recognition, development and teaching of non-technical skills during operative surgery has evolved.

The need for a better appreciation of the potential benefits and hazards accruing from interpersonal behaviours and the cognitive performance of the surgeon, as well as his/her ability to execute the technical tasks with precision and care, requires a different approach, a new way of thinking, a new language and way of speaking.

The RCSEd was therefore delighted to play host to this international workshop involving researchers in the human factors involved in surgery from across the globe. The college itself had organized the 'Advancing Patient Safety in Surgery' (APSIS) conference the previous day, which had set the scene for a paradigm shift in the way that surgeons lead, follow, communicate, act and think. This book is therefore a welcome contribution to the understanding of team performance in the operating theatre and how I, as surgeon, can maximize the contributions of those around me, at the same time ensuring my performance is to the best of my abilities in pursuit of the optimal outcome for my patient.

Chapter 1
Introduction

Rhona Flin and Lucy Mitchell

Background

This book is designed to present a state-of-the-art perspective on a new area of psychological and medical research where social scientists are engaged with clinicians in collaborative projects to study surgical teams at work in hospital operating theatres. Their goal is to improve understanding of the factors shaping safe and efficient operative performance. Given the importance of anaesthetic, theatre nursing and surgical tasks for patient safety during an operation, it is surprising how little scientific investigation of working life has taken place in this domain. There are very few reports of the culture and behaviour patterns in surgical and anaesthesia units, apart from some accounts from sociologists (Bosk 1979, Hindmarsh and Pilnick 2002, Millman 1976), journalists (Ruhlman 2003) and personal recollections from surgeons (e.g. Conley 1998, Miller 2009, Weston 2009). These provide rich descriptions of an unusual workplace, powerful professional cultures, considerable technical expertise and behaviours not always conducive for patient safety. Adverse events for surgical patients are undesirable but do sometimes happen (Manuel and Nora 2005). The Chief Medical Officer for England recently stated:

> Surgery has seen rapid improvements in recent years: however errors do still occur. Further improvements will need a more detailed understanding of the prevalence of harm, a change in culture and the use of innovative new tools, such as surgical checklists. (Donaldson 2008, p. 27)

Yet, compared to other high risk industrial settings, hardly any systematic research into workers' behaviour has been carried out in the hazardous task environment of the operating theatre. High risk workplaces do not provide the easiest of research subjects but they are an important domain for psychological research, as Wilpert (1996, p. 78) noted:

> Psychology in high hazard organizations is an unusual conception, a field which is only gingerly approached by our discipline. It requires a drastic expansion of received theoretical frameworks and demands incisive steps towards interdisciplinary cooperation. Barriers to more intensive involvement exist inside and outside psychology. Nevertheless enough theoretical and practical

– even survival – reasons exist for psychologists not to pass up the challenge of helping to contribute to safety and reliability of high hazard systems.

The chapters in this volume have been prepared by clinicians, research psychologists and other social scientists, working with clinicians in an attempt to develop our understanding of the behaviours of anaesthetists, surgeons, nurses and co-workers in the operating theatre and their consequences for patients. This unique collection is the result of a scientific meeting which was organized by the Industrial Psychology Research Centre of the University of Aberdeen and was sponsored by the Royal College of Surgeons of Edinburgh who hosted the event in November 2007. Research teams who were investigating the behaviour of operating theatre personnel were invited to participate and somewhat to our surprise (having anticipated that only a few UK delegates would take part), representatives from teams based in Australia, Canada, Denmark, Germany, Netherlands, Sweden, Switzerland and the USA also decided to attend. Travelling across the world in the middle of the northern winter for a one day meeting in Edinburgh was not possible for all those invited. Fortunately, three of the North American teams who could not be at the meeting, agreed to contribute chapters describing their latest work

Our aim in organizing the meeting was to provide an opportunity for researchers to exchange information on theoretical and methodological approaches suited to carrying out psychological investigations in the operating theatre, as well as to share emerging findings. The material presented demonstrated the range and quality of some of the most innovative and significant research being conducted in the service of surgical safety (the original presentations are available on www. abdn.ac.uk/iprc). The day was a considerable success with too little time for an adequate exchange or scientific discussion but a tantalizing array of data and methods was revealed. In an effort to capture the shared knowledge presented at this first gathering of operating theatre behavioural researchers, we decided (and acknowledge a suggestive email message from Andy Smith, author of Chapter 15) to produce this edited book.

Overview

The chapters to follow represent different conceptual approaches to the study of behaviour in operating theatres and they are typically describing work which has been published very recently or is still in progress. In some cases, authors are outlining their ideas for studies that are currently under development. They were all encouraged to provide full references to illustrate the supporting evidence for their theories and methods and, where possible, to include examples or sources for the measurement tools they were using to study behaviour.

Opening prefaces and closing commentaries have been contributed by surgeons, anaesthetists and psychologists, reflecting the multidisciplinary nature of the rest of the book. In Part I, Chapters 2 to 10 describe the latest research with new measurement tools that have been designed to record and rate the behaviours and skills of individuals and/ or teams when working in the anaesthetic room or the operating theatre. Many of these instruments, being developed for behavioural measurement and training in anaesthesia and surgery, have their roots in aviation practices. Part II, consisting of Chapters 11–24, presents a broader range of different kinds of observational studies of theatre teams or individual clinicians in action during the induction or recovery from anaesthesia or engaged in surgical operations. Chapter 25, by Musson, one of the very few physicians with a Ph.D. in aviation psychology, offers a cautionary perspective on the risks for medicine of generalizing too readily from the world of aviation.

We hope this collection will prove to be a valuable resource for both practitioners and researchers in their endeavours to improve safety for surgical patients.

Acknowledgements

We are particularly grateful for the support offered by Professors Rowley and Youngson of the Royal College of Surgeons of Edinburgh in offering to host the first scientific meeting of this new research community. A second, and equally beneficial, meeting was held at Oxford University in July 2008, hosted by Mr Peter McCulloch and Dr Ken Catchpole. The papers from that meeting are available from: <www.surgery.ox.ac.uk/research/qrstu/International%20workshop>.

Our thanks go to Guy Loft at Ashgate for all his support and advice during the preparation of this volume, and to all those who contributed chapters; we are specially appreciative of all the expert help we received from Wendy Booth in transforming multiple idiosyncratic interpretations of the Ashgate style manual into a coherent typescript.

References

Bosk, C. (1979) *Forgive and Remember: Managing Medical Failure.* Chicago: University of Chicago Press.

Conley, F. (1998) *Walking out on the Boys.* New York: Farrar, Straus and Giroux.

Donaldson, L. (2008) While you were sleeping. Making surgery safer. In *Chief Medical Officer's Report for England and Wales.* London: Department of Health, 27–33.

Hindmarsh, J. and Pilnick, A. (2002) The tacit order of teamwork: Collaboration and embodied conduct in anaesthesia. *Sociological Quarterly* 43, 139–64.

Manuel, B. and Nora, P. (2005) (eds) *Surgical Patient Safety.* Chicago: American College of Surgeons.

Miller, C. (2009) *The Making of a Surgeon in the 21st Century.* Nevada City, CA: Blue Dolphin.

Millman, M. (1976) *The Unkindest Cut. Life in the Backrooms of Medicine.* New York: Morrow Quill.

Ruhlman, M. (2003) *Walk on Water. Inside an Elite Paediatric Unit.* New York: Viking.

Weston, G. (2009) *Direct Red. A Surgeon's Story.* London: Jonathan Cape.

Wilpert, B. (1996) Psychology in high hazard systems: Contribution to safety and reliability. In J. Georgas, M. Manthouli, E. Besevegis and A. Kokkevi (eds) *Contemporary Psychology in Europe. Proceedings of the IVth European Congress of Psychology.* Seattle, WA: Hogrefe and Huber.

PART I
Tools for Measuring Behaviour in the Operating Theatre

Chapter 2

Development and Evaluation of the NOTSS Behaviour Rating System for Intraoperative Surgery (2003–2008)

Steven Yule, Rhona Flin, Nikki Maran, David Rowley, George Youngson, John Duncan and Simon Paterson-Brown

Introduction

In 2002, a number of surgeons in Scotland were intrigued by the development of the ANTS (Anaesthetists' Non-Technical Skills) system and the use of behaviour rating checklists in other industries such as nuclear power and civil aviation. There was a realization in the healthcare and medical literature that adverse events occurred in the operating theatre. Surgeons and their patients have also had to come to terms with the uncovering and analysis of the true nature and extent of surgical misadventure and failure. Ten years ago, it was not generally realized that a significant number of surgical patients were harmed not as a result of underlying illness or disease but as a result of their treatment (Vincent et al. 2001). Further analysis of this problem revealed that non-technical aspects of performance play a contributory role in the multifaceted nature of surgical adverse events; failures in decision-making, teamwork, coordination and leadership have all emerged from case reviews and studies of behaviour in the operating theatre (Gawande et al. 2003, Studdert et al. 2006, Christian et al. 2006). Non-technical skills are defined as the critical cognitive and interpersonal skills that complement surgeons' technical ability (Yule et al. 2006a). Despite the fact that the behavioural (Baldwin et al. 1999) and cognitive demands of surgery have been recognized as a critical part of surgical performance (Hall et al. 2002, Jacklin et al. 2008), and that effective leadership has been shown to improve team performance (Edmondson 2003), non-technical skills are often referred to as 'non-operative' and deemed not as important as clinical science in the surgical literature. Scant attention has been paid to the cognitive and social processes that underpin intra-operative performance in training as well: training and assessment in these skills are only conducted in a rather tacit and discretionary basis, and the surgical curriculum in the UK does not yet extend to non-technical skills.

Amid this backdrop, the surgical profession has also been rapidly changing to cope with internal and external pressures such as the European Working Time Directive, which restricts the working week to 48 hours; the challenges of new professional roles such as nurse practitioners (Kneebone and Darzi 2005), the modernization of training and education including Medical Training Application Service (MTAS) and new technology. These changes mean that trainees have fewer training opportunities than their trainers had, before reaching consultant level, so there is now a greater need to maximize the available learning opportunities.

Changes to the configuration of surgical training and education are currently underway in the UK to attempt to streamline development of doctors and ensure that they are skilled at communicating and working as effective members of a team. This approach recommends that progress through and completion of surgical training be based on competence; it has moved the emphasis of assessment away from set-piece examinations of knowledge towards learning and assessment of skills in the workplace (see Pitts and Rowley, Chapter 3 of this volume). Selection of trainees into surgical specialties has also been radically altered and provides an opportunity to formalize the role of non-technical skills in surgical education and assessment.

The main methods of workplace-based assessment of surgical trainees in the UK are observational tools which cover skills such as ability to work in a multi-professional team (Mini-PAT: Peer Assessment Tool) and communication (Mini-CEX: Clinical Evaluation Exercise). However, these tools are for the assessment of perioperative skills, often using interactions with patients as a basis for assessment. This is to be encouraged, but the skills assessed do not necessarily relate to those required for working with other professionals during a surgical procedure, commonly with an anaesthetized patient. The systems that are used to assess trainees' intra-operative competence, such as surgical DOPS (Direct Observation of Procedural Skills) and Procedure Based Assessment (PBA) are focused almost entirely on technical ability. However PBAs, which are written for specific index procedures, sometimes integrate non-technical aspects (see in this volume Chapter 3 by Pitts and Rowley, Chapter 4 by Marriott et al.).

The cognitive and social skills which underpin clinical and technical proficiency are recognized as requirements for surgical competency and rank highly as core competencies within organizations such as CanMeds (Frank 2005), the General Medical Council (GMC 2001), and the Royal Colleges of Surgeons in the UK (Youngson 2000, Giddings and Williamson 2007) but until recently there were no tools to reliably assess these skills in the workplace. To begin to address this, a behavioural observation and rating system called NOTSS (Non-Technical Skills for Surgeons) was developed and tested under funding from the Royal College of Surgeons of Edinburgh and NHS Education for Scotland, from 2003 to 2007. This chapter outlines the development and evaluation of the NOTSS system. Like similar systems in civil aviation and anaesthesia, the behaviour rating system was based on a skills taxonomy which was developed with subject matter experts.

NOTSS Project Design

The project was run by the University of Aberdeen, with a multidisciplinary steering group of surgeons, psychologists and an anaesthetist. The research drew on previous work in Scotland on surgical competence, professionalism and the skills surgeons required to operate safely and followed on from a similar project which developed a behaviour rating system for anaesthetists – the ANTS system (Fletcher et al. 2004, see Chapter 11 in this volume by Glavin and Patey). The aim of the NOTSS project was to develop and test an educational system for assessment and training based on observed skills in the intra-operative phase of surgery. The system was developed from the bottom up with subject matter experts (consultant surgeons), instead of adapting existing frameworks used in other industries. It was considered important to recognize and understand the unique aspects of non-technical skills in surgery, and not to assume that those non-technical skills identified for pilots, nuclear power controllers or anaesthetists would be exactly mirrored in, or be relevant to, surgery. The NOTSS system is in surgical language for suitably trained surgeons to observe, rate and provide feedback on non-technical skills in a structured manner. An adaptation of Gordon's (1993) model of systems design was used to guide the iterative development of NOTSS.

   This three-phase model maps the process from task analysis through system design to evaluation. The phases relate to the three objectives set by the NOTSS steering group in 2003: to identify the relevant non-technical skills required by surgeons, to develop a system to allow surgeons to rate these skills, and to test the system for reliability and usability. A fourth phase was added to cover a trial in the operating theatre using NOTSS to debrief surgical trainees over the course of an attachment (see Figure 2.1).

Phase 1: Task Analysis

In Phase 1 we used three main methods to collect data on individual surgeons' intra-operative non-technical skills, as follows:

1. Literature review on surgeons' non-technical skills (Yule et al. 2006a).
2. Survey of theatre personnel attitudes to teamwork, error and safety (Flin et al. 2006a).
3. Critical incident interviews with subject matter experts (Yule et al. 2006b).

   These methods were supported by field notes taken during observation sessions in the operating theatre during operative surgery and a review of surgical adverse event and mortality reports.

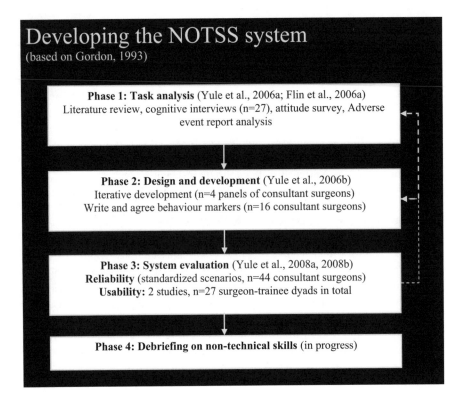

Developing the NOTSS system
(based on Gordon, 1993)

Phase 1: Task analysis (Yule et al., 2006a; Flin et al., 2006a)
Literature review, cognitive interviews (n=27), attitude survey, Adverse event report analysis

Phase 2: Design and development (Yule et al., 2006b)
Iterative development (n=4 panels of consultant surgeons)
Write and agree behaviour markers (n=16 consultant surgeons)

Phase 3: System evaluation (Yule et al., 2008a, 2008b)
Reliability (standardized scenarios, n=44 consultant surgeons)
Usability: 2 studies, n=27 surgeon-trainee dyads in total

Phase 4: Debriefing on non-technical skills (in progress)

Figure 2.1   Developing the NOTSS system

Literature Review

The aims of the literature review (Yule et al. 2006a) were to examine the surgical and psychological literature on surgeons' intra-operative non-technical skills in order to (i) identify the non-technical skills required by surgeons in the operating theatre, and (ii) assess the behavioural marker systems that have been developed for rating surgeons' non-technical skills. In order to achieve this, we searched the literature using defined search terms and a set of inclusion criteria. Databases searched included BioMed Central, Medline, Web-of-Knowledge, PsychLit, and ScienceDirect. Relevant studies were organized according to the source material used. This yielded published research from observational studies, questionnaires and interviews, adverse event analyses and papers on surgical education (including curricula and standards of competence). Within these, the review highlighted the main non-technical skill categories to be: anticipation, decision-making, teamworking, leadership and communication. At the time of the review (August 2005), there were three research tools in the literature which could be used to measure surgeons' non-technical skills. On closer examination, these existing frameworks were found to be deficient either in terms of their psychometric properties or suitability for assessing individual surgeons rather than a surgical team in theatre. On the basis of this review, we concluded that further research was required to develop a taxonomy of individual surgeons' non-technical skills for training and feedback.

Attitude Survey (ORMAQ)

The literature review highlighted the lack of basic data on cognitive and social skills in surgeons, and little was known about prevailing attitudes to teamwork and safety in the operating theatre. Attitude surveys of theatre personnel had been conducted in other countries and can provide useful diagnostic information relating to behaviour and safety in surgical units. There were no such data available in Scotland, so as part of our initial task analysis, we ran a baseline survey (Flin et al. 2006a) using a version of the Operating Room Management Attitudes Questionnaire (ORMAQ), initially developed by Helmreich et al. (1997) to assess surgical team members' attitudes to safety and teamwork in operating theatres. The ORMAQ was adapted from an instrument measuring pilots' safety attitudes in aviation. At the time (late 2005), it was the most extensively used attitudes questionnaire with operating theatre personnel with data collected from Israel, USA, Germany, Switzerland and Italy (Helmreich and Schaefer 1994, Helmreich and Davies 1996, Sexton et al. 2000). It was not clear to what extent these earlier findings would generalize to a British sample but the questionnaire topics of leadership, teamwork, stress and fatigue and error were shown to be relevant from our literature review. The ORMAQ was modified for language only by a panel of consultant surgeons and was distributed to surgical teams in 17 hospitals in Scotland. A total of 352 responses were analysed, 138 from consultant surgeons (response rate: 47 per cent), 93 from trainee surgeons (27 per cent) and 121 from theatre nurses (19 per cent). Respondents generally demonstrated positive attitudes to behaviours associated with effective teamwork and safety. Attitudes indicating a belief in personal invulnerability to stress and fatigue were evident in both nurses and surgeons. Consultant surgeons had more positive views on the quality of surgical leadership and communication in theatre than trainees and theatre nurses. While the ubiquity of human error was well recognized, attitudes to error management strategies (incident reporting, procedural compliance) suggest that they may not be fully functioning across hospitals. While theatre staff placed a clear priority on patient safety, against other business objectives (e.g., waiting lists, cost cutting), not all of them felt that this was endorsed by their hospital management. Discrepancies were found between the views of consultants compared to trainees and nurses, in relation to leadership and teamwork. While attitudes to safety were generally positive, there were several areas where theatre staff did not seem to appreciate the impact of psychological factors on technical performance. These results were taken into consideration in the design of the NOTSS system.

Observations

To provide context and meaning for the literature review and interviews, a psychology researcher conducted observations of surgical cases. Observations were made at three hospitals in a variety of specialisms: general, orthopaedic and cardiac surgery. No formal method was used for structuring observations because we did not want to narrow the observer's data collection at this stage. Field notes were taken. The observer also shadowed surgeons in the perioperative environment to understand how this stage impacted on operative performance. During this phase of the project, detailed field notes revealed that surgeons displayed a range of non-technical skills, communication was variable and there often seemed to be conflicting priorities between training and service delivery. There was no standard method of conducting a given operation, the atmosphere or climate in the operating theatre would change depending on which surgeon was operating that day, and the number of people in the operating theatre ranged from four to eighteen. In comparison with other industries, the formal work procedures, if they existed, were not explicit. Team members seemed to start critical tasks such as commencing the anaesthetic, positioning the patient and making the first incision to start the operation without speaking to other members. Often operations would start without critical team members in the operating theatre and without all the information being present. Distractions seemed to be commonplace and normal; on several occasions the operating surgeon had to answer questions about another ongoing operation or speak to someone on the telephone while in the middle of what appeared to be a complex part of the operation for which he or she was scrubbed. Despite all this, the observers were struck by how well the surgeon and the team performed under those circumstances. As with any observation study, it was not possible to plan to see surgeons perform under stress or to analyse surgical adverse events in a systematic manner during live cases. For this, we selected other methods, as will be discussed below.

Adverse Event and Mortality Reviews

The systematic analysis of near misses, incidents and accidents is an essential diagnostic process for safety management in industry (Reason 1997) and we thought that these data sets in surgery could provide us with a rich source of information on error and surgical failings that would credibly fit into the skills analysis for NOTSS. Surgical colleagues indicated that data were not usually collected on non-technical skills, so this would be a short task. In the end, we reviewed the Scottish Audit of Surgical Mortality (SASM) reports from 2001 (SASM 2003) and commented on them in the literature review. The nature of data fed back to individual hospitals and in case assessments highlights that SASM is strong on providing technical feedback and on reporting the proximal causes of error but provides relatively little in the way of human factors information and therefore offered limited insight into non-technical skills in surgery. There are two likely causes of this: (i) the forms used to collect data do not adequately capture human factors or non-technical contributions to incidents, and (ii) the coding framework used to analyse the incident reports does not adequately deal with non-technical skills. A similar situation emerged in the analyses of anaesthetic adverse event reports for the ANTS project (Fletcher et al. 2004). These conditions explain the current technical (e.g., what happened) bias in published audit reports in favour of non-technical (e.g., why it happened) causes of adverse events. The SASM forms since 2007 include non-technical skills categories.

Critical Incident Interviews

The critical incident technique (CIT) is a type of cognitive interview (Crandall et al. 2006, Flanagan 1954, Hoffmann et al. 1998) used to identify tacit knowledge about the way an expert manages a stressful or non-routine situation at work. CITs were conducted with 27 consultant surgeons in order to identify non-technical skills used by surgeons in the intra-operative environment. By focusing on a specific memorable incident, the interviews provided insight into the surgeon's use of information, strategies, meta-cognition, resources and interpersonal skills during an operative case (Yule et al. 2006b; see also Fletcher et al. (2004) who used this technique with anaesthetists). To summarize the method, surgeons were asked to recall events in theatre during a challenging, non-routine case and were probed about the course of events a further two times. After the surgeon described the case, the interviewer recounted the sequence of events back to the surgeon and asked for clarification and more explanation of the course of events. This second sweep of the case allowed for more detail to be gleaned. The case was then discussed for a third time with the addition of cognitive cues which recreate aspects of the case to elicit deeper-held tacit knowledge about the non-technical skills that were or were not being used. Examples of the cognitive cues used include: 'what cues were you using to help understand the situation' and 'how did you re-establish goals?' The interview questions were developed by a multidisciplinary group, based on work in other domains including anaesthesia and piloted with three consultant surgeons. The sample of surgeons interviewed were consultant surgeons (n=27) from 11 hospitals in Scotland in general surgery (n=13), orthopaedic surgery (n=10) and cardiac surgery (n=4). One of the participants was female. A variety of cases were discussed in the interviews which lasted around one hour each, including emergencies with duodenal ulcers, difficulties in hip and knee replacements, problems in transplant operations and difficulties with cardiac bypass. The interview transcripts were analysed using the line-by-line coding technique from grounded theory (Glaser and Strauss 1967) in order to explore the data and aid system development. Coders were asked to identify when non-technical skills were discussed in the interview and to interpret those specific skills. Three pairs of psychologists who were experienced at coding interview transcripts each coded six transcripts independently to an acceptable level of inter-rater reliability before the remaining transcripts were then coded. This process produced a list of 150 unsorted non-technical skills such as 'coordinates the team', and 'confirms understanding with assistant' as raw input data for system development in phase 2.

Phase 2: Development of the NOTSS System

The goal of Phase 2 was to develop a system that could be used by surgeons to rate other surgeons' behaviours *in vivo* in the operating theatre rather than to develop a comprehensive taxonomy or research instrument. The tri-level hierarchical format used for behavioural marker systems in anaesthesia (Fletcher et al. 2004) and European civil aviation (Flin et al. 2003) was adopted. This format structures skills into category and element levels with observable behaviours (markers) indicative of good and poor performance for each element. The prototype system was developed in three stages to (i) refine the skill set that emerged from phase 1, (ii) sort those skills into a skills taxonomy, and (iii) identify observable behaviours that were indicative of each skill in the taxonomy.

The aim of Stage 1 was to refine the skills that emerged from Phase 1 and remove duplication without diluting the conceptual breadth of the skills that emerged from the task analysis. This process was to form the basis of the system. To achieve this, the multidisciplinary research group reduced and refined the list of 150 skills extracted from the transcripts, considering the results of the literature review, survey, and observations in theatre. The skills taxonomy was developed according to design criteria derived from the JARTEL (Joint Aviation Requirements: Translation and Elaboration of Legislation) project (Flin et al. 2003), an expert panel on behavioural markers (Klampfer et al. 2001) and from Cognitive Task Analysis (Seamster et al. 1997).[1] The reduced skills list was then thematically organized and broad categories emerged broken down into component elements.

In Stage 2, an iterative process was used with four independent panels of consultant surgeons from four hospitals, who modified the structure into a skills taxonomy. The panels checked the wording and labelling of elements, and ensured that the framework was relevant to the surgical domain. This formed the basis for the behavioural marker system.

In stage three, observable behaviours (markers) indicative of good and poor performance were developed for each element by 16 consultant surgeons. The surgeons were asked to think of behaviours that could be either directly observed or inferred through communication. Two subsequent multidisciplinary review meetings refined this set of illustrative behaviours, all phrased as active verbs. This ensured that the system had cognitive and interpersonal functionality, was grounded in surgery, and complied with the guidelines on system design (Gordon 1993) and criteria for development of behavioural markers mentioned earlier.

---

1   See Table 1 in Yule et al. (2006b) for the full set of design criteria.

The NOTSS Rating Scale

The aim of the system is to allow surgeons to rate skills they observe. After considering the possible rating scale formats, a four-point scale was chosen, as follows: 4 good, 3 acceptable, 2 marginal, 1 poor, and N/A not applicable. The 'not applicable rating' applies when the behaviour was not required in a given clinical scenario. If the skill should have been observed but was not, then a rating of 1 (poor) should be given. Behaviours which potentially endanger patient safety should also be given this rating.

Phase 3: System Evaluation

The aim of Phase 3 was to evaluate the NOTSS v1.1 system, specifically to assess its psychometric properties of (i) sensitivity, (ii) inter-rater reliability, and (iii) internal structure and consistency. To exert some control over the evaluation and stimuli used, we used a pseudo-experimental design which involved 44 consultant surgeons rating standardized video clips of surgeons' intraoperative behaviour. To achieve this we filmed eleven video scenarios illustrating a range of surgeons' non-technical skills in general and orthopaedic surgery. The scenarios were filmed using a patient simulator in operating rooms with practising surgeons, anaesthetists and nurses acting the main roles. The scenarios were designed by surgeons, anaesthetists and psychologists who were experienced in non-technical skills training. From these, three scenarios were selected for training and six for the evaluation, the longest of which ran for 5 minutes and 40 seconds. The participating surgeons attended a half-day training session on how to use the NOTSS system, with some guidance on behaviour rating (Baker et al. 2001). They were instructed to watch each scenario and to rate the observed skills of the consultant surgeon using the NOTSS rating form. Participants were informed of the simulated nature of the scenarios.

Table 2.1 shows the criteria for each of the evaluation metrics used in this study and the corresponding results. For more details on the evaluation see Yule et al. (2008a) and Yule et al. (2009). This table shows that the system was moderately sensitive, but operated best when observers had to make a decision regarding whether the behaviour was acceptable or not. Within-group agreement was acceptable for the interpersonal skill categories but below acceptable criteria for cognitive skills. Internal reliability was high with an overall mean difference of 0.25 scale points between categories and elements.

There were also differences in the way the scenarios were rated, two scenarios yielded either floor or ceiling ratings as the behaviours were explicitly good or poor, and other scenarios displayed more ambiguous behaviours and were rated in the mid-range of the scale. Orthopaedic surgeons were found to agree on rated behaviours significantly more than general surgeons (Yule et al. 2008a).

Table 2.1   **Summary of NOTSS v1.1 evaluation results (see Yule et al. 2008a for detailed results)**

Type of evaluation	Why it is important	How calculated and criteria	Result of test
Sensitivity	This is a measure of how accurate the group of raters are in absolute ratings of behaviour compared with reference ratings	Mean number of scale point difference between raters and reference, represented as a decimal, usually <1	Mean sensitivity across all categories was .67
Within-group agreement (r_{wg})[18]	This is a measure of statistical agreement between a number of raters. In this study, it represents the degree to which the groups of participants agree on the absolute ratings they give to behaviours in the scenarios that reflect the NOTSS categories and elements	Scores lie between 0 (no agreement) and 1 (perfect agreement); scores above .7 are deemed acceptable. r_{wg} was calculated for the NOTSS categories and elements ratings for each of the 6 experimental groups	r_{wg} exceeded the criteria of >.7 for two categories: Leadership and Communication & Teamwork. r_{wg} for Decision-making and Task Management approached the criterion but the value of r_{wg} for Situation Awareness was .51
Internal reliability	There should be a high degree of consistency between the category rating and the ratings for the two or three underpinning elements due to conceptual overlap	The mean absolute difference between raters' element ratings and their rating for the corresponding category. Lower scores (tending to zero) indicate closer agreement	Mean difference for all categories was < 0.25 of a scale point between elements and category on a 4-point scale. Consistency between category and element deemed very high for all categories

On the basis of the evaluation a number of changes were made to the taxonomy, the most important being the removal of 'Task Management'. This was done because conceptually, many of the task management behaviours were actually more reflective of situation awareness; some reliability tests did not reach an acceptable threshold for the category and practically, removing a category and elements from the taxonomy reduced the cognitive load for raters who have a finite capacity for holding a number of categories and elements in working memory while engaged in a real-time observation and rating task (Yule et al. 2008a). This produced the NOTSS taxonomy version 1.2 (see Figure 2.2).

Category	Element
Situation Awareness	Gathering information Understanding information Projecting and anticipating future state
Decision-making	Considering options Selecting and communicating option Implementing and reviewing decisions
Communication and Teamwork	Exchanging information Establishing a shared understanding Coordinating team
Leadership	Setting and maintaining standards Supporting others Coping with pressure

Figure 2.2   NOTSS skills taxonomy v1.2

The NOTSS v1.2 Handbook

A user handbook (Flin et al. 2006b) was then written which contained background information on the development of NOTSS, advice for using system in clinical practice, definitions and behavioural examples of the NOTSS categories and elements, a set of rating forms for users, indicative good and poor behaviours for each element, and advice on how to use the rating scale. Practical tips to aid surgeons embed non-technical skills observations into clinical practice were included, as was advice for surgical trainers planning to use NOTSS with higher surgical trainees.

Phase 4: System Usability

A follow-up study was conducted to evaluate system usability with 22 surgical trainers and their trainees from three Scottish hospitals. The trainers were asked to use the NOTSS rating form and supporting handbook to rate and provide feedback to trainees as soon as possible after each of ten cases where the trainee had contributed significantly to the operation. Inguinal hernia repair and laparoscopic cholecystectomy were typical operations observed during this trial but it was recommended that specific use of NOTSS be determined by the educational needs of the trainees. For example, with junior trainees, the focus of training is on developing basic surgical expertise, so it was advised that the NOTSS system be used for general discussion of non-technical skills and their importance to clinical practice. For more senior trainees such as specialist registrars (SpRs), it was suggested that the NOTSS system be used to rate skills and provide feedback during increasingly challenging cases.

Most of the consultant surgeons had been trained to use the system in the three-hour group session for the system evaluation study reported previously. Those who did not participate in this session were given the same training course in a one-to-one setting. Trainees attended an information session about non-technical skills and the usability trial at their hospital. During this session, it was explained that the NOTSS system has been designed to aid the development of professional skills and that we were evaluating the system rather than assessing their skills during the study. An online post-trial questionnaire was used to establish if using NOTSS was of any value as an adjunct to the currently available surgical education and assessment methods. An initial invitation to complete it was followed up with a reminder after one month and a further reminder a month later. Self-report measures were selected as the most appropriate method of gathering data on user experiences although are not without limitations, as such data are by their nature subjective, and susceptible to memory decay and social desirability bias.

In total, eleven consultant surgeons completed the usability trial. Data on trainee surgeons were not tracked (to ensure that they were confident that the purpose of the study was solely to assess the usability of the tool, rather than their own competence) but analysis of completed feedback forms indicate that at least 12 trainees took part. The NOTSS system was used to observe and debrief on non-technical skills during a total of 43 cases (mean 4 per consultant, range 1–8 cases). In all cases, the trainee was lead surgeon. In some cases the consultant was an unscrubbed observer and on other occasions was scrubbed and assisting as well as observing. The majority of trainers (90 per cent) thought that they had received enough training to use the system and preferred to conduct the debrief immediately after the operation (81 per cent) in the operating theatre suite. The median length of debrief session was 3–5 minutes. See Figure 2.3 for an example of a NOTSS rating card completed after a laparoscopic cholecystectomy which mainly focused on the trainee's ability to gather information about the patient, communicate decisions to the team and work with the assistant and consultant surgeon in a coordinated manner.

All trainers used 'communication & teamwork', 90 per cent used 'situation awareness', 72 per cent used decision-making, and just over half (54 per cent) used the leadership category. Some categories were not used by some trainers due to the level of the trainee and the complexity of the procedure being completed. The majority of surgical trainers thought that the NOTSS system was useful for debriefing trainees and a valuable adjunct to currently available assessment tools. The trainers were all in agreement that NOTSS provided a common language to discuss non-technical skills and was useful to support reflective practice, but there were mixed opinions regarding the ease of rating non-technical skills. Although 45 per cent of trainers agreed that cognitive and interpersonal skills were easy

Hospital .... Trainer name .... Date ....

Trainee name .... JT .... Operation .... Lap chole ....

Category	Category rating*	Element	Element rating*	Feedback on performance and debriefing notes
Situation Awareness	3	Gathering information	2	Needs to get full history before sedating pt.
		Understanding information	4	Recognised common bile duct
		Projecting and anticipating future state	3	Think ahead more – ask scrub nurse for kit up in advance
Decision Making	3	Considering options	3	Discussed potential approaches
		Selecting and communicating option	2	Made appropriate decisions but needs to comm – them more to the team
		Implementing and reviewing decisions	3	
Communication and Teamwork	2	Exchanging information	2	Did not brief team at start of op
		Establishing a shared understanding	2	Stopped several times to adjust camera but did not tell assistant what was trying to achieve
		Co-ordinating team activities	2	
Leadership	3	Setting and maintaining standards	4	Was scrubbed + sterility rules respected
		Supporting others	3	Did not guide novice scrub nurse
		Coping with pressure	3	Kept calm but you were starting to 'clam up' – talk more about what is happening!

* 1 Poor; 2 Marginal; 3 Acceptable; 4 Good; N/A Not Applicable

1 Poor	Performance endangered or potentially endangered patient safety, serious remediation is required
2 Marginal	Performance indicated cause for concern, considerable improvement is needed
3 Acceptable	Performance was of a satisfactory standard but could be improved
4 Good	Performance was of a consistently high standard, enhancing patient safety; it could be used as a positive example for others
N/A	Not Applicable

NOTSS was funded by the Royal College of Surgeons of Edinburgh and NHS Education for Scotland

Figure 2.3 Completed NOTSS rating form

to rate, 27 per cent found interpersonal skills difficult to rate compared with only 9 per cent who felt cognitive skills were difficult to rate (Yule et al. 2008b). The remaining trainers were ambivalent regarding ease of rating. Time can be a precious commodity in the operating theatre but only 9 per cent of trainers thought using NOTSS to debrief added too much time to their operating list and 73 per cent thought that routine use of NOTSS would enhance safety in the operating theatre. All trainers thought that NOTSS has a place in surgical education and assessment. Comments from trainers indicated that positive aspects of the system for surgical education were the transparent structure; common language; ability to objectively assess skills; framework for providing feedback; ease of use in real-life situations, and that using the system made time to discuss aspects of surgical performance that are 'usually ignored'. Although some trainers reported no difficulties rating behaviours using NOTSS, four main problems were articulated. These related to understanding some descriptors in the NOTSS handbook; selecting an appropriate trainee and case; observing and rating behaviours while also scrubbed, and an over-reliance on communication to infer cognitive skills.

Discussion

The aims of the NOTSS project was to develop and evaluate a behavioural marker system for surgeons' non-technical skills using human factors methods and basing the system development and associated rating scale on a skills taxonomy. These aims were met and the prototype NOTSS system is being used by practising surgeons and research groups in Australasia, Japan, Europe, and North America. Further development of the tool is required and there remain some unanswered questions such as the amount of training required for a practising surgeon to be able to use the tool reliably, and whether observations and ratings have to be made by surgeons (as opposed to anaesthetists, nurses or even psychologists) to be valid and meaningful. A research group at Sheffield (see Chapter 4 of this volume) are attempting to answer some of these questions. Other research teams have developed tools to observe and rate the behaviours of surgical teams (Undre et al. 2007 – Imperial College) or have adapted the NOTECHS tool from civil aviation (Flin et al. 2003) for use with surgeons in operating theatre (Sevdalis et al. 2008 – Imperial College, Mishra et al. 2008 – University of Oxford). These lines of research differ in concept and approach but nonetheless enrich our understanding of non-technical skills in surgery.

The focus of surgical training still heavily favours technical skill acquisition, yet surgeons increasingly operate in teams with whom they may be unfamiliar, especially in an emergency setting. The adoption of specific training in non-technical areas of expertise is still done on an ad hoc basis although the Royal Colleges of Surgery in Great Britain and Ireland all provide training in this emerging area to some extent. These courses have so far been taken by enthusiastic surgeons, both consultant and trainee but are not compulsory aspects of surgical training. The Royal College of Surgeons of Ireland however, provides funding for all trainee surgeons to attend a human factors training course. As part of the NOTSS evaluation, it emerged that training in using the system was not sufficient for many users as they did not have background knowledge in psychology and human factors. Therefore, we developed and ran training courses for surgeons, introducing human factors and the basics of workplace assessment of behaviour. This developed into a two-day course, specifically on the NOTSS system in 2006, run with the Royal College of Surgeons of Edinburgh. This course was then further developed to include wider surgical safety issues to become the SOS (Safer Operative Surgery) courses which were run in 2007. These courses were designed for higher trainee and consultant surgeons only and were based on task analysis of surgeons' non-technical skills, the NOTSS behaviour rating system, and underlying psychology (Flin et al. 2007). In 2008/09 the Royal College of Surgeons of Edinburgh is developing these courses for a multidisciplinary audience.

The Future of Non-Technical Skills in Surgical Education

Although not formally achieved yet, the future of surgical training will need to encompass more than just clinical and technical skills (Davidson 2002). If the aviation model was to be adopted in surgery then experienced consultant surgeons would be taken off clinical work for a period to concentrate on assessing other consultants' non-technical skills. Assessments would be done using a framework such as NOTSS to rate observable skills in a simulated environment and during real cases in the operating theatre (similar to LOSA checks in aviation, see Chapter 25 in this volume by Musson). The assessors would be trained, calibrated, and their competence to rate others assured at an acceptable *a priori* level. Crucially, the assessments would be 'high stakes' and surgeons would have to pass the assessment by displaying appropriate behaviours in order to continue operative surgery. Surgeons who did not pass would be able to attend a remedial training course for those skills requiring attention. This would require courses to be developed (e.g., Flin et al. 2007), and the surgeon to then be assessed at a future point before being allowed back into clinical practice. This process would apply to consultant surgeons although senior trainee surgeons would be assessed and given feedback on their non-technical skills as part of their ongoing training and may have to pass a non-technical skills assessment as part of the selection process into consultant grades. Research teams may be involved in the training and assurance of assessors, instructors and practising surgeons, and would be interested in the development of measures of behaviour and performance.

This model may not be appropriate for surgery and competence assessment at this time, but in the near future, recertification will be introduced as a part of revalidation, which will require global assessment of professional performance including the skills referred to above. Moreover there are some promising advancements: research teams are developing, validating and collecting data with observational tools, appraisals are commonplace, and the introduction of Procedure-Based Assessment (PBAs) has demonstrated that there is more to surgery than technical skills, and that workplace assessment is the method by which consultant surgeons of the future will be assessed. Perhaps as important is that in some hospitals non-technical language is becoming common parlance both intra-operatively and in the coffee room. However, the surgeons who use behaviour rating scales and discuss non-technical skills with their trainees are still in the minority. In order for widespread change in practice, a trigger is required, such as official endorsement by the Postgraduate Medical Education and Training Board (PMETB) or the Intercollegiate Surgical Curriculum Programme (ISCP), or inclusion in the processes of revalidation of doctors which is currently being discussed.

The Future of NOTSS Research: Integrating Systemic Issues in the Operating Theatre

NOTSS has been widely cited in the clinical literature, adopted by professional bodies for training, and the system is being used by other research groups around the world. However, a reliance solely on individual skills or even those of the surgical team will not achieve the levels of safety required by patients. Feedback from users of the NOTSS system indicated that aspects of surgery such as scheduling, anaesthetic care, competence and experience of other staff, availability of equipment in theatre, new technology and training also have an impact on surgical performance and surgical outcomes. Attention to these components from systems-based thinking have been found to be particularly useful in understanding and improving the safety and reliability of complex systems in other high consequence industries such as power generation and aviation (Perrow 1999). There is emerging research on the impact of distractions (Sevdalis et al. 2007) and latent failures (Catchpole et al. 2007) on patient safety in the operating theatre, and tools for understanding the systemic causes of adverse events in the operating theatre (Taylor-Adams and Vincent 2004) but we do not yet have a complete understanding of the systems aspects that affect patient safety.

The Accreditation Council for Graduate Medical Education in the USA explicitly demands that resident trainee surgeons obtain specific knowledge, skills and attributes to demonstrate 'systems-based practice' (ACGME, 2007). Professional skills training needs to incorporate content on systems thinking in order to meet the demands of modern surgery, and this content should be based on research evidence. In addition to the dangers that systems pose for safety, there are also strengths embedded in surgical systems that make surgeons and surgical teams resilient in the face of dynamic, error-producing conditions. A new project, funded by the Royal College of Surgeons of Edinburgh is attempting to make these aspects of the surgical system explicit and measurable. With this research strategy, in time we will understand more about individual skills, the role of the team and how they interact with the system to protect or harm patients, and have evidence-based tools and training to support the surgeons of the future.

References

ACGME (2007) *Common Program Requirements: General Competencies* Accreditation Counsel for Graduate Medical Education. Available from: <www.acgme.org/outcome/comp/GeneralCompetenciesStandards21307.pdf> [accessed October 2008].

Baldwin, P.J., Paisley, A.M. and Paterson-Brown, S. (1999) Consultant surgeons' opinions of the skills required of basic surgical trainees. *British Journal of Surgery* 86, 1078–82.

Baker, D., Mulqueen, C. and Dismukes, R. (2001) Training raters to assess resource management skills. In E. Salas, C. Bowers and E. Edens (eds), *Improving Teamwork in Organizations*. New Jersey: LEA, 131–45.

Catchpole, K.R., Giddings, A.E.B., Wilkinson, M., Hirst, G., Dale, T. and de Leval, M. (2007) Improving patient safety by identifying latent failures in successful operations. *Surgery* 142, 102–10.

Christian, C., Gustafson, M., Roth, E., Sheridan T., Gandhi, T., Dwyer, K., Zinner, M. and Dierks, M. (2006) A prospective study of patient safety in the operating room. *Surgery* 139, 159–73.

Crandall, B., Klein, G. and Hoffman, R. (2006) *Working Minds: A Practitioner's Guide to Cognitive Task Analysis*. Boston: MIT Press.

Davidson, P. (2002) The surgeon of the future and implications for training. *ANZ Journal of Surgery* 72, 822–8.

Edmondson, A.C. (2003) Speaking up in the operating room: How team leaders promote learning in interdisciplinary action teams. *Journal of Management Studies* 40(6), 1419–52.

Flanagan, J. (1954) The critical incident technique. *Psychological Bulletin* 51, 327–58.

Fletcher, G., Flin, R., McGeorge, P., Glavin, R., Maran, N. and Patey, R. (2004) Rating non-technical skills: Developing a behavioural marker system for use in anaesthesia. *Cognition Technology and Work* 6, 165–71.

Flin, R., Goeters, K., Amalberti, R., et al. (2003) The development of the NOTECHS system for evaluating pilots' CRM skills. *Human Factors and Aerospace Safety* 3, 95–117.

Flin, R., Yule, S., McKenzie, L., Paterson-Brown, S. and Maran, N. (2006a) Attitudes to teamwork and safety in the operating theatre. *The Surgeon* 4, 145–51.

Flin, R., Yule, S., Paterson-Brown, S., Maran, N. and Rowley, D. (2006b) *The Non-Technical Skills for Surgeons (NOTSS) System Handbook (v1.2)*. Available at: <www.abdn.ac.uk/iprc/notss>

Flin, R., Yule, S., Paterson-Brown, S., Maran, N., Rowley, D.R. and Youngson, G.G. (2007) Teaching surgeons about non-technical skills. *The Surgeon* 5(2), 86–9.

Frank, J.R. (ed.) (2005) The CanMEDS 2005 Physician Competency Framework. Better Standards. Better Physicians. Better Care. Ottawa: The Royal College of Physicians and Surgeons of Canada.

Gawande, A.A., Zinner, M.J., Studdert, D.M. and Brennan, T.A. (2003) Analysis of errors reported by surgeons at three teaching hospitals. *Surgery* 133, 614–21.

Giddings, A.E.B. and Williamson, C. (2007) *The Leadership and Management of Surgical Teams*. London: The Royal College of Surgeons of England.

Glaser, B.G. and Strauss, A.L. (1967) *The Discovery of Grounded Theory*. Chicago: Aldine.

GMC (2001) *Good Medical Practice*. London: General Medical Council.

Gordon, S.E. (1993) Systematic Training Programme Design: Maximizing Effectiveness and Minimizing Liability. Englewood Cliffs, NJ: Prentice Hall.

Hall, J.C., Ellis, C. and Hamdorf, J. (2002) Surgeons and cognitive processes. *British Journal of Surgery* 90, 10–16.

Helmreich, R. and Davies, J. (1996) Human factors in the operating room: Interpersonal determinants of safety, efficiency and morale. In A. Aikenhead (ed.) *Balliere's Clinical Anaesthesiology* 10(2), 277–95.

Helmreich, R. and Schaefer, H. (1994) Team performance in the operating room. In M. Bogner (ed.) *Human Error in Medicine*. Hillsdale, NJ: LEA, 225–53.

Helmreich, R., Sexton, B. and Merritt, A. (1997) The Operating Room Management Attitudes Questionnaire (ORMAQ). *University of Texas Aerospace Crew Research Project Technical Report 97-6*. Austin, TX: The University of Texas.

Hoffmann, R., Crandall, B., and Shadbolt, N. (1998) A case study in cognitive task analysis methodology: The Critical Decision Method for the elicitation of expert knowledge. *Human Factors* 40, 254–76.

Jacklin, R., Sevdalis, N., Darzi, A. and Vincent, C. (2008) Mapping surgical practice decision making: An interview study to evaluate decisions in surgical care. *The American Journal of Surgery*, 195, 689–96.

Kneebone, R. and Darzi, A. (2005) New professional roles in surgery. *British Medical Journal* 330, 803–804.

Klampfer, B., Flin, R., Helmreich, R.L., Hausler, R., Sexton, B., Fletcher, G., et al. (2001) Group Interaction in High Risk Environments: Enhancing Performance in High Risk Environments, Recommendations for the use of Behavioural Markers. Berlin: GIHRE. Available on <www.abdn.ac.uk/iprc> [last accessed November 2008].

Mishra, K., Catchpole, K., Dale, T. and McCulloch, P. (2008) The influence of non-technical performance on technical outcome in laparoscopic cholecystectomy. *Surgical Endoscopy* 22, 68–73.

Perrow, C. (1999) *Normal Accidents: Living with High-risk Technologies.* Princeton, NJ: Princeton University Press.

Reason, J.T. (1997) Managing the Risks of Organizational Accidents. Aldershot: Ashgate.

SASM (2003) Scottish Audit of Surgical Mortality Annual Report – 2001 data. Glasgow: SASM.

Seamster, T., Redding, R. and Kaempf, G. (1997) *Applied Cognitive Task Analysis in Aviation.* Aldershot: Avebury.

Sevdalis, N., Healey, A.N. and Vincent, C.A. (2007) Distracting communications in the operating theatre. *Journal of Evaluation in Clinical Practice* 13, 390–4

Sevdalis, N., Davis, R., Koutantji, M., Undre, S., Darzi, A. and Vincent, C.A. (2008) Reliability of a revised NOTECHS scale for use in surgical teams. *The American Journal of Surgery* 196, 184–90.

Sexton, B., Thomas, E. and Helmreich, R. (2000) Error, stress, and teamwork in medicine and aviation: Cross sectional surveys. *British Medical Journal* 320, 745–9.

Studdert, D.M., Mello, M.M., Gawande, A.A., et al. (2006) Claims, errors, and compensation payments in medical malpractice litigation. *The New England Journal of Medicine* 354, 2024–33.

Taylor-Adams, S. and Vincent, C. (2004) Systems analysis of clinical incidents: The London protocol. *Clinical Risk* 10, 211–20.

Undre, S., Sevdalis, N., Healey, A.N., Darzi, A. and Vincent, C. (2007) Observational Teamwork Assessment for Surgery (OTAS): Refinement and application in urological surgery. *World Journal of Surgery* 31, 1373–81.

Vincent, C.A., Neale, G. and Woloshynowych, M. (2001) Adverse events in British hospitals: Preliminary restrospective record review. *British Journal of Medicine* 322, 517–19.

Youngson, G.G. (2000) *Surgical Competence: Acquisition, Measurement, and Retention.* Edinburgh: The Royal College of Surgeons of Edinburgh.

Yule, S., Flin, R., Paterson-Brown, S. and Maran, N. (2006a) Non-technical skills for surgeons: A review of the literature. *Surgery* 139, 140–9.

Yule, S., Flin, R., Paterson-Brown, S., Maran, N. and Rowley, D. (2006b) Development of a rating system for surgeons' non-technical skills. *Medical Education* 40, 1098–104.

Yule, S., Flin, R., Maran, N., Rowley, D. R., Youngson, G.G. and Paterson-Brown, S. (2008a) Surgeons' non-technical skills in the operating room: Reliability testing of the NOTSS behaviour rating system. *World Journal of Surgery* 32, 548–56.

Yule, S., Flin, R., Rowley, D., Mitchell, A., Youngson, G.G., Maran, N. and Paterson-Brown, S. (2008b) Debriefing surgical trainees on non-technical skills (NOTSS). *Cognition, Technology & Work* 10, 265–74.

Yule, S., Rowley, D., Flin, R., Maran, N., Youngson, G.G., Duncan, J. and Paterson-Brown, S. (2009) Experience matters: Comparing novice and expert ratings of non-technical skills using the NOTSS system. *Australian Journal of Surgery* 79, 154–160.

Chapter 3

Competence Evaluation in Orthopaedics – A 'Bottom-up' Approach

David Pitts and David Rowley

Introduction

The design and implementation of what we now know as Procedure Based Assessments (PBAs) began in the UK in the early 1990s. In 2008, PBAs are in use in all UK surgical specialties, embedded in all surgical curricula as the primary tool for evaluating perioperative competence in the middle and later years of surgical training. The motivation driving their development has been practical problem solving. In this respect their development has much in common with other 'need pull' innovations (Langrish et al. 1972) in that their wider foundations can only be seen retrospectively and although they have much in common with other surgical assessments, their early development occurred completely independently.

PBAs have been developed and introduced against a backdrop of transition in surgical training. Their development has involved not only the design of an assessment tool but also the battle to gain acceptance of the concept and practice of overt competence evaluation in the surgical workplace. This chapter describes the evolution of PBAs from instigation to practical usage and describes ongoing evaluation of the outcome in terms of the instrument and its use.

Surgical Training in Transition

Since the early 1990s UK surgical training has been in a state of constant transition. Not only have the regulations governing training changed radically but the political, social and healthcare environments in which training occurs have swung between extremes. A review of some of these changes will show why gaining acceptance by the surgical community for the use of a competence assessment tool such as the PBA has been so vital.

Changes in Structure and Regulation

Until the publication of the Calman Report (Department of Health 1993), surgical training in the UK involved a lengthy apprenticeship punctuated by knowledge tests but without any assessment of practical skills and no formal requirement to address non-technical areas such as communication or teamwork. Although the Calman reforms introduced some degree of structure, it was not until the Richards Report of 1997 (Richards 1997) and the subsequent report of the Competence Working Party of the Joint Committee for Higher Surgical Training (JCHST) in 2001 (Rowley et al. 2002) that assessments of practical ability or competence were openly recommended.

> Royal Colleges should give serious consideration to establishing innovative procedures, other than written exit examinations, to assess clinical competence of candidates for the award of a certificate of Completion of Specialist Training. (Richards 1997)

> It is essential that trainers and trainees extend their assessment of operative and clinical performance. Speciality Advisory Committees (SACs) in surgery should determine which operations should occur and to what extent, and what level of operative ability is required for a given stage of training. Simply recording a minimum number of operations is insufficient – the quality of the training experience is more important than the number of experiences. (Rowley et al. 2002: 21)

Following the publication of *Unfinished Business* (Donaldson 2002), a report on the current state of training, further reforms were introduced and the 'Modernizing Medical Careers' project coincided with the inception of the Postgraduate Medical Education and Training Board (PMETB) in 2003 which insisted on the introduction of comprehensive curricula for each specialty and principles established whereby regular assessment of practical skills was encouraged. PMETB's key task has been to establish standards defining medical education, training and assessment and to assure these standards (including competence based curricula) through external management of quality.

The Trauma and Orthopaedics surgical curriculum (the first time such a document has been produced in the specialty in the UK), in which competence-based training and assessment were enshrined, was approved by PMETB in September 2006 (Pitts et al. 2007). PBAs have been introduced against this changing structural backdrop.

Changes in Public Attitude

There is no doubt that the public attitude towards medicine in general, and to surgery in particular, has changed. This change was most notably precipitated by the Bristol (Kennedy 2001) and Shipman (Smith 2005) inquiries into high death rates in paediatric surgery and general practice respectively. High mortality rates in the Bristol Paediatric Cardiac Unit resulted in action from the Department of Health in 1994 and the suspension of operating in that unit in 1995. The subsequent inquiry's report into that unit (Kennedy 2001) coincided with the very public trial and eventual incarceration of Harold Shipman, a general practitioner, for actions resulting in the deaths of a number of his patients. The Shipman Inquiry, reporting from 2002–2005 (Smith 2005), revealed serious shortfalls in processes and procedures surrounding the use of controlled drugs, certification of death and the monitoring of clinical performance stretching back, in Shipman's case, to his time as a medical trainee. The Donaldson White Paper in 2007, for new revalidation processes in the UK for clinicians and other medical professionals (Department of Health 2007), has been one of the longer-term outcomes of the Shipman Inquiry which will undoubtedly culminate in the use of PBAs or similar tools in the revalidation process.

Changes in Time Available for Training

The European Working Time Directive introduced in 1998 reduced the number of hours a trainee might stay in the workplace to 58 in 2004 and are likely to reduce those hours further, to 48 in 2009. There have undoubtedly been benefits from this directive but it has significantly reduced the access to surgical experience for trainees, particularly with respect to unusual trauma cases arriving out of normal working hours.

Changes in Service Delivery

Recent years have seen the growth of Independent Sector Treatment Centres (ISTC). Such centres, normally operating outwith the control of NHS local management, have been used to reduce waiting lists, particularly for common surgical procedures conducted on anaesthetically less challenging patients. This has further reduced the access to routine surgical experience, particularly for more junior trainees.

PBAs have been developed against this background of sudden and discontinuous change with reduced access to surgical experience necessitating the introduction of training tools that help to derive maximum benefit from the time available. Facilitating positive change in such circumstances is (and always has been) difficult.

> The innovator has for enemies those who did well under the old system and only faint friends in those who might do well under the new (Machiavelli 1515, Chapter VI)

What is a PBA?

A PBA is a collection of behavioural markers (elements) for observing activities around a surgical operation set in seven domains covering the whole of a surgical procedure from consent to post operative management.

A PBA is a formal, structured assessment of a trainee's competence in performing surgery. An individual PBA provides a formative assessment to the trainee and evidence for the trainer on which to base their future input and level of supervision. A collection of PBAs (assembled over several years, conducted by a variety of trainers) provides summative evidence of the trainee's progress and competence in learning surgical procedures and techniques, performing them to the required protocol and quality.

A PBA happens in real time, in a real operating theatre with a live patient. It is normally undertaken, without pressure, between a trainee and their trainer (with whom a relationship is already established) surrounded by an operating team who will not take any unusual measures to support the trainee. A PBA will not normally be conducted on the first occasion a trainer and trainee operate together. It is normally conducted on a procedure with which the trainee is already familiar. There is no limit to the number of times a trainee may attempt a particular PBA so there is no pressure to succeed on a particular occasion. All of these conditions help the trainee to give a 'normal' performance and, more importantly, protect the patient.

PBAs in Practice – Applying the Seven Domains

Table 3.1   PBA domains

1.	Consent
2.	Pre-operative planning
3.	Pre-operative preparation
4.	Exposure and closure
5.	Intra-operative technique
6.	Post-operative management
7.	Global summary

Within each domain there are a number of related yet unique elements which identify activities which must be performed successfully in order to achieve a 'satisfactory' score. Most elements are identical across all procedures but in some domains there is opportunity for procedure-specific items which identify the trainee's grasp of the unique aspects of particular surgical procedures. Table 3.2 illustrates both generic and specific items.

Although superficially the structure of a PBA resembles a two-page checklist (see Figure 3.1) a PBA is not a schedule of how to perform the procedure, rather it identifies places in the procedure where competence is observable. In the same

Table 3.2 Example elements for total hip replacement PBA, taken from T&O curriculum (Pitts et al. 2007)

	Competencies and definitions	Score N/U/S	Comments
	Intra-operative technique		
IT1	Follows an agreed, logical sequence or protocol for the procedure		
IT2	Consistently handles tissue well with minimal damage		
IT3	Controls bleeding promptly by an appropriate method		
IT4	Demonstrates a sound technique of knots and sutures/ staples		
IT5	Uses instruments appropriately and safely		
IT6	Proceeds at appropriate pace with economy of movement		
IT7	Anticipates and responds appropriately to variation e.g. anatomy		
IT8	Deals calmly and effectively with untoward events/ complications		
IT9	Uses assistant(s) to the best advantage at all times		
IT10	Communicates clearly and consistently with the scrub team		
IT11	Communicates clearly and consistently with the anaesthetist		
IT12	Dislocates hip safely		
IT13	Cuts femoral neck appropriately to match design of implant		
IT14	Demonstrates familiarity and understanding of acetabular preparation including osteophyte trimming medially and at rim		
IT15	Broaches the femur properly and prepares the bony surface		
IT16	Uses trials and checks component orientation properly		
IT17	Fix acetabular component appropriately		
IT18	Implants femoral component appropriately		
IT19	Performs final reduction and checks for stability		

Trauma & Orthopaedics PBA 6: Total Hip Replacement [07 03 06]
APPROVED SURGICAL TEMPLATE Feb 06

Trainee:	Assessor:	Date:
Start time:	End time:	Duration:

Operation more difficult than usual? Yes / No (if yes, state reason)

Score: N = Not observed or not appropriate   U = Unsatisfactory   S = Satisfactory

Competencies and Definitions	Score N/U/S	Comments
I. Consent		
C1 Demonstrates sound knowledge of indications and contraindications including alternatives to surgery		
C2 Demonstrates awareness of sequelae of operative or non operative management		
C3 Demonstrates sound knowledge of complications of surgery		
C4 Explains the perioperative process to the patient and/or relatives or carers and checks understanding		
C5 Explains likely outcome and time to recovery and checks investigations		
II. Pre operative planning		
PL1 Ensures recognition of anatomical and pathological abnormalities (and relevant co-morbidities) and selects appropriate operative strategies/techniques to deal with these e.g. nutritional status		
PL2 Demonstrates ability to make reasoned choice of appropriate equipment, materials or devices (if any) taking into account appropriate investigations e.g. x-rays		
PL3 Checks materials, equipment and device requirements with operating room staff		
PL4 Ensures the operation site is marked where applicable		
PL5 Checks patient records, personally reviews investigations		
III. Pre operative preparation		
PR1 Checks in theatre that consent has been obtained		
PR2 Gives effective briefing to theatre team		
PR3 Ensures proper and safe positioning of the patient on the operating table		
PR4 Demonstrates careful skin preparation		
PR5 Demonstrates careful draping of the patient's operative field		
PR6 Ensures general equipment and materials are deployed safely (e.g. catheter, diathermy)		
PR7 Ensures appropriate drugs administered		
PR8 Arranges for and deploys supporting specialist equipment (e.g. image intensifiers) effectively		
IV. Exposure and closure		
E1 Demonstrates knowledge of optimum skin incision / portal / access		
E2 Achieves an adequate exposure through purposeful dissection in correct tissue planes and identifies all structures correctly		
E3 Completes a sound wound repair where appropriate		
E4 Protects the wound with dressings, splints and drains where appropriate		

Competencies and Definitions	Score N/U/S	Comments
V. Intra Operative Technique		
IT1 Follows an agreed, logical sequence or protocol for the procedure		
IT2 Consistently handles tissue well with minimal damage		
IT3 Controls bleeding promptly by an appropriate method		
IT4 Demonstrates a sound technique of knots and sutures/staples		
IT5 Uses instruments appropriately and safely		
IT6 Proceeds at appropriate pace with economy of movement		
IT7 Anticipates and responds appropriately to variation e.g. anatomy		
IT8 Deals calmly and effectively with untoward events/complications		
IT9 Uses assistant(s) to the best advantage at all times		
IT10 Communicates clearly and consistently with the scrub team		
IT11 Communicates clearly and consistently with the anaesthetist		
IT12 Dislocates hip safely		
IT13 Cuts femoral neck appropriately to match design of implant		
IT14 Demonstrates familiarity and understanding of acetabular preparation including osteophyte trimming medially and at rim		
IT15 Broaches the femur properly and prepares the bony surface		
IT16 Uses trials and checks component orientation properly		
IT17 Fix acetabular component appropriately		
IT18 Implants femoral component appropriately		
IT19 Performs final reduction and checks for stability		
VI. Post operative management		
PM1 Ensures the patient is transferred safely from the operating table to bed		
PM2 Constructs a clear operation note		
PM3 Records clear and appropriate post operative instructions		
PM4 Deals with specimens. Labels and orientates specimens appropriately		

Global summary

Level at which completed elements of the PBA were performed	Tick as appropriate	Comments
Level 0 Insufficient evidence observed to support a judgment		
Level 1 Unable to perform the procedure under supervision		
Level 2 Able to perform the procedure under supervision		
Level 3 Able to perform the procedure with minimum supervision (would need occasional help)		
Level 4 Competent to perform the procedure unsupervised (could deal with complications)		

Signatures:

Trainee:	Assessor(s):

Figure 3.1   Total hip replacement PBA T&O curriculum (Pitts et al. 2007)

way that a driving examiner looks for key behaviours (mirrors, signal, manoeuvre) the assessor is guided by the PBA to key performance points in the procedure.

Both the trainer and trainee may trigger a PBA. It is normally conducted with the trainer scrubbed (able to observe trainee's actions closely). The trainee conducts the agreed sections of the procedure taking care to verbalize their intentions (in order to not only enable more effective assessment but also to avoid any compromise in the quality of patient care). At any point, the trainer may step in and perform all or some remaining sections of the procedure, if there is the slightest risk that the trainee will provide less than optimal care.

After the surgery is complete the trainee and trainer review the PBA form and complete it. Each element of relevant domains assessed is scored as satisfactory or unsatisfactory according to whether there is sufficient evidence from the trainer's observation that the required standard was met. The final domain of the PBA is the global assessment (see Table 3.3).

The global assessment gives the trainer the opportunity to comment on the trainee's overall performance. Even though the individual elements may have been performed to a satisfactory finished quality, the trainer is still able to apply an overall expert judgement. For example, the trainee may have been slow or hesitant or struggled to deal with an unexpected complication.

The results of the PBA are transferred to a PBA summary sheet where they are seen alongside results from other PBA assessments. This document's key function is to demonstrate clearly, to the annual review panel, whether the trainee is making progress, to indicate if certain areas of competence require further attention or highlight whether there are serious causes for concern.

Table 3.3   Global assessment taken from T&O curriculum (Pitts et al. 2007)

Level at which completed elements of the PBA were performed		Tick as appropriate	Comments
Level 0	Insufficient evidence observed to support a judgement		
Level 1	Unable to perform the procedure under supervision		
Level 2	Able to perform the procedure under supervision		
Level 3	Able to perform the procedure with minimum supervision (would need occasional help)		
Level 4	Competent to perform the procedure unsupervised (could deal with complications)		

Which Procedure?

In order to guarantee a sufficiently wide range of assessment, each surgical specialty has selected a number of *index procedures*. These procedures are selected on the basis of their broad accessibility to trainees, observability and in most cases an aspect of the procedure which contributes something unique to the assessment range. In orthopaedics there is presently a collection of 14 index procedures (e.g., carpal tunnel decompression, total knee replacement, compression hip screw for intertrochanteric fracture neck of femur). A trainee may submit PBA assessments on any number of procedures but a successful example of all 14 must be included before the completion of training. By the end of training all the index procedures must be scored at the defined competence level of four. Naturally in the early years an intermediate score is inevitable for all or some domains. It is very important for both trainer and trainee to appreciate that it is progression towards competence which is being assessed primarily. Less than a score of four is to be expected early on in training, culminating in 'straight fours' towards the completion of training.

PBA and the Curriculum

It should be noted that PBAs are one element of a wider specialty curriculum. They are linked to the learning agreement and work in synergy with other tools that vary to some degree between specialties.

Designing and Developing PBA

Historically the roots of PBA go back in the authors' experience to the early 1990s[1] when a desire to evaluate the change in performance before and after a fracture fixation course lead to the development of a 20-item multisource feedback tool assessing performance in inserting a dynamic hip screw (DHS) into a fractured neck of femur. The potential of this approach went unrecognized until 2002 when the recommendations of the JCHST Competence Working Party (Rowley et al. 2002) made it possible to proceed with PBA development in orthopaedics, at which time it was referred to as a performance-based assessment. Parallel developments in other specialties led to the development of the Operative Competence (OPCOMP) tool by Jonathan Beard in vascular surgery (Thornton et al. 2003). In 2004, elements of both systems were integrated into what became the Procedure Based Assessment (PBA). In 2005 the tool was introduced to all surgical specialties through workshops conducted for the Specialist Advisory Committee Chairs (Pitts

---

1   The first PBA was designed in 1994 as a follow up to a project investigating the change in competence following a training course (Oliver et al. 1997) but was not published until the report of the JCHST Competence working party (Rowley et al. 2002), when it was included as an appendix.

and Rowley 2005) and minor amendments made to the wording of elements and domains to make them accessible to the widest possible user group. Since this time they have been embedded in both the trauma and orthopaedic (T&O) curriculum (Pitts et al. 2007) and the Intercollegiate Surgical Curriculum Project (ISCP 2008). In the latter case some minor changes have been made but the instruments remain broadly identical.

Design Considerations

Features and characteristics of the surgical workplace, alongside the personality of the surgical team and requirements of assessment have influenced the development of the PBA.

Surgical environment   The surgical environment is special and although many aspects of it may be simulated, there is at present no adequate simulation of the high stakes of a real operative procedure. In order to make a valid assessment of operative competence, the real world has to be used. This imposes considerable constraints on assessment, not the least of which is the central purpose of providing an overwhelmingly safe service to the patient. Each operation is unique. Not only do the physical circumstances of the operating environment vary but also the composition of the team, type of instruments in use (even for similar procedures) and most fundamentally the patients in whom there is a wide variation of largely similar anatomy and variation in the severity of disease.

Nature of the surgical task   The basic separation of surgical procedures into emergency and elective shows that some procedures are conducted on suitable patients who may be screened and selected for surgery by a variety of measures beforehand whereas others will arrive unscheduled with possibly life threatening conditions in a variety of states of ill health. The operating room is inevitably a stressful environment in which the formal assessment of trainees' competence is of secondary concern.

Characteristics of assessors (trainers) and trainees   An 'early years' specialist surgical trainee is by no means a novice. She/he will have undergone at least five years of medical school education followed by between two and five years of postgraduate training before she/he enter specialty training. A senior surgical trainee, towards the end of training, will be a widely experienced practitioner who regularly operates on her/his own with accessible supervisors who are never the less outside the room in which the surgery is being conducted. The trainer (a consultant surgeon) is primarily responsible for the care of the patient and often for the leadership of a large team of professionals during the operative procedure. The introduction of a novel activity such as conducting a PBA is (rightly) questioned in order to ensure it does not compromise the primacy of provision of patient care.

Scale of the community   The orthopaedic community is one of the largest in surgery comprising over 40 per cent of practising surgeons. In the UK this involves approximately 3000 surgeons (including trainees) in over 450 hospital locations. This imposes considerable demands on the innovation process, not the least of which being to provide effective assessor training for the entire community

Connecting to patients   All patients who undergo surgery in a UK teaching hospital consent to part of their care being undertaken by trainees under supervision. PBAs form a part of that patient care process and as such should ideally be understandable by patients and their representatives.

Curriculum requirements   The same principles that have guided the development of the orthopaedic curriculum as a whole also guided the design of PBA. These principles were derived from a series of centre case studies. The list below is adapted from the Trauma & Orthopaedic curriculum (Pitts et al. 2007):

- *A radical alternative* – PBAs have been introduced into an environment where there were no established assessment tools and no foundations on which to build. They have been designed with the intention of gaining as much support from the orthopaedic community as possible in order to facilitate their implementation.
- *Competence focused* – There are debates about the nature or meaning of the word 'competence'. One conceptual standpoint states that a competence is simply a demonstrable ability to do something, using directly observable performance as evidence. Another understands competence as being a holistic integration of understandings, abilities and professional judgments, where 'competence' is not necessarily directly observable, rather it is inferred from performance (Eraut 1994). The integration of these two aspects acknowledges a much greater level of complexity within surgical competencies and avoids the problem that individuals may well be able to demonstrate that they can 'do' something, but that does not necessarily mean that they understand what they are doing or why until they give evidence for it. Within our particular competence model we look not only for the three key domains i.e., knowledge, skills and attitudes, but also for the unique combination of those domains in areas such as professional judgement. The development of professional judgement is a key outcome of surgical training.
- *Flexible and easy (intuitive) to use* – PBAs have to fit a variety of specialties, situations and personnel (see above). It is intended that their design will recognize this, whilst providing a consistency of standard and outcome. The hospital environment, where many trainers do not have their own office space and distractions abound, is hostile to finding time and space to

meet and talk. Most surgeons join the profession to perform surgery. They acknowledge the need to train but appreciate the evaluation of training must be part and parcel of service delivery. With these factors in mind we have tried to keep PBA s straightforward and sympathetic to the paucity of time in rapidly changing settings to learn complex tools.

- *Able to adapt to new developments (open architecture)* – Many innovations, especially in social technology settings, have a lengthy gestation period. From the beginning every effort has been made to try to ensure that the PBA's architecture is sufficiently open to allow synergy with new developments and requirements.

- *Driven by the trainee* – The triggered nature of the PBA puts responsibility into the hands of those who hold largest stake in seeing training happen – the trainees. PBA require and enables the trainee to take the initiative and responsibility for her/his own training.

- *Valid* – Questions of validity (truth) may be addressed in several different ways. Does the implementation of the whole system make a valid improvement in the outcomes of training? Are the index procedures selected for assessments a valid choice? Is the internal structure of each assessment valid in terms of the measures of performance it proposes? A major problem in this area is the lack of previous measures of surgical competence. It is impossible to make comparison with anything other than examination results, which only measure a limited area of intellectual competence. Extensive efforts must be ongoing, within other constraints, to achieve detailed validation of index procedures and PBA.

- *Reliable* – PBA should be understood by all in the same way. Efforts have been made to link PBA closely to accepted practice so that a firm foundation of agreement can be laid for the future.

- *Usable* – The circumstances in which PBAs are used dictate that this area is of primary concern. 'It might be valid and reliable but can you use it in a practical situation?' Efforts have been made to ensure that PBAs can be used in real life contexts within the constraints of time, user skills and attitudes.

- *Holistic in approach* – It was clear from early observations that many problems encountered amongst trainees had their roots in the area of non-technical skills. Elements of the PBA address these skills (and highlight them for assessors as well as trainees). It is hoped that more elements of current non-technical advances will be incorporated into PBA in the future.

- *Formative and summative* – The notion of a summative assessment where a trainer (possibly external) observes a trainee's performance in a pass/fail scenario was rejected at an early stage after two pilot studies. On one hand there seemed to be insurmountable logistic and resource problems but more importantly, training in the workplace is an ongoing activity and assessment should resonate with its formative nature. It was decided that all workplace assessments should be formative, giving feedback to the trainee to inform and guide her/his future performance. It was noted, however, that such assessments would, as a whole, be a useful summary of the trainee's ability to learn and progress. The successful completion of a PBA is not seen as a licence to operate in that procedure but as a single component of a wider assessment of the trainee's ability to learn operative procedures and perform them on a variety of patients with differing degrees of severity and complexity in their condition.

- *Electronic application* – If data are to be gathered from workplace-based assessments then it must have an electronic application which would facilitate this. Sadly the levels of IT 'literacy' encountered in pilots trials were highly variable and, more importantly, access to IT resources in NHS Trusts is extremely patchy. PBAs have been developed in a paper-based format whilst maintaining the possibility of an easy transfer to a digital system.

Selection of a Rating Scale

In the 1994 PBA, it was envisaged that the rater/assessor could be a scrub nurse, senior colleague or peer. The rating of any element was made on the basis of how much evidence there was for the judgment. For example, one element of the instrument asked about skin preparation, with three options: 'Was it prepared aseptically/dry prior to draping procedure/ensure no pooling of antiseptic solutions below patient?' (NB: the early version posed the questions in a very different way.)

The available scores were:

1 = no evidence whatsoever that the stage/task/activity has been completed
2 = some evidence
3 = ample evidence

This approach was taken because we were uncertain at that time whether such observations were possible and in particular, we wanted to compare the scores from professionals with differing interests (e.g., nurses and surgeons) and how much impact a training event had on the trainee's behaviour in theatre.

For the early versions of the later PBAs, we chose a similarly simple scale but from a different assessment viewpoint. By this time we were not trying to measure the impact of training, we were attempting to capture a snapshot of the trainee's behaviour in order to assess competence. The rating scale chosen for this was:

0 = not assessed
1 = unsatisfactory
2 = satisfactory

Numbers were chosen initially with a view to producing an electronic version later. We considered the use of a Likert scale and there was considerable debate as to whether this would be beneficial in demonstrating degrees of progress that would have a motivational effect. We also considered the inclusion of an extra column that could be marked if a trainee showed excellence at particular points (star quality) but eventually concluded that the simplest rating options would be the most effective.

A number of factors influenced the choice of the simple scale.

The first was that we needed to cater for the possibility that not all items would be assessed. There could be no guarantee that the trainee would be able to complete the whole procedure for a variety of reasons and to complete part of the assessment would be of great benefit to more junior trainees (mirroring actual training practice).

Secondly, it was never considered feasible, given the numbers of assessments involved and the variety of locations, that an independent assessor would be present in theatre. Even if they were, their independence would prevent them entering the sterile area and so limit their observations. The consequence of this was that the detail of the observation would only be recorded by the assessor at the end of the procedure. The more detailed the rating scale, the more likely the assessor might be to enter an incorrect score, having remembered the performance inadequately.

Thirdly, the naturally competitive personality of surgical trainees suggests that there could be lengthy debates about whether their performance should score two or three on a larger scale and this would introduce an unwanted variable (trainer personality) into the assessment process.

The final change to the rating scale came after a meeting in which the PBA was discussed by individuals (surgeons, educators and administrators) who had not been part of the original design group. One person in particular found it difficult to grasp the *nominative* nature of the scores and insisted on trying to calculate a minimum average score for the PBA. To avoid such problems recurring, the scale was altered to:

N = not assessed
U = unsatisfactory
S = satisfactory

Since the acceptance of PBA by all specialties, some have insisted on changing the scale from *unsatisfactory* to *requiring further development*. The authors see no advantage in this and some potential problems including the danger of increasing uncertainty through lack of definition.

The inclusion of the global assessment at the end of the PBA was one of the elements acquired from the merger with the OpComp tool. The inclusion of this domain enables a qualitative triangulation of the other domains which has proved extremely beneficial for the reasons of adding an element of overall professional judgement as described above.

Validity and Reliability of PBAs

The power of the PBA assessment rests in part on the fact that the PBA assesses the same competencies in a variety of procedures with a broad range of suitably qualified assessors. An orthopaedic trainee will normally have at least eight trainers, in a series of six-month attachments, during her/his training. In addition, she/he will operate in emergency situations, through rostering, with an even wider set of trainers, all of whom may act as assessors for a PBA.

Internal Validity of PBA

The initial selection of PBA domains and elements came from two sources. One was the original 20-element tool (Pitts and Ross 1994) the other was a series of Delphic groups involving surgeons within the orthopaedic community selected for their expertise as both trainers and surgeons. At a later stage the PBA which related to specific procedures was reviewed by a further series of individuals and groups. These revisions were to establish that in a particular procedure all elements were easily observable in a particular procedure and so that examples of positive and negative descriptors, as well as negative-passive indicators (sins of omission) could be identified. As a result, all PBAs have been validated against a standard worksheet of these descriptors for every element of every domain, an extract from which is shown as Table 3.4. The worksheet offers the opportunity to articulate specific examples (in italics) of generic competences.

Validity of Index Procedures

Whilst the initial selection of index procedures was made by a small group, its work was corroborated using a further set of groups consisting of 50+ surgical trainers in all. In this exercise the trainers were required to produce lists of index procedures (to the agreed criteria) on which they had achieved consensus. After the outliers were removed from the group lists, a high degree of correlation was seen with the earlier Delphic group selection.

A further triangulation of the selection of index procedures was made using the orthopaedic electronic logbook to check that all selected procedures were accessible to trainees in sufficient numbers (Pitts et al. 2005). A final review of the procedures' list was made using a further group of surgeons, during a south east training conference, who reviewed the list from the point of view of procedures that they felt they would, in their practice, be able to use to assess trainees

Reliability

Establishing the inter-rater reliability of the PBA tools proved extremely difficult within the time and budgetary constraints of the PBA Orthopaedic Competence Assessment Project (OCAP) project. An early attempt at producing video material

Table 3.4   Validation worksheet example taken from T&O curriculum (Pitts et al. 2007)

Competences and definitions	Positive behaviours (doing what should be done)	Negative behaviours (doing what shouldn't be done)	Negative – passive behaviours (*not* doing what should be done)
Pre-operative planning			
Demonstrates recognition of anatomical and pathological abnormalities and operative strategy to deal with these	Articulates the realistic clinical findings against any investigative findings and achieves a balance between the two	Describes an operative plan without the full use of the clinical and investigative material	Fails to take into account specific medical conditions that might limit the technical choices
Ability to make reasoned choice of appropriate equipment, materials or devices (if any) taking into account appropriate investigations e.g., x-rays	Is able to draw, write or iterate a preoperative plan	Does not take into account investigative findings when planning or selecting the equipment	Fails to check the notes for relevant or unexpected findings
	Takes the x-ray and any templates and plans the operation on paper checking both AP and lateral	*Does not consult the x-ray at all. Makes all the decisions on the AP x-ray*	*Fails to check both AP and lateral x-rays and makes all the decisions on the AP x-ray*
Checks materials, equipment and device requirements with operating room staff	Either personally visits or rings up the operating theatre to check on equipment availability	Delegates the task to a more junior team member with no plans to check the instruction has been carried out	Fails to communicate with the theatre staff
Where applicable ensures the operation site is marked	Personally marks the site	Delegates the task of marking the site to a junior doctor or nurse	Fails to check that the site has been marked
Checks patient records	Ensures that the relevant information such as investigative findings are present	During the procedure asks theatre staff to look something up in the notes	Fails to check notes to ensure all information is available that is needed

for viewing by raters was abandoned due to the difficulty of obtaining sufficiently high quality footage of a lengthy procedure and persuading sufficient numbers of surgical trainers to spend time scoring it. Fortunately this area has now been revisited by a team at Sheffield (Beard, Purdie et al. – see Chapter 4 in this volume).

Innovation and Acceptability

The positioning of the PBA tool has, from its inception, been as a device 'designed by surgeons for surgeons'. The orthopaedic curriculum (OCAP) steering group has had some 22 members in its approximately six-year lifespan with all but one being practising surgeons. This has resulted in a high degree of face validity. We have further supplemented this with a number of audits in various aspects of the PBA (and curriculum) acceptance and adoption by the orthopaedic community and this is described below. It has as yet not been possible to replicate this work in other specialties.

Baseline Survey

Prior to the launch of the curriculum materials into the orthopaedic trainee population in 2005 a small survey was conducted of trainee activity using trainees attending the annual British Orthopaedic Association (BOA) congress. Amongst other results, the survey found the following:

- 10 per cent of respondents had no meeting with their trainer outside the operating theatre in their entire six month attachment;
- 40 per cent of respondents had no written aims or objectives (learning agreement) for their attachment;
- 55 per cent had no formal assessment of their operating skills during their attachment;
- although the results fitted the expected picture the number of respondents was small (50) but it provided a baseline against which future progress might be measured.

Acceptance Survey

In the process of introducing the PBA and other curriculum tools, a number of briefing meetings were held across the UK, with varying numbers attending. At each of these meetings a survey was issued with questions relating to different tools, including the PBA. Two questions were posed: 1. Is this a good idea? and 2. Will it work?

Whilst some doubts were expressed as to whether trainers would comply with the new system (or have time to do so) respondents clearly expressed the view that it was a good idea and, to a lesser extent, that it would work, although all the outcomes tended to the positive.

In addition to gathering broad response, the questionnaires highlighted areas of expected difficulty, many of which have proven to be valid.

RITA Questionnaire

The Regional In service Training Assessment (RITA) has been an annual or bi-annual event for UK surgical trainees. It is in the process of being replaced by the Annual Review of Competence Progression (ARCP). In October 2005, following the launch of OCAP in August of that year, a questionnaire was issued to all trainees and programme directors to be completed before the RITA. The questionnaire asked factual questions about how many PBAs had been conducted, who triggered them and if none or few had been conducted, what the reasons were. The primary purpose of this tool was to find out what was happening in the field. The secondary purpose was to send a clear message that the Specialist Advisory Committee (SAC) was taking note of progress and would (and did) investigate instances of non compliance in a low key way. The results have been invaluable in identifying areas where engagement has been weak and further intervention is necessary.

Subsequently, an internet survey has been conducted since 2006, annually open to all T&O trainees contacted via their electronic logbook. In January 2006 only 50 per cent of trainees had completed one or more PBA assessments but this has risen to 93 per cent by January 2008 (Boardman et al. 2008). The work will be submitted for publication shortly as a longitudinal audit study.

Latest Developments

PBA assessment tools are now embedded in all surgical curricula. Their development continues in a number of areas; particularly in orthopaedics but also in other specialties.

Later Years of Training

Orthopaedic trainees often specialise further in the later years of training preparing for a career in a sub-specialty such as spine, joint replacement, hand surgery etc. Debate is continuing as to whether there should be the same PBA assessment conducted on more difficult and specialised procedures or whether an 'advanced' PBA should be designed that would assess higher order surgical competencies.

OCAP Online

The online version of the orthopaedic curriculum (OCAP Online) was launched in August 2008. Details can be found on the website: <www.ocap.org.uk>. The system itself is located on a secure site at: <www.elogbook.org>. As well as giving considerable benefits by automating tedious aspects of recording PBA, the online version offers the opportunity to gather information in real time and capture it so that trainees will submit a realistic record of their progression rather than simply retaining those PBAs they deem 'their best' – which is counter to the core values of the system. Naturally, electronic data permit one to contrast and compare data from different training programmes and differing contexts of training so that, hopefully, an evaluation may be made of learning in surgical training.

International Compatibility

Considerable interest from overseas in the orthopaedic curriculum and in particular with the PBA tools has led to a number of proposed international pilot projects. International compatibility of surgical training systems is a key issue in relation to making it possible for trainees to complete part of their training overseas but, at a wider level, may have considerable consequences for the mobility of surgical labour. The PBA tool may offer a way of ensuring that widely differing training systems are producing compatible surgical skill sets.

NOTSS

It is hoped that we will, in the near future have the opportunity to combine the progress made in both the Non-Technical Skills for Surgeons (NOTSS) project (see Chapter 2 in this volume) and in PBAs by either producing a new assessment tool based on the PBA or to integrate behavioural markers from NOTSS into the existing PBA.

PowerPoint Guidance

For PBA, as for all elements of the orthopaedic curriculum, we have produced PowerPoint guides available through the website. The use of this technology, in preference to a user manual, enables a trainer and trainee to sit together and review the guidance and also for a programme director to present the guide in a group setting. These guides have been developed for all PBA applications to date and will be added to as work continues.

Conclusion

PBAs have been an attempt to maintain and improve the high quality of surgical training in the UK. Their development is still in its early stages compared to other, more established and practiced assessment methods. We will have to monitor their progress for some time before we will be able to see whether, in the midst of many other changes, they have been successful.

References

Boardman, D., Pitts, D. and Edge, J. (2008) *The Orthopaedic Curriculum and Assessment Project: A National Survey of SpR Views Two years after Introduction*. Poster presented at the British Orthopaedic Association Annual Congress, Liverpool, September 2008.

Department of Health (1993) *Hospital Doctors: Training for the Future*. The report of the Working Group on Specialist Medical Training (the Calman Report). London: Department of Health.

Department of Health (2007) *Trust, Assurance and Safety – The Regulation of Health Professionals in the 21st Century*. CM 7013. London: Department of Health.

Donaldson, L. (2002) *Unfinished Business – Proposals for Reform of the Senior House Officer Grade. A Paper for Consultation*. London: Department of Health

Eraut, M. (1994) *Developing Professional Knowledge and Competence*. London: Falmer Press.

ISCP (2008) *Intercollegiate Surgical Curriculum Programme*: Available at: <http://www.iscp.ac.uk> [accessed June 2008].

Kennedy, I. (2001) *Bristol Royal Infirmary Inquiry*. Retrieved from <http:/www.bristol-inquiry.org.uk/final_report/index.htm> [last accessed October 2008].

Langrish, J., Gibbons, M., Evans, W.G. and Jevons, F.R. 1(972) Linear models of innovation, in J. Langrish (ed.) *Wealth from Knowledge: Studies of Innovation in Industry*. London: Macmillan

Machiavelli, N. (1515) *The Prince*, trans. 1908 by W.K. Marriott. Available at: <http://www.constitution.org/mac/prince.txt> [last accessed October 2008].

OCAP Online (2008) Orthopaedic curriculum. Available at: <http://www.ocap.org.uk/orthocurriculum/Content/01_Intro_160707.pdf>

Oliver, C.W., Ross, E.R.S., Hollis, S. and Pitts, D. (1997) Impact of distance learning material on trauma surgeons, *Injury* 28(3), 245–245(1).

Pitts, D. and Rowley, D.I. (2005) Establishing consensus on PBA; Workshops for SAC chairs. Unpublished internal report for OCAP steering group.

Pitts, D., Rowley, D.I. and Sher, J.L. (2005) Assessment of performance in orthopaedic training. *Journal of Bone and Joint Surgery* (British) 87–B(9), 1187–91.

Pitts, D. and Ross, E.R.S. (2002) A competence assessment tool for the Dynamic Hip Screw. In D.I. Rowley, D. Pitts and C. Galasko *Competence Working Party report to the JCHST*. London: Joint Committee on Higher Surgical Training.

Pitts, D., Rowley, D.I., Marx, C., Sher, L, Banks, A.J. and Murray, A. (2007). *Specialist Training in Trauma and Orthopaedics – A Competency Based Curriculum 2007*. Available at: <http//:www.ocap.org.uk/curriculum> [last accessed October 2008].

Richards, R. (1997) Clinical academic careers: Report of an independent task force chaired by Sir Rex Richards. Available at: <http://www.rcgp.org.uk/docs/ISS_ SUMM97_14.DOC> [accessed November 2008].

Rowley, D, Pitts, D. and Galasko, C. (2002) *Competence Working Party report to the JCHST*. London: Joint Committee on Higher Surgical Training.

Smith, J. (2005) *The Shipman Inquiry*. Availably at: <http://www.the-shipman-inquiry.org.uk> [accessed June 2008].

Thornton, M., Donlon, M. and Beard, J.D. (2003) The operative skills of higher surgical trainees: Measuring competence achieved rather than experience undertaken. *Royal College of Surgeons of England* (bulletin), 85, 190–3.

Chapter 4

Implementing the Assessment of Surgical Skills and Non-Technical Behaviours in the Operating Room

Joy Marriott, Helen Purdie, Jim Crossley and Jonathan Beard

Introduction to the Study

The Sheffield Surgical Skills Study is currently evaluating the validity, reliability, feasibility and acceptability of three different workplace-based assessment tools for rating surgeons' technical and non-technical skills in the operating room. This chapter describes the design, methodology and implementation of the study. It focuses on the problem-solving approach taken by the research team to address the practical issues of implementing this broad study of behaviours, drawing upon some of the successes and barriers we encountered, to illustrate this. It is intended to provide valuable lessons for researchers in the field of surgical skills assessment, and for those involved in implementing workplace based assessment into surgical training.

Background to Surgical Skills Assessment

Traditionally, surgical training in the UK has been based upon an apprenticeship and examination model without formal assessment of technical or non-technical skills. Trainees undertook a set number of years of training and passed the Intercollegiate Examination of the Royal Colleges of Surgeons (FRCS) to achieve their Certificate of Completion of Specialist Training (CCST) for consultant practice. Progress in surgical competence was historically achieved through many years and long hours spent in the operating room. Although log books formed a useful record of surgical experience (Galasko and Mackay 1997), they did not provide evidence of competence (Thornton et al. 2003). However, opportunities to gain experience in the operating room have decreased due to shorter training time following the Calman Report (Calman 1999) and the changes in working practices following the European Directive on Hours of Work (Department of Health 2003). This has resulted in trainees having reduced access to surgical experience before their CCST (Katory et al. 2001).

Over the last 15 years there has been a move to competency-based surgical curricula in the UK, driven by the introduction of regulations for training by the Postgraduate Medical Education Board (PMETB). The transitions in surgical training have been described previously by Pitts and Rowley in Chapter 3 of this book.

Background to Surgical Skill Assessment Tools

The surgical skill assessment methods developed by the GMC Performance Procedures (Beard et al. 2005b) and by the medical royal colleges and specialty associations responsible for postgraduate surgical training, are based upon the demonstration of surgical competencies and standards of competence. The need for robust methods of assessment for technical and non-technical surgical skills is axiomatic, as they underpin the competency based assessment strategy and curricula for all UK surgical specialties.

Procedure Based Assessment (PBA) and Objective Structured Assessment of Technical Skill (OSATS) are two of the tools being considered in this study. They are the current workplace-based assessment tools being used by UK royal colleges and specialty associations for assessing the surgical competence of trainees and for informing objective feedback. The overall assessment strategies and individual assessment tools they have adopted conform to the assessment principles laid down by the Postgraduate Medical Education and Training Board (PMETB 2008), and the assessment tools are also designed to measure all the domains of *Good Medical Practice* (General Medical Council 1998).

PBAs are embedded within the Orthopaedic Curriculum and Assessment Project (OCAP – <www.ocap.org.uk>) and the Intercollegiate Surgical Curriculum Programme (ISCP – <www.iscp.ac.uk>). The development of the PBA with examples of the assessment tool is covered by Pitts and Rowley in Chapter 3. PBAs have been used by OCAP since 2005, and were introduced into the surgical specialty curricula by ISCP in August 2007. Therefore, this study is taking place alongside the implementation of PBAs for trainees who are required to register onto the ISCP curriculum.

Objective Structured Assessment of Technical Skill (OSATS) was introduced by the Royal College of Obstetricians and Gynaecologists (RCOG – <www.rcog. org.uk>) as a requirement of their New Training and Education Programme, launched in parallel with ISCP in August 2007. The OSATS tool was developed by Reznick's group in Toronto (Winckel et al. 1994, Martin et al. 1997).

Ensuring that our assessment methods are valid, reliable and feasible are the principal considerations of a well designed and evaluated assessment system (Van der Vleuten 1996). Evidence of validity and reliability are essential characteristics of fair and defensible assessments, particularly in identifying under-performing surgeons who could compromise patient safety (Schuwirth et al. 2002). The observation of real-time surgical performance in the workplace is essential in the authentic assessment of competence. Direct observation of skills and behaviours in the operating theatre has good authenticity for assessing surgical competence, since this method approximates to the 'real world' as closely as possible. In addition, the feasibility and acceptability of such assessments will influence the successful implementation of competency-based assessment, which is a key consideration for stakeholders with a responsibility for postgraduate surgical training.

Preliminary validation studies on PBA have been performed by Rowley and Pitts (see Chapter 3). Our study seeks to further examine the validity and evaluate the reliability of the PBA tool. OSATS has demonstrated inter-rater reliability and construct validity in assessing general surgeons performing common operations (Winckel et al. 1994). However, there have not been validity and reliability studies performed for the ten OSATS of obstetrics and gynaecology procedures used by the RCOG.

The third tool considered in this study is the Non-Technical Skills for Surgeons (NOTSS) tool (Yule et al. 2008) described in Chapter 2. This tool is not currently used in a formal way for training in the UK. However, there is increasing recognition of the need for training and assessment in non-technical skills because of the importance of these skills for patient safety.

Purpose of the Surgical Skills Study

The aim is to evaluate the validity, reliability, feasibility and acceptability of three different methods of rating the technical and non-technical skills of trainee surgeons in the operating room across a range of different procedures and surgical specialties.

The three tools under evaluation in the study are:

- PBA: Procedure-Based Assessment;
- OSATS: Objective Structured Assessment of Technical Skill;
- NOTSS: Non-Technical Skills for Surgeons.

The PBA forms for index procedures used by each UK surgical specialty can be downloaded from the ISCP (<www.iscp.ac.uk>) and OCAP websites (<www.ocap.og.uk>). The OSATS forms used by the RCOG can be downloaded from: <www.rcog.org.uk/resources/public/pdf/section6_at.pdf>. The NOTSS rating form and booklet are available from <www.abdn.ac.uk/iprc/notss>.

Design and Methodology

Timescale

The study commenced in April 2007 at a large UK teaching hospital NHS foundation trust and is due to be completed in June 2009.

Sample Size

Our intention is to perform between 400 and 500 assessments of surgical procedures. The first case was assessed in June 2007. To date we have completed 240 cases. Reliability estimates become more dependable as the evaluation includes more cases, assessors and trainees. However, there is no accepted equivalent of a power calculation to guide sample sizes.

Participants

We are assessing trainee surgeons using the tools for those cases which have the informed consent of the patient. The assessments on individual trainees are performed with as little delay as possible to avoid the confounding effect of training.

Procedures

We are assessing a total of 15 index procedures within six surgical specialties (see Table 4.1). Each case is judged for complexity by the supervising consultant.

Observation and Assessment

Within each specialty, the aim is to assess each trainee performing at least two cases of each relevant index procedure. Assessments of their technical and non-technical

Table 4.1   Index procedures within the surgical specialties

Specialty	Index procedures
Upper Gastrointestinal	Laparoscopic cholecystectomy Open hernia repair
Orthopaedics	Primary hip replacement Primary knee replacement
Obstetrics & Gynaecology	Elective Caesarean section Urgent Caesarean section Diagnostic laparoscopy Surgical evacuation of uterus
Vascular	Saphenofemoral ligation Carotid endarterectomy Abdominal aortic aneurysm repair
Colorectal	Open right hemicolectomy Open anterior resection
Cardiac	Coronary artery bypass grafting Aortic valve replacement

skills are undertaken across the cases by as many supervising consultants (one for each case) and independent assessors (up to three in one case) as is practicable.

Methods of Observation

1. Direct observation by assessors in the operating room.
2. Video observation.

We are currently filming approximately 20 per cent of the cases using a picture in picture technique which records the operating field and the operating room. Filming is performed by medical illustration technicians with audio provided by microphones fitted to the trainee surgeon and supervising consultant. During the consent process, patients have the option to decline videoing, with consent only for the direct observation of their operation. We will be able to compare the fidelity and reliability of video observation with direct observation. The videos will also provide rich data on the non-technical skills of trainee surgeons in the operating room for collaborative work with the NOTSS team.

Process of Study Implementation and Assessments

The implementation of the study within a surgical specialty is illustrated by the flowchart in Figure 4.1.

Progress to Date

The original proposal for recruitment was 400–500 surgical cases from three teaching hospitals but it soon became clear that this would be logistically impossible without dedicated research staff at each hospital trust. We have therefore recruited from a single teaching hospital's NHS trust, including two hospital sites with an independent assessor based at each hospital. At the time of writing (June 2008), we have completed 240 cases in 5 surgical specialties, with a further 11 months of study time for recruitment. Provided recruitment continues at the same pace, we will be on target to complete 400 to 500 assessments.

Relating the Study Design to the Research Aim

The study aim encompasses several research questions. We have outlined the main questions below, showing how they have driven the overall study design, and provided examples of how we have addressed them within the study. Our research questions take into account the assessment characteristics proposed by Van der Vleuten (1996) in his model of assessment *utility*.

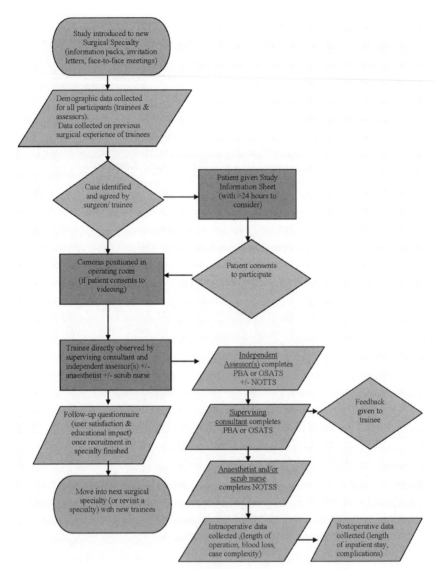

Figure 4.1   Flowchart of the study implementation

Are the Tools Valid?

Validity can be described in a number of ways depending on the context of the assessment. For us, it refers to evidence presented to support or refute the interpretation of assessment scores, i.e., the degree to which the scores of the assessment reflect the *intention of the assessment*. In the case of the assessment tools included in this study, the intention is for the assessment scores to reflect the technical and non-technical surgical competence of the trainee being assessed.

Validity requires multiple sources of evidence to allow a meaningful interpretation of assessment scores (Downing 2003). Our study design provides many sources of validity evidence and these will all be used to support or refute the validity of the three assessment tools. As one example, if the assessment tools are valid for the assessment of surgical competence, we would expect scores to increase with the trainee's level of training and experience. We have ensured that the study includes all grades of trainees and that our demographic questionnaires include questions addressing years of surgical experience and the number of index procedures previously performed by the trainee.

Are the Tools Reliable?

Reliability refers to the reproducibility of assessment scores. Indicators of test score precision (e.g., Standard Error of Measurement) and indicators of reliability (e.g., G co-efficient) are both based upon estimates of measurement error.

Reliability within this study is a measure of how well an assessor's score of the surgical competence for a particular trainee would reflect any assessor's score when the trainee carried out the operation on any patient. To be able to generalize the construct of 'surgical competence' to all of its possible measurements requires that all sources of error (termed 'variability') are quantified. Therefore, its calculation depends on comparing the effect of assessor-to-assessor variability and case-to-case variability in scores with overall trainee-to-trainee variability in scores. The use of generalizability theory for the analysis of assessment scores within the study is fundamental in providing the most elegant estimates of assessor variability and case variability, which represent the greatest threats to the reliability of real time assessments in the workplace (Downing 2004).

Within each surgical specialty, we have aimed to assess each trainee performing two cases of each relevant index procedure, providing four to eight assessments overall for each trainee. Assessing a particular trainee performing several index procedures of varying complexity with different assessors provides a broad sample of observations for assessing surgical skill. Assessment scores from observations on a number of occasions by different assessors provides the most dependable reliability data (Crossley et al. 2002).

Are the Assessment Tools Feasible *in Practice?*

Feasibility governs the likelihood of implementing an assessment method. There are a number of strands to consider within the scope of assessment feasibility, including the time and resources required for implementation as well as cost effectiveness of the assessment strategy.

Our study views feasibility as a key assessment characteristic and it is formally considered within the study's design. Following each case, the supervising consultant completes a PBA or OSATS before giving feedback to the trainee. We observe this process and record the time taken to complete the assessment form and the duration of feedback. The follow-up questionnaires which we distribute to trainees and assessors approximately one month after completing assessments, in the relevant specialty, include questions to address feasibility issues, e.g., time added to operating list, available room for feedback, ease of use of tools. We have not directly addressed cost effectiveness in this study, although the data could inform future research.

Are the Assessment Tools Acceptable to Stakeholders?

User acceptability is the extent to which an assessment tool or method is accepted by the stakeholders involved in the assessment. It is a crucial factor in the design and successful implementation of assessment programmes.

The acceptability of the assessment tools to trainees and assessors is being evaluated during the study's implementation, as the future direction of competency-based assessment in the UK will be influenced by the opinions of surgical trainees and trainers. After each feedback session and in the follow-up questionnaires we address the acceptability of the assessments and the assessment tools.

There is some overlap of user acceptability issues with feasibility and validity. For example, an assessment tool which is very complex and time-consuming to complete is likely to have low face validity and low feasibility as well as having inferior acceptability. However, we consider acceptability from the overall perspective of the people directly involved in the assessments. We ask supervising consultants and trainees to rate their overall satisfaction with the assessment tools immediately after feedback. The subsequent questionnaires provide an opportunity for trainees and assessors to express their views on the ease or difficulty of using the tools, their perspectives on the value of assessment and feedback and the impact of assessment on training and patient safety.

Thematic Analysis of the Problem-solving Approach to the Study Implementation

We have used a number of themes below to illustrate the problem-solving approaches we have adopted during the study implementation. We have identified lessons learnt and made some practical suggestions which may be of use to those undertaking similar work.

1. Matching the Research Team to the Study Design

We have assembled a research team which has the skills required to evaluate assessment in the operating room. The team includes surgeons, a research coordinator with surgical experience and a psychometrician whose particular area of expertise is workplace-based assessment and generalizability theory. All three independent assessors are practising surgeons with expertise in many of the surgical specialities, having received training in assessment and feedback through the 'Training the Trainers' course at the Royal College of Surgeons, and NOTSS training facilitated by the NOTSS research team, in Edinburgh.

Lessons learnt and suggested learning points   Whilst it is impossible to outline all the skills and attributes required from a research team in this field, we consider the following to be essential:

- expertise in surgical knowledge, skills, attributes and competence;
- familiarity and confidence with working in the operating room environment;
- firm research governance knowledge and 'good clinical practice' training;
- statistical expertise independent from the grass roots researchers;
- diplomacy in negotiating the socio-political surgical frameworks;
- tenacity towards recruitment of cases and engagement of trainees and trainers;
- flexibility towards workload and research schedule;
- consistent communication and organization between team members to use the team's resources to their full potential.

Our aim was to bring together a multidisciplinary team of researchers with a mix of skills and attributes to complement the design and implementation of our study.

2. Engaging and Informing Clinicians

We are carrying out research in real time in the workplace. However, surgical environments are both busy and rapidly changing. One of the challenges we faced in implementing the study was ensuring that we used a timely and appropriate method to inform the surgical teams involved. We used the following methods of communication, often in combination, to disseminate the purpose and design of the research study:

- email information packs;
- written information packs;
- presentations at departmental meetings;
- face-to-face discussions.

Our main aim in the advance communication was to familiarize staff with the study before we moved the research into their specialty. This approach recognized that research and assessment in the operating room could be viewed by staff as threatening or unnecessary, unless we clearly explained the aims of the study within the context of work-place based assessment and the surgical curricula. The information packs include an overview of the study and examples of the assessment tools with guidance on their use for assessment and feedback. As the study has rolled out, we have recognized the need to support email communication with meetings, written information and face-to-face discussion. We have been able to use formal meetings at times but this has often been constrained by practical considerations, for example the size, organizational structure and availability of the target audience. Presentations at specialty meetings for surgeons and surgical trainees have proved useful in some specialties but impractical in others. It has not been feasible to organize formal presentations within work time for scrub team and anaesthetic staff, which we have managed by arranging smaller ad hoc meetings. Overall we have found that trainee and assessor engagement has been best achieved using face-to-face discussions in the field with supporting written information, having provided a background to the study by email communication and presentations where possible.

Lessons Learnt and Suggested Learning Points

- Identify the most effective way to communicate and disseminate your research to all interested parties.
- Consider your resources and the feasibility of your approach to communicate and disseminate the study.
- Be flexible and revise your approach to overcome time constraints and structural barriers in the workplace.

3. Training of Assessors

Further to communicating and disseminating the study methodology, there was the need for us to familiarize and train staff involved in assessing and/or giving feedback. We experienced wide variations in staff engagement and attitude towards the research, which challenged our ability to provide consistent training for all staff. The breadth of the personnel involved in the study and the feasibility of providing training within work time were also significant barriers to the study implementation.

Staff for whom training was required included:

- *consultant surgeons*: PBA and OSATS assessment tool and feedback training;
- *consultant/senior anaesthetists*: NOTSS training;
- *scrub nurses*: NOTSS training.

We have made great efforts to train all assessors to ensure confidence in and credibility of the assessor ratings. We have provided all assessors with information packs, including the relevant assessment tools, guidance on their use and access to web-based training which we have usually supported with one to one familiarization before they have undertaken any assessments.

We acknowledge that we have been unable to achieve an entirely level playing field for training assessors in the use of workplace assessment tools, which reflects the reality of the surgical workplace. Consultant assessors differ in their educational interest and awareness, as well as their uptake of assessment training, including web-based training and the Training the Trainers course. However, the study design includes several 'quality measures' of training. Supervising consultants are asked at the time of giving feedback to trainees and in a subsequent questionnaire what type of training they have received in assessment. This will be incorporated in the data analysis. Furthermore, our data analysis using generalizability theory will enable an examination of the variance in ratings for different assessor designations, for example a comparison of NOTSS ratings between independent assessors, anaesthetists and scrub nurses. Despite training all assessors in the appropriate use of the tools, we have observed some inconsistencies in the way the tools are used:

- prompting trainees too readily;
- being unable to allow trainees to lead the case *within* their level of competence, taking over decision-making, or the surgical instruments;
- directing trainees to operate using their preferred surgical sequence and/or technique;
- being reluctant to score competencies negatively (and/or give difficult feedback), particularly for senior trainees.

We recognize that these training styles may influence ratings of trainee skills and behaviours. For example, if a trainee is directed to operate using a different technique, they are unlikely to be as smooth in its delivery, affecting PBA/OSATS scores. We found it very difficult to rate skills and behaviours where a trainer repeatedly intervened and in some cases we used 'not applicable' to rate these skills and behaviours.

The most successful assessments and training opportunities are during cases where the consultant trainer permits the trainee to operate within their limits of competence, and grants them the leadership to carry this out, prompting or intervening only when required or requested. Supervisor training to this level is beyond the scope of our study, but is what will be required of trainers in the future if training is to become more effective.

Lessons Learnt and Suggested Learning Points

- Providing training in the workplace requires flexibility and tenacity to ensure full coverage.
- Identify the most effective and suitable method for training different assessors.

- Consider consistency in the training approach you adopt, taking into account differences in staff engagement and attitude.
- Be prepared to abandon assessments or preclude assessors if an authentic assessment is compromised.

4. Consenting and Recruitment of Patient Participants

To successfully recruit a surgical case requires the favourable alignment and accurate timing of many factors which are beyond our control. These factors are often not confirmed until the day of the operation and the case cannot go ahead as part of the study if any one of them is missing:

- an appropriate case;
- a consenting patient;
- a surgical/HDU bed;
- a suitable and consenting surgical trainee;
- an available consultant for providing supervision, assessment and feedback;
- an independent assessor;
- theatre staff for the list;
- sufficient operating time for the case;
- a suitable training list (some lists are for service provision only).

Furthermore, the ethical requirement of the study is that patients receive a Patient Information Sheet 24 hours before they are approached for consent to give them time to consider. This requires us to provide patients with an Information Sheet before their admission, with the corollary that we need to identify suitable cases for recruitment at least three working days ahead to allow for postage time. Our selection of cases in advance is affected by a number of other last-minute changes such as lack of beds, insufficient operative time or there being no available trainee for assessment. This results in a number of cases which cannot be recruited as planned, with patient consent rarely being the determining factor.

For the few cases in which patients declined to participate, we found that their decision was often surrounded by misconceptions regarding trainee involvement in performing supervised elective surgery. For some patients this was a reflection of heightened concern for their surgery and a wish for a consultant to perform the operation. For some others, there was simply an expectation that a consultant would be performing the operation. We provided an open discussion of the training system, acknowledging the role of supervised operating in training. In some cases, this open discussion resulted in patients deciding to consent to participate.

Lessons Learnt and Suggested Learning Points

- Consider the complexity of consenting and recruiting patient participants for observational studies in the surgical environment and the resources required.
- Appreciate the patient's perspective towards surgical systems and training, which will inform your consent process.
- Communicate at all levels to make full potential of the team's resources and to maximize the recruitment of suitable cases.
- Consider contingency lists, so that if a surgical case 'goes down', there may be other suitable cases for assessments.

5. Surgical Trainees as Study 'Participants'

Ethical approval for the study dictates written consent from patients as participants but not from trainees. However, from a training perspective and during the implementation of the study, we have also considered surgical trainees to be study participants. It could be argued that competency-based assessment of surgical skills is now a requirement of surgical training. However, this does not extend to the additional research conditions, including independent assessors, video and NOTSS assessments. Our approach has been to seek verbal consent from surgical trainees before their involvement in the study. We provide all trainees with an invitation letter before introducing the study into a new surgical specialty and give them an opportunity to discuss the research with the study coordinator, thereby ensuring participation without duress. There have been a handful of trainees across the specialties, usually senior trainees approaching their CCT (certificate of completed training), who have declined to take part.

We have experienced initial hesitancy from some trainees regarding their involvement in the study, often centred on misunderstanding the purpose of the study and concerns that research data could affect their training, for example in the event of a critical incident occurring. One of the clear messages we have conveyed is that the study is designed to assess the assessment tools themselves, in particular their validity and reliability across different surgeons, cases and specialties, and it is not assessing an individual's level of surgical skill or competence. The majority of trainees, who decided to participate, have increasingly engaged with assessments. (See Theme 6, 'Research versus Training Agenda', for a fuller discussion.)

We have continued in our attempts to collect data to suit the statistical model employed for the study, the optimal data being different combination of trainees and assessors across the cases. Some trainees operate more frequently, some senior surgical trainees perform complex procedures which are not covered by the study and some consultant lists have more index procedures. These differences generate unbalanced data. However, moving trainees across lists for assessments in the operating room proved unworkable. Some trainees were resistant to movement, preferring training and assessment by their regular consultant. We also realized that assigning a particular trainee to perform a surgical case assessed their behaviour as 'technical operators', rather than reflecting the complete role of a holistic surgical practitioner. For the same reasons, if there were late changes to the trainee covering a particular list, we decided to exclude the case to focus the study on authentic workplace assessments.

Lessons Learnt and Suggested Learning Points

- Consider the ethics of trainees as participants in observational surgical education studies.
- Engage trainees in the process of assessment by communicating effectively the research purpose and the role of their involvement.
- Respect the working surgical system in place: research needs to work *with* the surgical system rather than *adapt* the system to suit the research.

6. Research versus Training Agenda: A Dichotomy or Collaboration?

The study protocol includes the validation of assessment tools which are in current use in the workplace for surgical training. (See the earlier background of this chapter for an overview of PBA and OSATS tools within surgical training programmes.) There are opportunities for educational research to form collaborations or conflicts with the training agenda, and this is illustrated by discussing our role as independent assessors in the study.

Examples of collaboration   Providing opportunities for training in workplace-based assessment has moved beyond the research agenda to provide trainees and trainers with valuable, timely training on the tools which are integral to the new surgical curricula.

The study has provided ring-fenced opportunities for training and assessment, which has resulted in the increasing engagement of trainees in the study. Trainees have made comments such as, 'I'm happy to take part; it means I get to operate' and 'It'll guarantee some assessments for my portfolio'. Participation in the study has also encouraged a number of trainers and trainees to use the PBA tool for the first time. We have been able to show trainers and trainees that suitable cases for workplace training can be identified opportunistically, and that the process of assessment and feedback is feasible, adding little time to an operating list. Highlighting the role of formative assessment in driving learning has encouraged appropriate use of the PBA within the curriculum. For example, use of parts of the PBA for trainees not ready to complete the whole operation under supervision.

Our 'field testing' of the assessment tools has generated suggestions for tool modification which have been forwarded to the relevant bodies for consideration. For example, carotid endarterectomy and caesarean section are performed under local or regional anaesthetic. The trainee's communication with the patient therefore becomes an important assessment item which was not part of the original template.

Examples of dichotomy All assessors score independently without conferring or discussion until the assessment tools for the case are completed. There is no discussion of scoring *between* cases, either between independent assessors or with trainers, which could have a convergent effect on assessor ratings. However, it is inevitable in the clinical setting for some discussion to take place with the presence of trained independent assessors who are facilitating cases for assessment purposes. Assessment in the operating theatre is a relatively new training method, and the research team are seen to represent a body of expertise in assessment and feedback.

We have found that our role as a *complete observer* in the independent assessment of skills and behaviours in the operating room is both unrealistic and unworkable. We suggest that our role within this study is more aligned to *observer-as-participant*, part way along the continuum from complete observer, to observer-as-participant, onto participant-as-observer, then to complete participant (Gold 1958). The process of assessment itself prompts discussion; for example, what constitutes a good surgical technique and why? Judgements on skills and behaviours are rated independently between assessors, although discussion surrounding the subjectivity of skills and behaviours is seen as a necessary outcome of the study implementation.

Another area of conflict we have recognized relates to the quantity and quality of the research data. The supervising consultant is often not present in the operating room until the case commences, which omits the pre-operative preparation section of the PBA and equivalent sections on the OSATS. Do we prompt consultants to be present at the whole case to maximize data quantity or is the research question most accurately answered by the researchers assuming the observer role? Do we encourage consultants to allow trainees to lead the case, which provides the most authentic assessment of surgical performance or observe the real-life training situation?

We have found it challenging, particularly when new trainees and/or trainers become involved in the study, to provide sufficiently general information to support the assessments and the use of the assessment tools, without introducing specific prompts which would affect the assessment ratings and overall data quality. We have made compromises to uphold the research agenda, as from a training standpoint, independent assessor(s) would prompt trainers on the appropriate use of the assessment tools, such as to address the inconsistencies in tool use highlighted above in Theme 3.

Lessons Learnt and Suggested Learning Points

- Educational research can engender collaboration and conflicts between the research and training agendas.

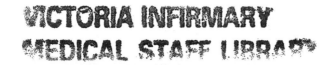

- Consider your role as researchers in upholding the research agenda whilst drawing upon collaborations with the training agenda.
- Some discussions surrounding the assessment of skills and behaviours are a necessary condition for implementing workplace assessments.

7. Developments in Study Design and Methodology during Implementation

Developments to the study design and methodology have arisen to meet the requirements of the study aim and to promote future research directions. It is only when the study design and methodology are subjected to field testing during their implementation that the full requirements of the study protocol can be realized. These developments have been driven by the foresight of the research team and with guidance from the Studys Steering Committee. External review of the original study protocol advised us to consider more than two assessment tools (originally PBA and OSATS). The development of rating non-technical skills in the operating room, supported by the literature evidence for the relationship of these skills to surgical skills and safety, stimulated the addition of NOTSS to the study protocol.

We originally recruited patients from one specialty at a time because of the logistical difficulties in working in multiple specialties simultaneously. However, in order to improve recruitment and maximize the reliability data it has been essential for us to recruit from two, sometimes three specialties at any one time. This has been achieved by securing funding for a further independent assessor who has also taken responsibility for coordination of cases within her own specialty of obstetrics and gynaecology. An early ethics amendment approved the addition of obstetrics and gynaecology as a surgical specialty with the inclusion of four extra index procedures. This has provided the opportunity to compare PBA with OSATS in a specialty that uses OSATS as the current workplace assessment tool. We needed to collect a larger dataset of assessments in this specialty compared to the others to allow a comparison of the tools. However, recruiting cases in obstetrics and gynaecology has been very successful because it lends itself to providing large numbers of suitable cases (see Theme 8, 'The Significance of Context', for a full discussion). The addition of this specialty has included a *non-elective* index procedure, urgent caesarean, which provides an opportunity for video assessment and use of the NOTSS tool in urgent surgical cases.

The completion of more than one assessment tool has a potential to confound each assessment. The best case scenario is for each independent assessor to complete one tool per case. However, the number of cases required to obtain sufficient data to test each of the assessment tools would be very large, certainly unachievable within this study. The final study protocol accepts that there will be completion of more than one tool by independent assessors (PBA or OSATS and NOTSS). We recognize that differences exist between the assessment tools which make their simultaneous use in assessment problematic. For the PBA tool, there is an expectation that trainees should verbalize their intentions throughout, also advised in the PBA validation document for training assessors. The NOTSS tool has been designed for use in as naturalistic a setting as possible, without prompting trainee communication or decision-making. Our concern surrounding the completion of two tools was raised with the Steering Committee and the decision has been to minimize the completion of two tools. For example, if there are two independent assessors observing a case, both complete the PBA or OSATS but only one completes a NOTSS assessment. Where two tools have been completed, the impact of this can be considered using a post hoc analysis.

Recruitment has been better in some specialties than in others. In specialties where we realized that recruitment would not improve, we decided to move on rather than risk a training effect by remaining in the speciality. Our intention is to return to specialties to capture another cohort of trainees next year, prioritizing the specialties in which further recruitment is needed.

Lessons Learnt and Suggested Learning Points

- Developments to study design may be required to meet the research aim or to take advantage of new research directions.
- Preliminary fieldwork can require changes to be made to the study design and methodology, which may involve ethics amendments.
- A flexible team approach with good foresight encourages the negotiation of study developments.

8. The Significance of Context: Inter-specialty Differences

The individual surgical specialties have offered different advantages and disadvantages to the study implementation. The obstetrics and gynaecology specialty has leant itself well to the study methodology. Index cases occur frequently on operating lists, for example between three to four elective caesareans every weekday. All the index cases are relatively short so it is feasible to obtain several trainee assessments per list. The specialty uses a team consultant structure, with each trainee assigned to a team of three to four consultants, which enables each trainee to operate with several consultants each week. Other specialties presented significant problems for study implementation. Within orthopaedics, operating lists were often amended at short notice, giving insufficient time to inform patients about the study. Staff structuring, with each consultant allocated a single trainee limited the combinations of trainees to trainers for assessment.

We also found the culture of surgical assessment and training within each surgical specialty significantly different. In obstetrics and gynaecology there is an established culture for objective assessments of surgical competence and a requirement of consultants to provide assessment and feedback to trainees, which facilitated our introduction of the study. The RCOG has phased in the use of

OSATS over the last two years prior to the formal requirement of OSATS within the new training and education programme. In other disciplines, there has been some cynicism towards competency based surgical assessment which has required our concerted efforts to overcome in implementing the study. However this does appear to be changing over time and with the opportunities provided by the study for training assessors and trainees.

The method we used to fully understand the systems and processes adopted by each specialty has been to spend several weeks working *with* the specialty in advance of assessments. This has enabled us to maximize recruitment of cases, not only through an appreciation of the practical listing of surgical cases, but by engaging with the working practices and culture of each surgical team.

Lessons Learnt and Suggested Learning Points

- Consider the specific nature of context for implementing studies in the surgical workplace.
- Spend time working with surgical teams to maximize the success of the research.

Future Research Directions

The use of video recordings has potential in providing trainees with additional feedback on their surgical performance. Feedback using videos is well established within general practice. Videotaped patient consultations are used for training (Pendleton et al. 1984) and assessment purposes, with videotaped consultations forming part of the current summative assessment for GP training, the new Membership of the Royal College of General Practitioners (Royal College of General Practitioners 2008). They have been shown to be valid and reliable as an assessment method for trainees (Campbell et al. 1995), and for practising general practitioners (Ram 1999).

We aim to develop the use of videoed operative cases for providing surgical trainees with feedback. There is reliability evidence for video assessment of some surgical procedures. Beard et al. (2005a) showed good inter-rater reliability between direct and video assessment of saphenofemoral ligation. There is also evidence that giving trainees feedback on their surgical performance improves their surgical skill (Grantcharov et al. 2007). Our study is investigating the fidelity and reliability of video recordings in different specialties. If we can show sufficient reliability of video recordings for these index procedures, we will be able to formally evaluate videos as a tool for providing feedback and additional training. Our premise is that video feedback, as an adjunct to verbal feedback from a trainer, will provide a feasible improvement to surgical training.

Summary

The intention of this chapter has been to provide a study overview to demonstrate the alignment of the study design and methodology to the study aim and main research questions. We have illustrated the implementation of the study using a descriptive analysis of our problem-solving approach. It is hoped that valuable lessons from our team experience can be drawn upon by researchers in the field, or trainers with a responsibility for workplace assessment.

Acknowledgements

The research team was the successful applicant for a grant provided by the NHS Research and Development Programme for research into the assessment of surgical skills in the UK.

References

Beard, J.D., Jolly, B.C., Newble, D.I., Thomas, W.E.G., Donnelly, J. and Southgate, L.J. (2005a) Assessing the technical skills of surgical trainees. *British Journal of Surgery* 92, 778–82.

Beard, J.D., Jolly, B.C., Southgate, L.J., Newble, D.I., Thomas, E.G. and Rochester, J. (2005b) Developing assessments of surgical skills for the GMC Performance Procedures. *Annals of the Royal College of Surgeons* 87, 242–7.

Calman, K.C., Temple, J.G., Naysmith, R., Cairncross, R.G. and Bennett, S.J. (1999) Reforming higher specialist training in the United Kingdom – a step along the continuum of medical education. *Medical Education* 33, 28–33.

Campbell, L.M., Howie, J.G. and Murray, T.S. (1995) Use of videotaped consultations in summative assessment of trainees in general practice. *British Journal of General Practice* 45, 137–41.

Crossley, J., Davies, H., Humphris, G. and Jolly, B. (2002) Generalisability: A key to unlock professional assessment. *Medical Education* 36, 972–8.

Department of Health (1993) *Hospital Doctors: Training for the Future*. The report of the Working Group on Specialist Medical Training (the Calman Report). London: Department of Health.

Department of Health (2003) *HSC 2003/001 – Protecting Staff; Delivering Services: Implementing the European Working Time Directive for Doctors in Training*. Available at: <http://www.dh.gov.uk/en/publicationsandstatistics/lettersandcirculars/healthservicecirculars/DH_4003588> [accessed March 2009].

Downing, S.M. (2003) Validity: On the meaningful interpretation of assessment data. *Medical Education* 37, 830–7.

Downing, S.M. (2004) Reliability: On the reproducibility of assessment data. *Medical Education* 38, 1006–12.

Galasko, C. and Mackay C. (1997) Unsupervised surgical training: Logbooks are essential for assessing progress. *British Medical Journal* 315, 1306–1307.

General Medical Council (1998) *Good Medical Practice*. London: General Medical Council.

Gold, R.L. (1958) Roles in sociological field observations. *Social Forces* 36, 217–23.

Grantcharov, T.P., Schulze, S., Kristiansen, V.B. (2007) The impact of objective assessment and constructive feedback on improvement of laparoscopic performance in the operating room. *Surgical Endoscopy* 21, 2240–3.

Katory, M., Singh, S. and Beard, J.D. (2001) Twenty Trent trainees: A comparison of operative competence after BST. *Annals of the Royal College of Surgeons* 83, 328–30.

Martin, J.A., Regehr, G. Reznick, R., Macrae, H., Murnaghan, J., Hutchison, C. and Brown, M. (1997) Objective structured assessment of technical skill (OSATS) for surgical residents. *British Journal of Surgery* 84(2), 273–8.

Pendleton, D., Schofield, T., Tate, P. and Havelock, P. (1984) *The Consultation: An Approach to Learning and Teaching*. Oxford: Oxford University Press.

PMETB (2008) *Standards for Curricula and Assessment Systems*. Available at: <http://www.pmetb.org.uk/fileadmin/user/Standards_Requirements/PMETB_Scas_July2008_Final.pdf> [accessed March 2009].

Ram, P. Grol, R., Rethans, J.J., Schouten, B., van der Vleuten, C. and Kester, A. (1999) Assessment of general practitioners by video observation of communication and medical performance in daily practice: Issues of validity, reliability and feasibility. *Medical Education* 33, 447–54.

Royal College of General Practitioners (2008) *Curriculum and Assessment Site*. Available at http://www.rcgp-curriculum.org.uk/nmrcgp/wpba.aspx.

Schuwirth, L.W.T., Southgate, L., Page, G.G., Paget, N.S., Lescop, J.M.J., Lew, S.R., Wade, W.B. and Baron-Maldonado, M. (2002) When enough is enough: A conceptual basis for fair and defensible practice performance assessment. *Medical Education* 36, 925–30.

Thornton, M., Donlon, M. and Beard, J.D. (2003) The operative skills of higher surgical trainees: Measuring competence rather than experience undertaken. *Annals of the Royal College of Surgeons* 85, 190–3.

Van der Vleuten, C.P.M. (1996) The Assessment of Professional Competence. *Advances in Health Sciences Education* 1, 41–67.

Winckel, C.P., Reznick, R.K., Cohen, R and Taylor, B. (1994) Reliability and construct validity of a structured technical skills assessment form. *American Journal of Surgery* 167(4), 423–7.

Yule, S., Flin, R., Maran, N., Rowley, D., Youngson, G.G. and Paterson-Brown, S. (2008) Surgeons' non-technical skills in the operating room. Reliability testing of the NOTSS behaviour rating system. *World Journal of Surgery* 32, 548–56.

Chapter 5

Scrub Practitioners' List of Intra-Operative Non-Technical Skills – SPLINTS

Lucy Mitchell and Rhona Flin

Modern surgery requires a group of people with a variety of skills to work together effectively to deliver patient care. In addition to their technical expertise, members of an operating theatre (OT) team will utilize a range of 'non-technical' skills. These are the cognitive and social skills that complement technical skills to achieve safe and efficient practice. Taxonomies of these non-technical skills have already been identified for anaesthetists' (see Glavin and Patey, Chapter 11 in this volume, Fletcher et al. 2004) and surgeons' performance (see Yule et al., Chapter 2 in this volume, Yule et al. 2006b) in the intra-operative phase of surgical procedures. Another key member of the theatre team is the scrub (or instrument) nurse, practitioner or technician,[1] who works directly with one or more surgeons while they are operating on the patient. As there was no taxonomy of non-technical skills for this member of the scrub team, a research project (funded 2007–2009 by NHS Education Scotland) was established to identify these skills and this chapter will describe the findings of the SPLINTS project to date.

Background

The aviation industry lead the way in the non-technical skills approach by developing special research programmes to identify pilots' cognitive and interpersonal skills that influenced fight safety. These skills are trained in special courses called Crew Resource Management (CRM) with the aim of reducing human error and improving the performance of flight crews (see Musson in Chapter 25, Wiener et al. 1993). The effectiveness of CRM training can be evaluated by using attitude surveys or observing and rating individuals' performance during task execution to establish whether training has resulted in knowledge transfer and improved skill execution (O'Connor et al. 2008). To increase the reliability and objectivity of these observations, behavioural assessment tools have been developed by listing the observable non-technical skills taught in these courses and devising a rating system to assess them. Other high risk work settings such as nuclear power, shipping and military have also accepted that human factors impact on safety and production and have also developed

---

1 Although this project focussed on scrub nurses, the resulting skills taxonomy will be relevant to the scrub role whether that is performed by a nurse, practitioner or technician.

this type of training and assessment method (Flin et al. 2008). In recent years, there have been efforts to extend the research and training in non-technical skills into areas of acute healthcare services, such as surgery, trauma centres and intensive care units (ICUs) (Baker et al. 2007). A recommended tool for rating individual airline pilots' behaviour called NOTECHS was developed by European pilots and psychologists (see O'Connor et al. 2002) and it has been adapted to rate teamwork in the operating theatre (see Catchpole et al. in Chapter 7, Undre and Sevdalis in Chapter 6). Rather than adapt tools designed for airline pilots, some other research teams have taken a task analysis approach to identify non-technical skills, e.g., in anaesthesia (Fletcher et al. 2004), surgery (Yule et al. 2006a; 2006b), ICU (Reader et al. 2006) and neonatal resuscitation (Thomas et al. 2004). These investigators have then devised behavioural rating systems, to evaluate the identified skills and these are now being used in professional training and formative assessment (see for example, Yule et al. in Chapter 2). Some of the team-based tools include behavioural ratings of nurses (e.g., Catchpole et al. 2008, Undre et al. 2006a) but, despite nurses being a key member of the operating theatre team, their particular non-technical skills have not been formally identified. The first task of our research project was to search the nursing and psychology literature for any studies of nurses' non-technical skills.

Literature Review

We searched electronic databases including BioMed Central, NHS e-library, Web-of-Science; publications from the Association for Perioperative Practice (AfPP), Association of peri-Operative Registered Nurses (AORN) and university library catalogues and bibliographies from related research papers. The skill categories searched for included communication, teamwork, situation awareness, leadership, decision-making and additional search terms such as *lead*, *trust*, *discussion* and *relationships* were included to keep the search as broad as possible.

The literature search identified very few studies, in fact from an initial total of 424 publications identified, only 13 papers had data pertaining to non-technical skills of scrub nurses (for full details see Mitchell and Flin 2008). Those papers only discussed the skills relating to scrub nurses' communication, teamwork and situation awareness (see Table 5.1).

There were no behaviours identified from this literature which could be classified as scrub nurses' leadership or decision-making although these may be skills which scrub nurses also require. Leadership might be displayed when assisting/advising junior team members and decisions could be made in relation to timing requests. For example, deciding when to ask the circulating nurse to bring warm saline to the table because if it is brought too soon, it will be cooled by the time the surgeon requires it and if this request is made too late, the surgeon will have to wait. The identified studies of scrub nurses' communication, teamwork and situation awareness are now briefly summarized in order to illustrate the types of behaviours which have received research attention.

Table 5.1 **Non-technical skill categories examined in the 13 included papers**

Paper	Non-technical skill				
	Communication	Teamwork	Situation Awareness	Leadership	Decision-making
Awad et al. (2005)	X	X			
Baylis et al. (2006)		X			
Edmondson (2003)	X	X			
Flin et al. (2006)	X	X			
Nestel and Kidd (2006)	X	X			
Riley and Manias (2006)	X	X	X		
Saunders (2004)	X				
Sevdalis et al. (2007)	X				
Sexton et al. (2000)	X	X			
Silen-Lipponen (2005)	X	X			
Tanner and Timmons (2000)		X			
Timmons and Reynolds (2005)		X			
Undre et al. (2006b)	X	X			

Categories of Scrub Nurses' Non-technical Skills

Communication

Communication is seen as fundamental to all types of nursing but the focus has mainly been on communicating with the patient as opposed to with colleagues. Despite the recognition that all members of a team require effective communication skills to enable the smooth running of the operating theatre (OT) (Taylor and Campbell 2000), insufficient or ineffective communication between team members in the OT setting has been recognized as a contributing factor to some adverse events (Helmreich and Schaefer 1994). This has lead to the development of checklists to promote team communication between the disciplines in the OT (see Lingard et al. 2005). Studies of nurses have shown general dissatisfaction with communication in the OT (Nestel and Kidd 2006). Case-irrelevant communications for example, questions about a previous patient, telephone calls or bleeps within the OT, particularly those which are intended for the nurse or anaesthetist were also found to be distracting to the OT team (Sevdalis et al. 2007).

In the USA, CRM principles were used in an attempt to improve communication through medical team training which included didactic instruction, interactive participation, training films, role-play and team briefings. After this intervention surgeons and anaesthetists reported that communication had improved although there was no significant improvement in nurses' perception of team communication (Awad et al. 2005). In another study (Edmondson 2003), the ability of team members to voice concerns or speak up within the hierarchical structure of the OT was examined during implementation of new technology in cardiac surgery. Since use of the new equipment required interdisciplinary communication, difficulties staff reported were more behavioural than technical. Nurses reported that nursing staff in the team had not been accustomed to speaking up – in the past, they would not have dared do so – but that surgeons had become more amenable to being questioned and team members listened more to others despite this being contrary to the previous power-based communication norms. Studies such as these illustrate that nurses' communication is obviously a key component of effective teamwork in this domain.

Teamwork

The composition of perioperative teams can vary, for example, the number of personnel, individual levels of experience, competence and familiarity of working together. We identified teamwork papers that mentioned nurse behaviours intended to aid teamwork such as memorizing surgeons' preferences and sharing information. There was also research on the effect on performance of stable versus flexible theatre teams. Attitudes to teamwork and hierarchy were also common themes discussed in these nursing articles.

Researchers have examined teamwork in the field of medicine to try to develop ways to enhance patient safety and increase team cohesion to reduce error. Perceptions of teamwork have been found to differ between disciplines. Nurses largely felt that the theatre team was a single unit, in contrast with surgeons' impressions of being a member of a team which comprised several highly specialized sub-teams (Undre et al. 2006b). Sexton et al. (2000) found low ratings of teamwork by surgical nurses in the USA and Europe when they rated interactions with consultant surgeons. In a Scottish study, surgeons rated their quality of relationships with other consultants and nurses equally, whereas nurses rated teamwork and communication with other nurses higher than between themselves and surgeons (Flin et al. 2006). Since Stein's classic paper (Stein 1967), in which the working relationship between doctor and nurse was described as a 'game' which involved nurses learning the art of making suggestions to doctors without appearing to do so, several researchers have considered how this relationship has evolved (e.g., Hughes 1988, Mackay 1993, Porter 1991, Stein et al. 1990, Svensson 1996). They have offered differing views as to why the relationship has changed, but the general consensus is that the relationship has become more informal over time. Still, ten years later, scrub nurses perceived their main responsibility as 'not upsetting' the surgeon or 'keeping the surgeons happy' (Timmons and Reynolds 2005).

Teams in the OT can either be flexible, where personnel are rotated, or stable, where members become used to working together as a unit. However, even within stable theatre nurse teams, members may alternate between scrub and circulating roles if they are multi-skilled. A study in Finland, UK and the USA by Silen-Lipponen et al. (2005) found stable OT teams helped combine team members' skills, enabled advance planning and promoted safety. When interviewed, less experienced nurses admitted that in a strange team they felt unable to prepare or participate in the planning of the surgery. There was also frustration from nurses towards the attitude of some surgeons, who seemed unaware that their operating style differed from that of their colleagues when they assumed that nurses would automatically know what equipment they required, resulting in the nurses becoming flustered and liable to make errors, causing concern for patient safety. Baylis et al. (2006) concluded that staff on unplanned leave being replaced in the team by temporary staff resulted in a higher incidence of complications. Familiarity with a surgeon's way of working helps the scrub nurse to anticipate what the surgeon will need and in what order. This cognitive skill, called 'situation awareness', was considered from the scrub nurses' perspective in only one paper.

Situation Awareness

Situation awareness is defined as 'the perception of the elements in the environment within a volume of time and space, the comprehension of their meaning and the projection of their status in the near future' (Endsley 1995, p. 36). The term was initially coined in military aviation, but is now being adopted by many other professions. Perceptual and anticipatory cognitive skills are clearly critical for scrub nurses as an element of their expertise is to 'think ahead of the surgeon'. The scrub nurse uses situation awareness, in addition to technical knowledge, to assess the stages of the surgical task correctly in order to select the appropriate instrument for the next phase of the operation. Situation awareness is not a term which has been used in the nursing literature, although an Australian study observing theatre nurses used the term 'judicial wisdom' to describe the way nurses combine their personal expertise, ability to read surgeons' demeanour and knowledge of surgical procedures to make sense of situations rather than interrupting surgery by asking questions. This unobtrusive manner of assessing the situation without interrupting was labelled 'prudent silence' (Riley and Manias 2006, p. 1548).

Surgeons' preference cards are used as an aide memoire for theatre nurses to gather the instrumentation the surgeon has indicated in the past that s/he prefers to use while performing the different procedures within his or her surgical speciality. In one study, the cards were often altered or unclear and sometimes included a choice of instruments for a single procedural element (Riley and Manias 2006). This was taken as indicative of the changeable nature of surgeons' requirements, making anticipating their needs much more difficult. That paper was the only one found directly studying scrub nurse situation awareness but since situation awareness has only recently been investigated in relation to surgeons (Way et al. 2003) this is not surprising. There have, however, been studies of situation awareness in other areas of nursing such as neonatal intensive care (Militello and Lim 2006). Scrub nurses were also interviewed about surgeons' non-technical skills during non-routine procedures and they referred more often to surgeons' interpersonal skills than cognitive skills as being important to the success of the procedure. Nurses said they were able to judge the mood and concentration level of the operating surgeon by observing and understanding their behaviour, and nurses also demonstrated situation awareness by reporting that they were able to comprehend that a patient's state was deteriorating by perceiving changes on physiological readouts (Yule et al. in preparation).

Decision-making and Leadership

The literature review did not uncover any papers specifically related to decision-making by scrub nurses during operations although they are obviously required to make decisions during interactions with surgeons and other team members whilst engaged in intra-operative problem-solving. Similarly, nurses' leadership was a skill which although studied in other areas of the hospital; for example, emergency departments and critical care (Nembhard and Edmondson 2006) did not appear to have been examined for scrub nurses. It is possible that leadership is not required by scrub nurses, yet this would be a skill displayed in a situation where an experienced scrub nurse is working with a less experienced or trainee circulating nurse or with an inexperienced surgeon.

So, from the literature we could see that although there was some evidence of the non-technical skills of scrub nurses having been examined, they were usually extracted where nurses had been interviewed or observed with regard to the theatre team as a whole or as a consequence of investigating surgeons' skills, improving safety or reducing error within the OT. Since such a small number of papers identified scrub nurses' non-technical skills in the course of the literature review, the next step in the project, to provide more examples, was to use a different method of task analysis (see Flin et al. 2008). Observing task execution and semi-structured interviews with experienced scrub nurses were two of the methods available. The project team consisting of experienced theatre nurse practitioners, a consultant surgeon and research psychologists chose the latter. Interviews with 25 scrub nurses and 9 consultant surgeons, to obtain a surgical perspective, were conducted. Ethics approval was granted from both UK National Health Service and University School of Psychology Ethics Committees.

Scrub Nurse Interviews

Semi-structured interviews with scrub nurses (n = 25) (mean scrub nurse experience of 15 years; range 2–33 years) were conducted at three Scottish hospitals to extract the non-technical skills required to do their job effectively. The interview protocol consisted of general questions designed to elicit responses which would provide details of non-technical skills used in general, day-to-day working as a scrub nurse during surgery. These questions were designed by drawing on knowledge of the generic non-technical skill categories (e.g., communication, decision-making, leadership, situation awareness) which had emerged from previous skill taxonomy development (Flin et al. 2008). Table 5.2 gives a sample of the questions asked in the interviews. For example, question 4 asks about what decisions the scrub nurse thinks s/he makes, questions 6 and 7 are designed to tease out situation awareness skills and question 8 elicited responses about teamwork and communication.

There were also questions where the interviewee was asked to recall a challenging case, to extract skills necessary to facilitate bringing a case to its conclusion on occasions where a diversion from the original plan is necessary. The interviews were conducted during the nurses' working shift in a quiet area and were digitally recorded before being transcribed and coded independently by LM and a psychology PhD student using QSR International's *NVivo* 8 software (NVivo 2008).

Table 5.2   Examples of scrub nurse interview questions

No.	General questions
4	What sort of decisions do you have to make during surgery?
6	How do you keep track of the status of an operation?
7	What factors affect the working atmosphere in the operating theatre?
8	What do you do to keep others in the team informed of what you are doing or requiring?
No.	**Case-related questions**
10	What did you contribute to making that operation end successfully?
11	Describe how your relationship with the circulating nurse helped you perform your role.

Results and Discussion

It quickly became apparent that the nurses were very keen to talk about their work and the interviews produced extremely rich data. At the time of writing, analyses of the data were ongoing but examples are now given of some coded segments in the identified non-technical skill categories. During coding, phrases fitting several different skill categories were regularly coded in answer to a question designed to capture one skill.

Communication

For example question 4, designed to elicit decision-making data, elicited a response coded as communication:

> If I hand over a suture which is short, maybe because the surgeon has already used it, I would say to him 'that's a short length' to make him aware of it otherwise he could get half way through using it before realising.

The reasoning behind this type of communication is so the nurse feels she has given the surgeon enough information for him/her to decide whether this will be a long enough suture for the immediate task. If it is not, she expects that the surgeon will tell her so that she can mount a full-length suture instead. This is to minimize the chance of causing the surgeon to become frustrated were s/he to discover, during the task, that the suture is shorter than expected and to prevent a confrontation with that surgeon, or delay in the procedure, while that is rectified. A number of items were coded referring to the different manner in which nurses speak to or communicate with different surgeons. For example:

> There are certain surgeons that if certain things happened, I feel able to say, 'Would this [piece of equipment] help?' and there are also surgeons who I would never suggest anything to.

The scrub nurse regularly communicates with all members of the theatre team; examples of communication items between the nurse and surgeon, circulating nurse and anaesthetist are shown in Table 5.3.

Teamwork

The data produced by the questions relating to teamwork were interesting. Generally, when asked to 'Describe the team that you work in when in theatre', the nurses named the other nursing team members, for example, team leader and circulating nurse, rather than describing members of the whole theatre team. Further questioning by the interviewer resulted in the surgical and anaesthetic team members also being described indicating that, in this sample of nurses, they

Table 5.3   Interviewee responses categorized as communication

Communication
If you can't see it [swab], you have to ask [the surgeon] what they've done with it. Sometimes they'll say, 'there's one inside' but they don't always.
If there are specimens to go off, I might say to the circulating nurse, 'go and get the registrar, he's [in another room], so that he can take these away in a minute'.
If there's a lot of blood loss, especially if that wasn't expected, I'll ask them [anaesthetist] if they want them [swabs] weighed because he's the one who'll be replacing the fluid.

did not automatically associate themselves as members of the whole theatre team, but rather as belonging to the nursing subteam. This contrasts with the majority view of nurses in the Undre (2006b) study who thought that OT professionals all belong to a single team whereas surgeons and anaesthetists perceived the OT as comprising multiple highly specialized teams. However, in our study, the nurses were advised that the interview was about their duties and skills as a scrub nurse which may have suggested that their role within the nurse subteam was under scrutiny. Additionally, they are very conscious that their ability to do their job efficiently depends largely on the working relationship with their circulating nurse.

It is unsurprising that a common theme to emerge was their relationship with the circulating nurse. The scrub nurse is the member of the team who is responsible for providing the surgeon with the equipment necessary for the procedure and once scrubbed can not leave the table. So, for the partnership between scrub and circulating nurse to work, the circulating nurse must be attentive and also follow the procedure. S/he must be able to anticipate the scrub nurses' needs so that s/he, in turn, is able to provide the surgeon with the equipment in a timely fashion.

> You are ultimately dependent on them [circulating nurse] because you are stuck at the table and can't get anything.

> I like to think we [scrub nurses] really do make a contribution to the end result. The people who are scrubbed at the table are useless without everybody else [in the team].

One underlying element of teamwork from the nurses' perspective appears to be coordination, i.e., that exchanges of information and equipment or instruments passing between team members must be smoothly executed, for example:

> I am really pleased if I have been able to make everything flow in a challenging case.

...so that they're [surgeon] not having to wait when they ask for something.

This means that if the scrub nurse is 'one step ahead' of the surgeon then the circulating nurse has to be two steps ahead in order to enable this information/ system to flow smoothly.

Situation Awareness

Situation awareness is most certainly a non-technical skill required by scrub nurses for effective performance. Available clues in the environment include listening to conversation exchanges between other team members, listening to and understanding changes in patient monitors, as well as observing changes in other team members' tone of voice, body language or demeanour:

> Listening, being aware of the other stuff round about you. I am always tuned into the pulse sats or the ECG or something so I'm instantly aware of the changes because I might have to stop ...

> You just know when something is going wrong, it's either ... you can physically see that something's happened but sometimes you can't see. You can just recognize the surgeon's body language, or see them clenching their jaw, that things are not going well.

These are skills which develop with experience and anticipation is an underlying element of situation awareness which one nurse enunciated:

> The longer you are a scrub nurse, the more you are able to not just react to what the surgeon does, you can anticipate what the surgeon is going to do.

Decision-making and Leadership

As was found in the literature review, there were minimal data in the interviews coded as decision-making or leadership skills. Some phrases coded as decision-making included those relating to choosing which instrument to hand to the surgeon, the quantity of supplies (e.g., swabs) or when to ask for things to be taken onto the trolley. However, most of these items are driven by the nurses' knowledge of the surgeons' preferences or stages of the procedure.

Leadership was not seen as a role which the scrub nurse felt they had in the theatre team. The question 'who do you see as the leader in the team?' was answered with a mixture of responses but the senior nursing team leader on duty or a fluctuating leadership role between consultant anaesthetist and consultant surgeon as the procedure progresses were responses.

Consultant surgeon interviews   In order to obtain a surgical perspective on what scrub nurse behaviours assist or hinder the surgeon to perform his/her task, interviews were conducted with nine consultant surgeons from four Scottish hospitals. The nurses' ability to anticipate and hand the surgeon instrumentation in a timely fashion were skills they appreciated:

> She should watch me and be ahead of me, a step ahead ... when I say knife she will hand me the knife and she should know what I'm going to ask next ...

> A lot of what you need arrives in your hand without you actually having got as far as asking for it, it's almost telepathy, it's smooth, it runs.

The scrub nurses' knowledge of surgical procedures and instrumentation were also skills which emerged as being important in the surgeons' view:

> They [scrub nurse] don't ask if I'm going to need a mounted suture or a mounted tie – it will come mounted because they know I'm working deep and they know I'll not be able to reach. They don't hand me short scissors when I'm in the pelvis, they're going to give me long scissors.

One behaviour identified as negatively affecting the surgeons was when the scrub nurse is distracted by other people or issues in the theatre:

> They need to have the ability to be quite focused on the procedure and not be distracted by what else is going on.

Although this was a common complaint from the surgeons, it should be acknowledged that the ability of the scrub nurse to assist the surgeon effectively seems largely as a consequence of their ability to absorb the conversations and cues in the rest of the theatre whilst still maintaining concentration on the procedure and the likely requirements of the surgeon. One surgeon acknowledged this point:

> It requires the female thing, the multi-tasking, able to do all of those things simultaneously and still give you what you need.

A communication issue which emerged in interviews with both nurses and surgeons was on occasions where the surgeon can not bring to mind the name of the instrument that s/he requires the scrub nurse to hand over:

> I find particularly when I am deeply concentrating and stressed out I can't find the names of the instruments.

One nurse explained how she compensates for that:

> When they ask for something and you give them what you think it is that they
> need and it's not the thing they said but you know it is what they actually want.

Surgeons do seem to prefer scrub nurses to possess a certain degree of 'mind reading' ability although this skill appears to be a combination of knowledge of the procedure, familiarity with surgeons and their preferred methods and use of instrumentation. This knowledge, combined with the ability to listen and process sources of available information, for example, conversations and monitors in the operating theatre environment, enables them to assist the surgeon efficiently and seemingly effortlessly. These skills also appear to contribute to the satisfaction derived by experienced scrub nurses when a procedure 'flows', particularly when they have planned well, have all possible equipment available and have anticipated his/her requirements so that the surgeon does not have to wait for anything.

Future Direction for Project

The next step in the project is for expert panels comprising three to four theatre nurse team leaders to review the data segments (example described in Table 5.3). These panels will be tasked with labelling the skill categories and also with providing labels for the underlying categories within those skills. In previous taxonomies, for example, within the 'Situation Awareness' category of the behavioural rating system for surgeons' non-technical skills (NOTSS) (see <www.abdn.ac.uk/iprc/notss>), the three elements are:

- gathering information;
- understanding information;
- projecting and anticipating future states.

Although the component elements of these skill categories remain to be determined for scrub nurses, it is likely that they will be similar to those previously identified for anaesthetists and surgeons however, it is critical that they are identified and labelled in terminology recognizable to scrub nurses if the rating system is to be valid for use by individuals in that domain.

Conclusion

There are a number of key non-technical skills required for effective and safe task performance by scrub nurses. One of the most important skills of the scrub nurse is situation awareness, that is, to monitor the actions of the surgeon, anticipate the surgeon's technical requirements and using coordination skills to enable the smooth flow of the operative procedure. In addition, scrub nurses' ability to identify and cope with different surgeons' personalities and changing preferences is a skill which enables them to assess surgical situations, particularly when a procedure is not going according to the original plan. They appear able to identify the changing behaviour of surgeons as well as absorbing audible and visual clues in the theatre environment, so that they can adjust their own performance to assist surgeons effectively. This project will produce a prototype rating tool for use by nurses to rate observations of performance by them in the operating theatre. Currently, training and assessment of trainee nurses is by subjective assessment and a formal rating tool, such as SPLINTS, would be of benefit to both trainees and trainers as well as for ongoing training and assessment for scrub nurses, practitioners or technicians.

References

Awad, S.S., Fagan, S.P., Bellows, C., Albo, D., Green-Rashad, B., De La Garza, M., et al. (2005) Bridging the communication gap in the operating room with medical team training. *American Journal of Surgery* 190, 770–4.

Baker, D.P., Salas, E., Barach, P., Battles, J. and King, H. (2007) The relationship between teamwork and patient safety. In P. Carayon (ed.), *Handbook of Human Factors and Ergonomics in Health Care and Patient Safety* (pp. 259–71). Mahwah, NJ: Laurence Erlbaum Associates.

Baylis, O.J., Adams, W.E., Allen, D. and Fraser, S.G. (2006) Do variations in the theatre team have an impact on the incidence of complications? *BMC Opthalmology* 6(13): doi: 10.1186/1471-2415-6-13.

Catchpole, K., Mishra, A., Handa, A. and McCulloch, P. (2008) Teamwork and error in the operating room: Analysis of skills and roles. *Annals of Surgery* 247, 699–706.

Edmondson, A.C. (2003) Speaking up in the operating room: How team leaders promote learning in interdisciplinary action teams. *Journal of Management Studies* 40(6), 1419–52.

Endsley, M. (1995). Toward a theory of situation awareness in dynamic systems. *Human Factors* 37, 32–64.

Fletcher, G., Flin, R., McGeorge, P., Glavin, R., Maran, N. and Patey, R. (2004) Rating non-technical skills: Developing a behavioural marker system for use in anaesthesia. *Cognition Technology and Work* 6, 165–71.

Flin, R., O'Connor, P. and Crichton, M. (2008) *Safety at the Sharp End. A Guide to Non-Technical Skills*. Aldershot: Ashgate.

Flin, R., Yule, S., McKenzie, L., Paterson-Brown, S. and Maran, N. (2006) Attitudes to teamwork and safety in the operating theatre. *The Surgeon* 4, 145–51.

Helmreich, R. L. and Schaefer, H.G. (1994) Team performance in the operating room. In M. Bogner (ed.), *Human Error in Medicine* (pp. 225–53). New Jersey: Lawrence Erlbaum Associates.

Hughes, D. (1988) When nurse knows best: Some aspects of nurse/doctor interaction in a casualty department. *Sociology of Health and Illness* 10, 1–21.

Lingard, L., Espin, S., Rubin, B., Whyte, S., Colmenares, M. and Baker, G.R. (2005) Getting teams to talk: Development and pilot implementation of a checklist to promote interprofessional communication in the OR. *Quality and Safety in Healthcare* 14, 340–6.

Mackay, L. (1993) *Conflicts in Care. Medicine and Nursing.* London: Chapman & Hall.

Militello, L. and Lim, L. (2006) Patient assessment skills: Assessing early cues of necrotizing enterocolitis. *Journal of Perinatal and Neonatal Nursing* 9, 42–52.

Mitchell, L. and Flin, R. (2008) Non-technical skills of the operating theatre scrub nurse: Literature review. *Journal of Advanced Nursing* 63, 15–24.

Nembhard, I.M. and Edmondson, A.C. (2006) Making it safe: The effects of leader inclusiveness and professional status on psychological safety and improvement efforts in health care teams. *Journal of Organizational Behavior* 27, 941–66.

Nestel, D. and Kidd, J. (2006) Nurses' perceptions and experiences of communication in the operating theatre: A focus group interview. *BMC Nursing* 5(1) doi: 10.1186/1472-6955-5-1.

NVivo qualitative data analysis software (2008) QSR International Pty Ltd. Version 8.

O'Connor, P., Hormann, H.J., Flin, R., Lodge, M., Goeters, K.M. and the JARTEL Group (2002) Developing a method for evaluating Crew Resource Management skills: A European perspective, *International Journal of Aviation Psychology* 12, 265–88.

O'Connor, P., Campbell, J., Newon, J., Melton, J., Salas, E. and Wilson, K. (2008) Crew Resource Management training effectiveness: A meta-analysis and some critical needs. *International Journal of Aviation Psychology* 18, 353–68.

Porter, S. (1991) A participant observation study of power relations between nurses and doctors in a general hospital. *Journal of Advanced Nursing* 16, 728–35.

Reader, T., Flin, R., Lauche, K. and Cuthbertson, B.H. (2006) Non-technical skills in the intensive care unit. *British Journal of Anaesthesia* 5, 551–9.

Riley, R.G. and Manias, E. (2006) Governance in operating room nursing: Nurses' knowledge of individual surgeons. *Social Science and Medicine* 62, 1541–51.

Saunders, S. (2004) Why good communication skills are important for theatre nurses. *Nursing Times* 100(14), 42–4.

Sevdalis, N., Healey, A.N. and Vincent, C.A. (2007) Distracting communications in the operating theatre. *Journal of Evaluation in Clinical Practice* 13, 390–4.

Sexton, J.B., Thomas, E.J. and Helmreich, R.L. (2000) Error, stress, and teamwork in medicine and aviation: Cross sectional surveys. *British Medical Journal* 320, 745–9.

Silen-Lipponen, M., Tossavainen, K., Turunen, H. and Smith, A. (2005) Potential errors and their prevention in operating room teamwork as experienced by Finnish, British and American nurses. *International Journal of Nursing Practice* 11, 21–32.

Stein, L., Watts, D.T. and Howell, T. (1990) The doctor-nurse game revisited. *New England Journal of Medicine* 322, 546–9.

Stein, L.I. (1967) The doctor-nurse game. *Archives of General Psychiatry* 16, 699–703.

Svensson, R. (1996). The interplay between doctors and nurses: A negotiated order perspective. *Sociology of Health and Illness* 18, 379–98.

Tanner, J. and Timmons, S. (2000) Backstage in the theatre. *Journal of Advanced Nursing* 32(4), 975–80.

Taylor, M. and Campbell, C. (2000) Communication skills in the operating department. In D. Plowes (ed.), *Back to Basics: Perioperative Practice Principles*, (pp. 50–3). Harrogate: National Association of Theatre Nurses.

Thomas, E.J., Sexton, J.B. and Helmreich, R.L. (2004) Translating teamwork behaviours from aviation to healthcare: Development of behavioural markers for neonatal resuscitation. *Quality and Safety in Healthcare* 13, 57–64.

Timmons, S. and Reynolds, A. (2005) The doctor-nurse relationship in the operating theatre. *British Journal of Perioperative Nursing* 15(3), 110–15.

Undre, S., Healey, A.H., Darzi, A. and Vincent, C.A. (2006a) Observational assessment of surgical teamwork: A feasibility study. *World Journal of Surgery* 30, 1774–83.

Undre, S., Sevdalis, N., Healey, A.N., Darzi, S. and Vincent, C. (2006b) Teamwork in the operating theatre: Cohesion or confusion? *Journal of Evaluation in Clinical Practice* 12(2), 182–9.

Way, L.W., Stewart, L., Gantert, W., Liu, K., Lee, C.M., Whang, K., et al. (2003) Causes and prevention of laparoscopic bile duct injuries. *Annals of Surgery* 237, 460–9.

Wiener, E., Kanki, B. and Helmreich, R. (eds) (1993) *Cockpit Resource Management*. San Diego: Academic Press.

Yule, S., Flin, R., Paterson-Brown, S. and Maran, N. (2006a) Non-technical skills for surgeons: A review of the literature. *Surgery* 139, 140–9.

Yule, S., Flin, R., Paterson-Brown, S., Maran, N. and Rowley, D. (2006b) Development of a rating system for surgeons' non-technical skills. *Medical Education* 40, 1098–104.

Yule, S., Reader, T. and Flin, R. (in preparation) Nurses' reflections of surgeons' behaviour during non-routine operations.

Chapter 6

Observing and Assessing Surgical Teams: The Observational Teamwork Assessment for Surgery© (OTAS)©

Shabnam Undre, Nick Sevdalis and Charles Vincent

Introduction

Until relatively recently, surgical performance and surgical outcomes were mostly understood and modelled as a function of, first, the surgical patients' risk factors and, second, the expertise and ability of the operating surgeon. In turn, surgical expertise was conceptualized predominantly in terms of the surgeon's visuo-motor (or technical) skills. In the last few years, however, a shift in the conceptualization of surgical competence has emerged in the literature, as well in training curricula for junior surgeons. The shift involves a systems-oriented approach to surgery, in which multiple determinants of surgical outcomes are considered (Calland et al. 2002, Healey and Vincent 2007, Vincent et al. 2004). These determinants include the surgeon's technical (Beard 2007, Fried and Feldman 2008), cognitive and behavioural skills (Yule et al. 2006a), the operative environment (Healey et al. 2006a, Sevdalis et al. 2008b), and teamwork in the operating theatre (Healey et al. 2006b). The focus of this chapter is on teamwork.

Teamwork in surgical teams refers to the way the operating surgeon interacts with other members of the operating theatre team – including assistant surgeon(s) and members of the anaesthetic and nursing sub-teams. Recent surgical publications have highlighted the importance of teamwork for the delivery of safe, high quality surgical care (e.g., Davenport et al. 2007, Gawande et al. 2003, Greenberg et al. 2007). Moreover, in the United States, the Joint Commission on Accreditation of Healthcare Organizations (JCAHO) has highlighted poor teamworking as a regular contributing factor to medical error (JCAHO 2000). Furthermore, in recent, high profile errors (e.g., wrong-sided surgery) the involvement and contribution of the rest of the team have been questioned in addition to that of the operating surgeon, thus highlighting a shift towards more emphasis on teamwork in the delivery of surgical care (Kaufman 2003).

In this chapter, we report the development and initial empirical exploration of the Observational Teamwork Assessment for Surgery© (OTAS©). In order to assess quantitatively the impact, direct or indirect, of teamwork on surgical performance, it is necessary to have a comprehensive and robust tool that assesses teamwork of an entire operating theatre team in real time. OTAS© aims to be such a comprehensive and robust measure of teamwork in surgery. We report, in detail, the conceptual background, initial development and empirical application, revision and further testing of the OTAS©. We conclude with an outline of ongoing empirical work and future directions in OTAS©-related research.

Conceptual Background

Components of Teamwork

Systematic study of teamworking started in the 1950s and 1960s, with an emphasis on military teams. The focus of this work was military teams functioning in demanding, stressful conditions and the ultimate aim was to understand the constituents of an effective team and to feed this understanding into team training (Paris et al. 2000). Subsequently, empirical study of teamwork extended to high risk industries outside the military (e.g., commercial aviation, nuclear industry) and, soon the conclusion was reached that effective teamwork is fundamental to safety and efficiency in high-risk environments (Helmreich and Foushee 1993). Team communication emerged as a particularly critical aspect of teamwork, which allows the fulfilment of other dimensions of teamwork, such as team coordination.

Numerous studies on teamwork were eventually reviewed and organized in a conceptual framework or model of teamwork by Dickinson and McIntyre (1997). These authors proposed that, from the existing literature, seven components of teamwork can be identified: team orientation, team leadership, communication, monitoring, feedback, backup behaviour and coordination.

Dickinson and McIntyre's (1997) model of teamwork and its components was an important step in conceptually clarifying what teamwork consist of (i.e., the sampling domain of the construct). The logical next step is how to best measure and assess the components of teamwork in real-world teams.

Measuring Teamwork in Real-World Teams

Since, historically, the study of teamwork started from teams of experts carrying out complex tasks in complex work environments it is perhaps not surprising that assessment of teamwork has been traditionally done through observation. Observation might be carried out within the actual work environment in real time, or in a simulated scenario or via recording teams while they are at work and retrospective analysis of video and audio recordings. Various tools have been developed for observation and assessment of teamwork – a sample of them is reviewed below:

- *TARGETS (Targeted Acceptable Responses to Generated Events or Tasks)*: this method was originally developed to evaluate team performance in complex environments such as air crew coordination training (Fowlkes et al. 1994). Specific 'focal' events are inserted into training scenarios, each one with a range of acceptable behavioural responses as criteria. An observer can then assess observed responses against the preset criteria. This method is ideally suited for assessment of teamwork during training, as focal events can be scored reasonably objectively (Dwyer et al. 1997). Disadvantages of the method include the need for development of large numbers of scenarios and lack of applicability to real-life teamworking, in which there is much less control compared to training.

- *Behavioural markers systems*: these are typically used in commercial aviation. A number of teamwork components are defined and observable behaviours are attached to each one of them in the form of behavioural statements. Observers rate team-members depending on whether the relevant behaviours were exhibited or not (or to what extent). Assessment can be done in real time, or retrospectively, using video/audio recordings. Perhaps the most well-known such tool is the Non-Technical Skills (NOTECHS), used to assess cockpit crews (Avermate van 1998, Flin et al. 2003, Klampfer et al. 2001, O'Connor et al. 2002). NOTECHS assesses leadership and management, decision-making, cooperation and situation awareness.
- A similar tool is the *Line Operations Safety Audit (LOSA)*: this system utilizes trained observers riding in cockpit jump seats to evaluate several aspects of crew performance and collect safety-related data. Observers record threats encountered by aircrew and types of errors committed, and they record how flight crews manage these situations to maintain safety (Helmreich et al. 2002, Klinect et al. 2003).

Early Observational Studies of Teamwork and Safety in Surgical Teams

At the early stages of OTAS development, we sought to identify empirical studies that had attempted to assess teamwork in operating theatres. Early attempts to empirically assess teamwork in surgical environments were evidently influenced by the principles of teamwork assessment tools and the relevant research approaches used in the context of (mostly) commercial aviation. Teamwork was assessed via observation and the key working hypothesis was that teamwork is implicated in the safety and quality of surgical care.

Roth et al. (2004) studied team performance using a field notes technique. Two observers, one surgeon and one human factors expert studied ten complex operations in an exploratory study to identify latent factors that could compromise patient safety and potentially lead to adverse events. Two key themes emerged from these observations: (i) multitasking and the ensuing pressure on operating theatre staff's attention; and (ii) multiple conflicting goals that the staff had to achieve. From a methodological perspective, Roth et al. concluded that retrospective analysis of video recordings could be an alternative to real-time observation in the operating theatre (Roth et al. 2004).

Carthey (2003) evaluated the role of structured observations in theatre. Data were collected from 173 neonatal arterial switch operations in paediatric cardiac units across 16 centres in the UK. Trained observers noted errors, problems and notable aspects of good performance. The observer's interpretation was checked with the operating theatre team after each case. Carthey (2003) concluded that structured, well-defined observational measures are needed for rapid training of observers, better inter-observer reliability, and clearer understanding of what should be observed.

An observational study of errors during paediatric cardiac surgery was conducted by de Leval et al. (2000). They found that surgeons' diagnostic skill, knowledge of strategies to correct problems and communication with the rest of the team were important for error compensation. The authors concluded that error recovery strategies are just as important as error prevention measures. In another study of paediatric cardiac operations, Catchpole et al. (2006) used a single observer in the operating theatre, who was making notes as well as recordings of the procedures (to be reviewed at a later stage). Although the study focused primarily on threats and errors associated with surgical failures, communication and coordination did emerge from it as components of teamwork (see Chapters 7 and 19 of this volume).

Mackenzie et al. (1996) used video studies to observe emergency intubations. They found that in stressful situations knowledge-based errors were committed (including drug dosage errors) and that not all observed errors were actually reported. The authors concluded that team training might be beneficial for improving team communication. In another study, Mackenzie, Xiao and the IPO Group (2003) used recordings of trauma resuscitations to study team performance in emergency medicine. They found that recordings had some advantage over observation in that they could be analysed iteratively and in more depth – however, they were more time consuming (see Chapter 23 in this volume).

Helmreich et al. (1995) developed a checklist to assess teamwork in the operating theatre. Their Operating Room Check List is based on behavioural markers developed for aviation and consists of observable behaviours that are divided into three sections: (i) team concerns; (ii) decision-making and communication; and (iii) management of the work situation. These are scored on four-point scales. Initial results using the checklist in a European hospital showed that there was wide variability in the behaviours observed with up to 40 per cent being below standard (Helmreich and Davies 2007).

Guerlain et al. (2002, 2005, 2007) developed the Remote Analysis of Team Environments (RATE) tool. RATE is a recording and analysis system that captures communication and team performance in operating theatres. The authors reported a successful application of the RATE in ten laparoscopic cholecystectomies and concluded that RATE has the potential to identify areas for improvement in teamwork (such as pre-operative briefing) (see Chapter 8 in this volume).

Finally, Lingard and her colleagues carried out a series of observational studies with a strong focus on communication (Lingard et al. 2002, Lingard et al. 2004a, 2004b, Chapter 17 in this volume). Five core communication themes in the operating theatre emerged from these studies: (i) time; (ii) resources; (iii) roles; (iv) safety and sterility; and (v) situation control. Lingard et al. (2002) recorded between one and four communication events where tension was high, typically between surgeons and nurses. In another study (Lingard 2004a), 421 communication events from 48 operations were analysed for failures and 129 failures (31 per cent) were found. These were related to the occasion of the communication, its content, its purpose, or its audience. They found that 23 of these failures resulted in some inefficiency, 16 triggered tension between staff, 10 caused a delay, 3 resulted in the bending of a rule, 2 in the waste of resources, 2 in inconvenience for the patient, and, finally, one failure resulted in a visible operating error. On the whole, 36 per cent of the failures affected teamwork negatively.

The empirical work that we reviewed above was or was becoming available at the early stages of OTAS© development. Upon review and evaluation of the findings and the methods/assessment tools that are reported in these papers, we concluded that:

1. assessment of surgical teamwork is feasible and acceptable to surgical teams;
2. direct observation appears to be a well-suited methodology for such assessment;
3. a theory-driven, robust observational tool that is specific to surgery needs to be developed.

This rationale guided the initial development of the OTAS© tool.

Initial OTAS© Development and Empirical Piloting (Healey et al. 2004, 2006c, Vincent et al. 2004, Undre et al. 2006a, 2006b, Undre and Healey 2006)[1]

We set out to develop OTAS© using real-time observations in the light of the conceptual framework and assessment issues and approaches summarised above. In designing and piloting OTAS©, we aimed for:

- a surgery-specific tool, based on a sound conceptual framework and appropriate rationale for assessment;
- a tool that assesses concurrently *what* surgical teams do and *how* they do it;
- a tool that assesses teamwork across the entire surgical team;
- a generic tool, designed to assess teamwork in routine procedures in real time across surgical specialities (but also amenable to subsequent adaptation for use, for instance, in emergency surgery or for team training purposes).

---

1 For the sections on OTAS© development, refinement and empirical testing, readers are referred to the original publications (cited in the text) for additional detail.

Surgical teams are usually comprised of four generic disciplinary groups: surgeons, nurses, anaesthetists and Operating Department Practitioners (ODPs: in the UK, they fulfil the role of an anaesthetic nurse/assistant). Depending on the procedure, other specialists can be part of the team (e.g., radiographers). Tasks and behaviours required in the team process might be carried out by individuals, or by several members within a disciplinary subgroup (e.g., anaesthetist and ODP), or, finally, between two or more subgroups, simultaneously or sequentially.

We adopted the approach that an observational assessment of teamwork should account for essential routine tasks relating to team process and patient safety. Thus the first component of the OTAS© is a task checklist. In addition, however, OTAS© also comprises behaviour ratings. The distinction between the checklist and the behaviour ratings is important: we took the stance that elements of team performance that are captured by checklists or very narrowly defined markers are only a part of the level of teamwork achieved by a team. Simply put, teams that carry out similar routine tasks may still appear very different to an external observer – due to significant differences in their communication and coordination patterns. Hence, in the initial development of OTAS© we chose to supplement the (more objective) task checklist with (more subjective) behaviour ratings, with an open format for recording of field observations.

Assessment Timeline: OTAS© Operative Phases and Stages

In order to facilitate the scoring of tasks and the rating of behaviours, OTAS© divides the surgical process into three meaningful phases (see Table 6.1):

1. *pre-operative phase*: includes everything up to the point of the actual operation;
2. *intra-operative phase*: from the point of incision (knife to skin) to the point of closure;
3. *post-operative phase*: from the point of closure to patient being transferred to recovery/ward.

Table 6.1   Operative phases and stages of OTAS©

Phase	Stage 1	Stage 2	Stage 3
1. PRE-OP	pre-op planning and preparation	patient sent for to anaesthesia given	patient set-up to op-readiness
2. INTRA-OP	opening/access to contact of target organ	op-specific procedure	from prepare to close to complete closure
3. POST-OP	anaesthetic reversal to exit from theatre	transfer to recovery/ recovery to ward	feedback and self-assessment

Within each phase, there are distinct stages. These are distinguished by concrete events that require teamwork – such as, for instance, patient entering the operating theatre under anaesthesia for transfer to the operating table.

Development of Task Checklist

The checklist was constructed for each phase/stage of the operation. Existing operating theatre protocols, recommendations for good practice, domain knowledge and expert advice were inputs to the development process. The initial list consisted of 203 tasks – plus checks for presence of staff in theatre. Tasks fall within one of three categories:

1. *patient tasks* comprise either actions or information associated directly with the patient, such as safe transfer to operating table and patient notes present;
2. *equipment/provisions tasks* include checking and counting of surgical instruments;
3. *communication tasks* include information such as confirmation of operative site laterality.

Items on the checklist are marked 'yes/no'. For example, under the category of equipment tasks, diathermy preparation is marked 'yes' if the diathermy machine is switched on and tested prior to the operation.

Development of Behaviour Rating Scales

Choice of behaviours to be observed followed Dickinson and McIntyre's (1997) model of teamwork. Of their seven dimensions we retained five, namely:

1. *communication* refers to the quality and the quantity of the information exchanged among members of the team;
2. *coordination* refers to the management and to the timing of activities and tasks;
3. *cooperation/back-up behaviour* refers to assistance provided among members of the team, supporting others and correcting errors;
4. *leadership* refers to the provision of directions, assertiveness and support among members of the team;
5. *monitoring/awareness* refers to team observation and awareness of ongoing processes.

Team orientation (which refers to the attitudes that team members have towards each other and to the team task) was deemed hard to assess by observation and also closely related to cooperation/back up behaviour – hence we incorporated it into that dimension. Similarly, team feedback (which refers to providing and receiving information about performance) was viewed as a component of communication. The five retained behaviours are rated on 0–6 point, behaviourally anchored scales.

The OTAS© Assessment Process

Two observers (surgeon and psychologist), enter the operating theatre before the patient arrives. Thereafter, both surgeon and psychologist observer record each stage start-time, they confirm stages in the procedure, serving as a double check on times. The surgeon observer begins checking tasks using a PDA (tasks in Excel spreadsheet, arranged by phase/stage). The psychologist observer begins observing and noting teamwork behaviours as they occur using a paper form. Towards the end of each stage, the psychologist observer uses the OTAS behaviour summary scales to provide ratings for the overall impression of each behaviour construct displayed by the team.

Initial Empirical Application: General Surgical Cases (Undre et al. 2006a)

This study aimed to assess the feasibility and practicality of systematic teamwork observations in real time in real procedures and also to test the OTAS© tool.

Prior to data collection, operating theatre staff were informed and notices about the study were displayed inside and outside the operating theatre. We took care to reassure staff that data would be used for research purposes only and not as surveillance of individuals' performance.

Methods

Data were collected from 50 general surgery operations (29 open, 21 laparoscopic) in a single operating theatre in our institution (central London teaching hospital). The data were collected from the operating lists of three consultant (attending) surgeons, but the research team did not have control over staff variation between cases (anaesthetists, trainee/assisting surgeons, nurses). Data were collected from procedures that lasted between 30–240 minutes. Tasks and behaviours were assessed from Pre-op Stage 1 to Post-op Stage 2. The last OTAS© stage was not feasible to assess.

Results and Comments

Task completion   Table 6.2 (general surgery columns) presents the task completion rates. Overall, task completion was higher at post-op than in pre- or intra-op phases. Moreover, task completion was higher for patient tasks than for either equipment/provisions tasks or communications tasks. Some more specific findings:

- anaesthetists had not checked their machines themselves in 20 per cent of the cases;

- suction was checked prior to the operation in just 37 per cent of cases;
- procedures were confirmed verbally in 32 per cent of cases;
- patient notes were absent in 12 per cent of cases;
- there was no communication regarding readiness to start procedure in 35 per cent of the cases;
- delays and changes to the case-list occurred in over 70 per cent of cases.

Table 6.2   Task completion rates in general surgery (first study) versus urology (second study)

Task type	Pre-operative		Intra-operative		Post-operative	
	General Surgery	Urology	General Surgery	Urology	General Surgery	Urology
Equipment/ provisions	56%	61%	82%	91%	89%	95%
Communication	61%	71%	55%	57%	90%	84%
Patient	90%	94%	93%	93%	97%	92%
Overall	69%	77%	77%	80%	92%	90%

Behaviour ratings   These were relatively high, with scores of four or higher (on a seven-point scale). Of significance were the findings that communication was rated significantly lower than the other behaviours and it was lower in the pre- and intra-operative phases.

The key finding of the study is that team observations in real procedures in real time are feasible. Moreover, we felt that the OTAS© does capture significant aspects of teamwork and that the format of the tool (task checklist and behaviour ratings) does allow for capturing some of the richness of surgical teamwork in a robust, replicable manner. Furthermore, the findings were not dissimilar to previous studies that have highlighted communication issues as well as problems with equipment in surgical teams. Importantly, this initial experience of using OTAS© revealed a number of ways in which the tool could be improved. These were addressed by refining and retesting the tool.

OTAS© refinement and further empirical testing (Healey et al. 2006c, Undre et al. 2006a, 2007b)

In the light of the findings and our experience with the first 50 observed cases, a number of revision points for OTAS© emerged:

- There were redundancies in the task checklist.

- The scoring of behaviours was relatively blunt, in that it did not allow any discrimination between the different sub-teams (anaesthetic, surgical, nursing) that make up a full operating theatre team.
- In addition, the scoring of the behaviours was too much reliant on the psychologist observer's impression of the team. Although the relative subjectivity of this part of the tool was intended, it was felt that it should be reduced to allow novice as well as non-psychology trained observers to be trained in using the tool.

In what follows, we report in detail how each one of these issues was addressed.

Revision of Task Checklist

Structured interviews with nine expert operating theatre staff (three anaesthetists, three nurses, three surgeons) were conducted. Participants were given the original checklist and the following criteria:

Inclusion criteria (any of the below)

1. Task contributes to patient safety or quality of care.
2. Task contributes to surgical outcome positively or its omission would contribute adversely to surgical outcome.
3. Task is essential for teamwork or enhances teamworking.
4. Task makes an important contribution to the whole system.

Exclusion criteria (any of the below)

1. Task which is duplicated or covered by another task.
2. Task which is irrelevant to any of the above inclusion categories.
3. Tasks which are inherent to the procedure.
4. Task which is not clinically important.

For each task, participants indicated whether it should be included/excluded, or whether they were not sure. This process of systematically eliciting expert agreement was used as input to the checklist revision. Working in parallel, two surgeons (consultant and trainee) who were blind to the interview findings prepared a revised version of the list.

No perfect agreement was reached for task exclusion or inclusion. We used the following cut off criteria:

1. Tasks where 9/9 respondents agreed should be included (31) were included.
2. Tasks where 8/9 respondents agreed should be included (55) were included.

3. Tasks where 6–7/9 respondents agreed should be excluded (15) were excluded.
4. Tasks where 4–5/9 respondents agreed should be excluded (25) were mostly excluded; these decisions were made with input from the consultant and trainee surgeons involved in the checklist revision.

The process furnished a revised, easier to use checklist of 115 tasks (significantly reduced from the original 203). The tasks still corresponded to the three operative phases as originally defined (pre-, intra- and post-operative). Importantly, virtually all tasks that the two blind surgeon reviewers included in their checklist were indeed included in the list (thus suggesting reliability in the reviewing process).

Modification of Behavioural Ratings to Assess Sub-Teams

In the initial assessment, one rating per behaviour was allocated to the entire surgical team. In the process of allocating ratings, however, it was noted that discrepancies existed at times between sub-teams (nursing, surgical and anaesthetic) and, as a result, single ratings for the entire team did not convey an accurate picture of that team's teamwork. The rating scheme was, therefore, revised to provide separate ratings for each one of the five behaviours to each one of the three theatre sub-teams. With this amendment to the rating scheme, the psychologist observer now generates 45 behavioural ratings per procedure (5 behaviours × 3 operative phases × 3 sub-teams).

Development of Behavioural Scoring Aids

In order to assist the scoring of the behaviours, demonstrative scenarios and behavioural exemplars were developed for each of the five behaviours.

- *Exemplar behaviours*: exemplar behaviours are items that serve to guide the observer in 'looking for behaviours' that indicate effective teamwork. Exemplar behaviours may be checked for their occurrence, in support of overall behaviour ratings – thus serving as reminders for the psychologist observer. Exemplar behaviours were constructed for each of the five behaviours, for each phase of the procedure, and, finally, for each of the three key sub-teams. For example, during the Intra-op Phase, the surgeon asks the team if they are ready and asks the anaesthetist if it is OK to start the procedure.
- *Demonstrative scenarios*: scenarios are particularly useful for calibrating the rating of behaviour to a standardized scale. Scenarios provide a context in which behaviours are related to levels of teamwork effectiveness and demonstrate that certain patterns of team behaviour are associated with certain levels of team effectiveness. For example, the anaesthetist gives clear and audible instructions to the team about the latest blood results and that s/he will be transfusing the patient with two units of blood.

Exemplar behaviours and demonstrative scenarios for each sub-team/stage of a procedure are fully described in the OTAS user manual (Undre and Healey 2006, freely available for research use at: <http://www.csru.org.uk>).

Further Empirical Testing: Urological Cases (Undre et al. 2007a)

This study aimed to further assess:

- feasibility of the revised OTAS© tool;
- usefulness of the revisions;
- reliability in the behavioural scoring.

The study also aimed to compare general surgery with urology elective procedures. As in the previous study, care was taken to inform staff about the study and to reassure them that data would be used for research purposes only.

Methods

Data were collected in 50 urological surgery operations in two operating theatres, one in our own institution (central London teaching hospital) and the other at a treatment centre. Twenty operations were the first operation of the list; the remaining 30 operations were the second or subsequent operation. The typical mix of operations contained cystoscopy, ureteroscopy, ureterorenoscopy, transurethral resection of the prostate (TURP) and short procedures such as orchidectomy, vasectomy and circumcisions. Data were collected from procedures that lasted 30–240 minutes. Tasks and behaviours were assessed from Pre-op Stage 1 to Post-op Stage 2. The last OTAS© stage was not feasible to assess.

In six additional procedures, behavioural ratings only were collected by two psychologist observers to assess inter-observer reliability.

Results and Comments

Task completion   Table 6.2 (urology columns) presents the task completion rates. Overall, task completion was higher in urology than in general surgery. The pattern of task completion rates between different types of tasks was strikingly similar, with patient tasks showing highest completion rates, followed by equipment/provisions and communication tasks. In addition, some variability was observed in urology theatres too, with significantly lower levels of equipment tasks in the Pre-op Phase than in the other two phases and significantly higher levels of communication tasks in the Pre- and Post-op Phases than in the Intra-operative Phase.

Behaviour ratings As in the previous study, these were relatively high (scores above four on a seven point scale). Of significance:

- Anaesthetists' and nurses' ratings were highest on cooperation and lowest on communication, with no significant different across operative phases.
- Surgeons' ratings exhibited a similar pattern, but, in addition, their scores were significantly lower in the post-operative phase.
- The Pearson r correlation coefficients between the two psychologists' ratings were as follows:
  - communication: 0.35, $p < 0.05$;
  - coordination: 0.72, $p < 0.001$;
  - cooperation/back up behaviour: 0.64, $p < 0.001$;
  - leadership: 0.62, $p < 0.001$;
  - monitoring/awareness: 0.53, $p < 0.001$.

In conclusion, team assessment appeared feasible in urology theatres. Importantly, the revised OTAS© application was successful. The revised tool replicated some of the findings of the initial version in both task completion and behaviour ratings. The acceptable reliability of the behavioural scoring suggests that the addition of exemplar behaviours and demonstrative scenarios did assist the behavioural assessment, as intended.

Current Work and Future Directions

Comprehensive and robust assessment of teamwork in the context of surgery is becoming increasingly important. It has been shown that poor teamworking in surgical teams is associated with the occurrence of adverse events to patients (e.g., Davenport et al. 2007, Gawande et al. 2003, Greenberg et al. 2007, JCAHO 2000). Recent increases in shift-working in the delivery of surgical services mean that operating theatre staff are now much less likely than in the past to be working in stable teams, in which individuals know each other as well as their strengths and weaknesses (Royal College of Surgeons of England 2007). Such changes have been followed by an increased emphasis on teamwork skills in the modern surgical training curriculum (ISCP 2005). Taken together, such developments are likely to increase the importance of robust teamwork assessment.

The aim of this chapter was to present in detail the development and initial application of the Observational Teamwork Assessment for Surgery© (OTAS©). The origins of OTAS© can be traced in the empirical work on teamwork in complex work environments that started more than 40 years ago with a focus on military teams. Conceptually, OTAS© is grounded on (Dickinson and McIntyre 1997) a model of teamwork. Empirically, it follows attempts to assess teamwork in expert teams that work in complex environments via observation. These attempts include the work on development of behavioural markers systems for assessing cockpit crews, as well as early work related to healthcare and surgery with a focus on teamwork or communication, threats and errors, or error recovery strategies in operating theatres.

Building on this work, our research team constructed the initial version of the OTAS©, which consisted of a task checklist (to be completed by a surgeon observer) and five behavioural scales (to be scored by a psychologist observer). Empirical testing of this first version suggested that team observations and assessment is indeed feasible and also led to modifications, aiming to assist the behavioural scoring – thus enhancing reliability and also allowing new observers to be trained. Subsequent testing supported empirically the feasibility, applicability and reliability of OTAS©.

At present, we are conducting more developmental as well as validation work using OTAS©. Regarding the validation process, three aspects are currently under investigation. First of all, we are in the process of assessing effects of observer's expertise in the behavioural scoring of OTAS©. The hypothesis is that ratings obtained from expert OTAS© users should exhibit higher correlations than those obtained by expert and novice users. Initial empirical evidence is consistent with this hypothesis. Secondly, we are in the process of using OTAS© to analyse teamwork in simulated crises-ridden procedures (Undre et al. 2007a). Procedures have been carried out, they have been video/audio-recorded and analysed using OTAS©. Initial evidence from the ratings of these procedures suggests that OTAS© can be used to rate teams retrospectively, in addition to its original real-time usage. Thirdly, we are using OTAS© alongside other observational tools that we have developed and that assess aspects of surgical process other than teamwork – including interruptions and disruptions to surgical workflow. Meaningful correlations between aspects of teamwork as captured by OTAS© and other surgical processes will contribute to the cross-validation of all tools involved.

Regarding the developmental work that is being carried out, we are in the process of producing a version of OTAS© to be used in simulation-based team training. Current work carried out by members of our group suggests that simulation-based training with formative feedback/debriefing has potential application to training surgeons how to cope most effectively with stressors that occur during procedures (Arora et al. 2009). Such stressors include technical difficulties (e.g., unexpected bleeding), but also lack/failure of equipment, unnecessary distractions and uncooperative team members. This work builds on previous team training modules addressed to the entire operating theatre team that we have piloted successfully (Moorthy et al. 2005, 2006, Undre et al. 2007a). Successful application of OTAS© in a training context will expand the domain of application of the tool and will contribute to its further validation.

OTAS© is one of the first assessment tools to be designed exclusively for surgical teams. In addition to OTAS©, we have also developed and tested a version of the NOTECHS (Avermate van 1998, Flin et al. 2003) to be used in surgical teams (Sevdalis et al. 2008a). In the past five years, other research groups working in parallel have developed tools that also aim to capture teamwork skills – including the Anaesthetists' Non Technical Skill ((ANTS) Fletcher et al. 2003), the Non Technical Skills for Surgeons ((NOTSS) Yule et al. 2006b, 2008) and the Mayo High Performance Teamwork Scale (MHPTS) (Malec et al. 2007 – see Chapters 2, 11 and 12 in this volume). The proliferation of tools with a focus on operating theatre teams signals an increasing recognition of the importance for teamwork in surgery. The uniqueness of OTAS© lies in that it captures the entire team, instead of individual members of it (i.e., the NOTECHS-based approach). Thus OTAS© offers a holistic, non-threatening assessment that can be used to assess teamwork via observation (as opposed to self-report) in any operating theatre. Importantly, it can also be used to provide formative feedback as part of a crisis management training module; such modules are becoming increasingly embedded in surgical training. Taken together with other tools and complementary measures, OTAS© can contribute to our understanding of surgical teamwork and is a potentially useful tool in attempts to improve teamwork, train surgical teams and, ultimately enhance surgical patient care.

Acknowledgements

This chapter is based on a large and long-lasting research programme on teamwork in surgical teams that is being carried out by our research group. Dr Andrew N. Healey, former member of the group, played an instrumental role in the shaping and development of the OTAS© since its inception and over a number of years. Dr Mary Koutantji and Mr Peter McCulloch also contributed significantly to this work – especially to the refinement of the tool.

The authors would like to thank the Department of Health: Patient Safety Research Programme (CAV), the BUPA Foundation (CAV), the Smith and Nephew Foundation (CAV), the British Academy (NS) and the Economic and Social Research Council (ESRC) Centre for Economic Learning and Social Evolution (NS) for funding for the work reported in this chapter.

References

Arora, S., Sevdalis, N., Nestel, D., Tierney, T., Woloshynowych, M. and Kneebone, R. (2009) Managing intra-operative stress: What do surgeons want from a crisis training programme. *American Journal of Surgery* 197, 537–543.

Avermate van, J.A.G. (1998) NOTECHS: The Evaluation of Non-technical Skills of Multi-pilot Air Crew in Relation to the JAR-FCL Requirements. Research Report for the European Commission. Amsterdam: National Aerospace Laboratory, DGVII NLR-CR-98443.

Beard, J.D. (2007) Assessment of surgical competence. *British Journal of Surgery* 94, 1315–16.

Calland, J.F., Guerlain, S., Adams, R.B., Tribble, C.G., Foley, E. and Chekan, E.G. (2002) A systems approach to surgical safety. *Surgical Endoscopy* 16, 1005–14.

Carthey, J. (2003) The role of structured observational research in health care. *Quality of Safety in Health Care* 12, Suppl 2, ii13–ii16.

Catchpole, K R., Giddings, A.E.B., de Leval, M.R., Peek, G.J., Godden, P.J., Utley, M., Gallivan, S., Hirst, G. and Dale, T. (2006) Identification of systems failure in successful paediatric cardiac surgery. *Ergonomics* 49, 567–88.

Davenport, D.L., Henderson, W.G., Mosca, C.L., Khuri, S.F. and Mentzer, R.M. (2007) Risk-adjusted morbidity in teaching hospitals correlates with reported levels of communication and collaboration in surgical teams but not with scale measures of teamwork climate, safety culture or working conditions, *Journal of the American College of Surgeons* 205, 778–84.

de Leval, M.R., Carthey, J., Wright, D.J., Farewell, V.T. and Reason, J.T. (2000) Human factors and cardiac surgery: A multicenter study, *Journal of Thoracic and Cardiovascular Surgery* 119, Pt 1, 661–72.

Dickinson, T.L. and McIntyre, R.M. (1997) A conceptual framework for teamwork measurement. In M.T. Brannick, E. Salas and C. Prince (eds) *Team Performance Assessment and Measurement*, 1st edition (pp. 19–44). New Jersey: Lawrence Erlbaum Associates, Inc.

Dwyer, D.J., Fowlkes, J.E., Oser, R.L., Salas, E. and Lane, N.E. (1997) Team performance measurement in distributed environments: The TARGETs methodology. In M.T. Brannick, E. Salas and C. Prince (eds) *Team Performance Assessment and Measurement*, 1st edition (pp. 137–54). New Jersey: Lawrence Erlbaum Associates, Inc.

Fletcher, G., Flin, R., McGeorge, P., Glavin, R., Maran, N. and Patey, R. (2003) Anaesthetists' Non-Technical Skills (ANTS): Evaluation of a behavioural marker system. *British Journal of Anaesthesia* 90(5), 580–8.

Flin, R., Martin, L., Goeters, K., Hoermann, J., Amalberti, R., Valot, C. and Nijhuis, H. (2003) Development of the NOTECHS (non-technical skills) system for assessing pilots' CRM skills. *Human Factors and Aerospace Safety* 3, 95–117.

Fowlkes, J.E., Lane, N.E., Salas, E., Franz, T. and Oser, R.L. (1994) Improving the measurement of team performance: The TARGETs methodology. *Military Psychology* 6, 47–61.

Fried, G.M. and Feldman, L.S. (2008) Objective assessment of technical performance. *World Journal of Surgery* 32, 156–60.

Gawande, A.A., Zinner, M.J., Studdert, D.M . and Brennan, T.A. (2003) Analysis of errors reported by surgeons at three teaching hospitals. *Surgery* 133(6), 614–21.

Greenberg, C.C., Regenbogen, S.E. and Studdert, D.M. (2007) Patterns of communication breakdowns resulting in injury to patients. *Journal of the American College of Surgeons* 204, 533–40.

Guerlain, S., Shin, T., Guo, H., Adams, R. and Calland, J.F. (2002) *A Team Performance Data Collection and Analysis System*. Proceedings of the Human Factors and Ergonomics Society, 46th Annual Meeting.

Guerlain, S., Adams, R.B., Turrentine, F.B., Shin, T., Guo, H., Collins, S.R. and Calland, J.F. (2005) Assessing team performance in the operating room: Development and use of a 'black-box' recorder and other tools for the intraoperative environment. *Journal of the American College of Surgeons* 200(1), 29–37.

Guerlain, S., Shin, T., Guo, H., Adams, R. and Calland, J.F. (2007) *A Team Performance Data Collection and Analysis System*. Proceedings of the Human Factors and Ergonomics Society 51st Annual Meeting, Baltimore, USA.

Healey, A.N., Undre, S. and Vincent, C.A. (2004) Developing observational measures of performance in surgical teams. *Quality of Safety in Health Care* 13, Suppl 1, i33–i40.

Healey, A.N., Sevdalis, N. and Vincent, C. (2006a) Measuring intra-operative interference from distraction and interruption observed in the operating theatre. *Ergonomics* 49, 589–604.

Healey, A.N., Undre, S. and Vincent, C.A. (2006b) Defining the technical skills of teamwork in surgery. *Quality of Safety in Health Care* 15(4), 231–4.

Healey, A.N., Undre, S., Sevdalis, N., Koutantji, M. and Vincent, C.A. (2006c) The complexity of measuring interprofessional teamwork in the operating theatre. *Journal of Interprofessional Care* 20(5), 485–95.

Healey, A.N. and Vincent, C. (2007) The systems of surgery, *Theoretical Issues in Ergonomic Science* 8, 429–43.

Helmreich, R.L. and Davies, J. (2007) Human factors in the operating: Interpersonal determinants of safety, efficiency and morale. In A.R. Aitkenhead (ed.) *Clinical Anaesthesiology: Safety and Risk Management in Anaesthesia*. London: Balliere Tindall.

Helmreich, R.L. and Foushee, H.C. (1993) Why crew resource management? Empirical and theoretical basis of human factors training in aviation. In E.L. Weiner, B.G. Kanki and R.L. Helmreich (eds) *Cockpit Resource Management* (pp. 3–45). New York: Academic.

Helmreich, R.L., Schaefer, H.G. and Sexton, B. (1995) *The Operating Room Checklist*. Technical Report 95-10. Austin, TX: NASA, University of Texas, FAA.

Helmreich, R.L, Klinect, J.R., Wilhelm, J.A., Tesmer, B., Gunther, D., Thomas, R., Romeo, C., Sumwalt, R. and Maurino, D. (2002) *Line Operations Safety Audit (LOSA)*. DOC 9803-AN/761. Montreal: ICAO.

ISCP (2008) *Intercollegiate Surgical Curriculum Programme*. Available at: <http://www.iscp.ac.uk> [last accessed November 2008].

JCAHO (2000) The Joint Commission: Operative and post-operative complications: Lessons for the future. *Sentinel Events Alert* 12. Available at: <http://www.jointcommission.org/sentinelevents/sentineleventalert/> [last accessed January 2008].

Kaufman, L. (2003) The wrong nephrectomy. *Bulletin of the Royal College of Anaesthetists* 7, 848–9.

Klampfer, B., Flin, R. Helmreich, R, Häusler, R., Sexton, B., Fletcher, G., Field, P., Staender, S., Lauche, K., Dieckmann, P. and Amacher, A. (2001) *Enhancing Performance in High Risk Environments: Recommendations for the Use of Behavioural Markers.* Report from the behavioural markers workshop, Zürich, June. Berlin: Damler Benz Foundation.

Klinect, J.R., Murray, P., Merritt, A.C. and Helmreich, R.L. (2003) Line Operations Safety Audit (LOSA): Definition and operating characteristics. *Proceedings of the 12th International Symposium on Aviation Psychology* (pp. 663–8). Dayton, OH: The Ohio State University.

Lingard, L., Reznick, R., Espin, S., Regehr, G. and DeVito, I. (2002) Team communications in the operating room: Talk patterns, sites of tension, and implications for novices. *Academic Medicine* 77(3), 232–7.

Lingard, L., Espin, S., Whyte, S., Regehr, G., Baker, G.R., Reznick, R., Bohnen, J., Orser, B., Doran, D. and Grober, E. (2004a) Communication failures in the operating room: An observational classification of recurrent types and effects. *Quality of Safety in Health Care* 13(5), 330–4.

Lingard, L., Garwood, S. and Poenaru, D. (2004b) Tensions influencing operating room team function: Does institutional context make a difference. *Medical Education* 38, 691–9.

Mackenzie, C.F., Jefferies, N.J., Hunter, W.A., Bernhard, W.N. and Xiao, Y. (1996) Comparison of self-reporting of deficiencies in airway management with video analyses of actual performance. LOTAS Group. Level One Trauma Anesthesia Simulation. *Human Factors* 38(4), 623–35.

Mackenzie, C.F., Xiao, Y. and The IPO Group (2003) *Observational Analysis of Video Records of Team Performance.* Proceedings of the Human Factors and Ergonomic Society 47th Annual Meeting, Denver, Colorado, 1493–7.

Malec, J.F., Torsher, L.C., Dunn, W.F., Weingmann, D.A., Arnold, J.J., Brown, D.A. and Phatak, V. (2007) The Mayo high performance teamwork scale: Reliability and validity for evaluating key crew resource management skills. *Simulation in Healthcare* 2, 4–10.

Moorthy, K., Munz, Y., Adams, S., Pandey, V. and Darzi, A. (2005) A human factors analysis of technical and team skills among surgical trainees during procedural simulations in a simulated operating theatre. *Annals of Surgery* 242(5), 631–9.

Moorthy, K., Munz, Y., Forrest, D., Pandey, V., Undre, S. and Vincent, C. (2006) Surgical crisis management skills training and assessment: A simulation-based approach to enhancing operating room performance. *Annals of Surgery* 242, 631–9.

O'Connor, P., Hormann, H.J., Flin, R., Lodge, M. and Goeters, K.M. (2002) Developing a method for evaluating crew resource management skills: A European perspective. *International Journal of Aviation Psychology* 12(3), 263–85.

Paris, C.R., Salas, E. and Cannon-Bowers, J.A. (2000) Teamwork in multi-person systems: A review and analysis. *Ergonomics* 43(8), 1052–75.

Roth, E.M., Christian, C.K., Gustafson, M., Sheridan, T.B., Dwyer, K., Gandhi, T.K., Zinner, M.J. and Dierks, M.M. (2004) Using field observations as a tool for discovery: Analysing cognitive and collaborative demands in the operating room. *Cognition, Technology & Work* 6(3), 148–57.

Royal College of Surgeons of England (2007) Safe Shift Working for Surgeons in Training: Revised Policy Statement from the Working Time Directive Working Party. London: Royal College of Surgeons of England.

Sevdalis, N., Davis, R., Koutantji, M., Undre, S., Darzi, A. and Vincent, C. (2008a) Reliability of a revised NOTECHS scale for use in surgical teams. *American Journal of Surgery* 196(2), 184–90.

Sevdalis, N., Forrest, D., Undre, S., Darzi, A. and Vincent, C. (2008b) Annoyances, disruptions and interruptions in surgery: The Disruption in Surgery Index (Disi). *World Journal of Surgery* 32(8), 1643–50.

Undre, S. and Healey, A.N. (2006) Observational Teamwork Assessment for Surgery© OTAS© User Manual. Available at: <http://www.csru.org.uk> [accessed June 2008].

Undre, S., Healey, A.N., Darzi, A. and Vincent, C.A. (2006a) Observational assessment of surgical teamwork: A feasibility study. *World Journal of Surgery* 30(10), 1774–83.

Undre, S., Sevdalis, N., Healey, A.N., Darzi, S.A. and Vincent, C.A. (2006b) Teamwork in the operating theatre: Cohesion or confusion? *Journal or Evaluation in Clinical Practice* 12(2), 182–9.

Undre, S., Koutantji, M., Sevdalis, N., Selvapatt, N., Williams, S., Gautama, S., McCulloch, P., Darzi, A. and Vincent, C. (2007a) Multi-disciplinary crisis simulations: The way forward for training surgical teams. *World Journal of Surgery* 31, 1843–53.

Undre, S., Sevdalis, N., Healey, A.N., Darzi, A. and Vincent, C.A. (2007b) Observational teamwork assessment for surgery (OTAS): Refinement and application in urological surgery. *World Journal of Surgery* 31(7), 1373–81.

Vincent, C., Moorthy, K., Sarker, S. K., Chang, A. and Darzi, A.W. (2004) Systems approaches to surgical quality and safety: From concept to measurement. *Annals of Surgery* 239(4), 475–82.

Yule, S., Flin, R., Paterson-Brown, S. and Maran, N. (2006a) Non-technical skills for surgeons in the operating room: A review of the literature. *Surgery* 139(2), 140–9.

Yule, S., Flin, R., Paterson-Brown, S., Maran, N. and Rowley, D.R. (2006b) Development of a rating system for surgeons' non-technical skills. *Medical Education* 40, 1098–104.

Yule, S., Flin, R., Maran, N., Rowley, D. R., Youngson, G.G. and Paterson-Brown, S. (2008) Surgeons' non-technical skills in the operating room: Reliability testing of the NOTSS behaviour rating system. *World Journal of Surgery* 32, 548–56.

Chapter 7

Rating Operating Theatre Teams – Surgical NOTECHS

Ami Mishra, Ken Catchpole, Guy Hirst, Trevor Dale and
Peter McCulloch

Introduction

In this chapter we discuss the development of a tool for rating operating teams, and sub-teams of surgeons, anaesthetists and nurses, on their non-technical performance in the operating theatre. Validated in laparoscopic cholecystectomy (LC) and carotid endarterectomy (CEA), this work built upon earlier studies of behaviour and process in orthopaedic and paediatric cardiac surgery, where the importance of non-technical skills was identified through direct observation of behaviour and process in the operating theatre (Catchpole et al. 2005, 2006, 2007). No operation observed was performed perfectly, and, in all, deviations from the optimal course of the operation were found. In some, these small deviations escalated into more serious situations that compromised the safety of the patient or the success of the operation. Often these problems derived from threats in the system of surgery that originated from outside the operating theatre – or at least could not be attributed solely to errors by the teams. As our understanding of how small events can escalate to more serious problems, and the role that non-technical skills may play in reducing or increasing the chances of harm, our methods of measuring those skills have been refined, and in turn our understanding has become more sophisticated. In this chapter, we attempt first to describe the process of intellectual and methodological development, and to provide a substantive analysis of our current tool for assessing non-technical skills in the operating room.

A Model of Error Causation in Surgery

Early work by the research team in orthopaedic and paediatric cardiac surgery at Great Ormond Street Hospital, London (Catchpole et al. 2005, 2006) set out to examine why errors in operating theatres occurred using a model similar to that proposed by Helmreich and colleagues for aviation (Helmreich and Musson 2000, Helmreich et al. 1999). The model adapted for surgery (see Figure 7.1) suggests that system threats can predispose and lead to human errors, revealing further

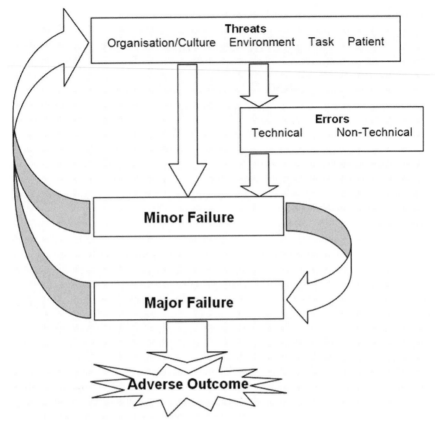

Figure 7.1   Escalation model of surgical error

threats and increasing the likelihood of further error, creating a cascade that leads
to more serious surgical problems, and subsequently to harm or adverse event.
Threats either predispose errors that cause minor failures in process, or directly
cause minor failures themselves. These minor failures either lead to more threats,
and so to more errors, or lead directly to more serious or potentially dangerous
major failures. Major failures may expose more threats, create more errors and can
lead directly to an adverse outcome (Catchpole et al. 2005).

Though we did not directly measure surgical outcomes or observe any death,
in more than 40 cases the Great Ormond Street team observed over 500 minor
problems and 8 major problems that represented considerable lapses in the quality
of care given, and a serious threat to the safety of the patient. The reader is
directed to our accompanying chapter (Catchpole, Chapter 19) in this volume that
describes the results in orthopaedic surgery. The multidisciplinary, cross-industry
team wondered why some operations went more smoothly than others, and why in
some operations even a large number of small problems did not result in serious
problems. In part, the research team observed that the escalation from small,

seemingly innocuous problems to these sometimes life-threatening situations was dependent upon the type of operation performed, and the risk (or complexity) of the operation. Some operations had more critical stages, and so the coincidence of a minor problem at a critical time might also be more likely, and also certain operations would be more demanding and thus might be more likely to result in human errors, or were more sensitive to the overloading of individual mental and physical capacity. The Great Ormond Street team therefore concluded that non-technical skills, which are specifically trained for in aviation to address these types of situations, might also have an influence in surgical care, and thus sought at first to derive a simple scale for evaluating this hypothesis.

NOTECHS was designed through a pan-European collaboration between airlines and academics to provide a generic structure for non-technical skills in aviation training and to allow consistent assessment across different national and organisational cultures (Avermaete and van Kruijsen 1998). It was this broad applicability, demonstrated utility (Avermaete and van Kruijsen 1998, Flin et al. 2003), operational validation (O'Connor et al. 2002, Lodge et al. 2001) and the success with which the method of developing the scale had been adapted to specialties in medicine previously (Fletcher et al. 2003, 2004) that this behavioural marker methodology was selected for adaptation to the surgical environment. The NOTECHS system consists of elements of behaviour grouped into four categories, which can be further grouped into two social skill categories (teamwork and cooperation, leadership and management) and two cognitive skills categories (situation awareness and problem-solving and decision-making), and was adapted for use with surgical teams following consultation with two cardiac surgeons, one vascular surgeon, one orthopaedic surgeon, one human factors researcher and two aviation non-technical skills trainers who regularly used NOTECHS in civil airline simulation. In this first iteration of the Surgical NOTECHS system, the changes from aviation to surgery largely related to alterations in language used, in the types of behaviour that were defined as markers, and the structure of the situation awareness dimension. The Surgical NOTECHS scale was applied to the whole team in each operation by assigning a score from 1 to 4 to each of the four dimensions (Table 7.1).

This was conducted once each for three pre-defined periods of the operation. The first phase, described as the access phase, started with the first incision, and lasted until the site of the surgical treatment had been exposed. The second phase, known as the treatment phase, followed directly afterwards, and lasted until the completion of the surgical treatment. The final phase, known as the closure phase, lasted from the completion of the surgical treatment, to the moment that the final suture in the closure of the incision was tied off. The human factors (non-clinically trained) observer (KC) recorded his observations on the scoring sheet, using ticks, crosses and notes, in order to promote consistency and balance of judgement intra-operatively and inter-operatively, and then made a global estimate of his overall impression of performance. For paediatric cardiac surgery, the Surgical NOTECHS evaluation was conducted entirely from the videotaped operation. In orthopaedic surgery, it was conducted by the observers *in situ*. Operations were then ranked

Table 7.1   Summary of first iteration of the surgical NOTECHS scoring system

LEADERSHIP and MANAGEMENT	
Leadership, planning and preparation, workload management, authority and assertiveness	
TEAMWORK and COOPERATION	
Team building/maintaining, support of others, understanding team needs, conflict solving	
PROBLEM-SOLVING and DECISION-MAKING	
Definition and diagnosis, option generation, risk assessment, outcome review	
SITUATION AWARENESS	
Notice (patient, procedure, people), understand (patient, procedure, people), think ahead (patient, procedure, people)	
Below standard = 1	Behaviour directly compromises patient safety and effective teamwork.
Basic standard = 2	Behaviour in other conditions could directly compromise patient safety and effective teamwork.
Standard = 3	Behaviour maintains an effective level of patient safety and teamwork.
Excellent = 4	Behaviour enhances patient safety and teamwork. A model for all other teams.

Source: Catchpole et al. 2005

from best to worst according to the number of 'below standard' Surgical NOTECHS scores obtained in each operation, then the number of 'basic standard' scores, then 'standard' and finally 'exceed' scores. This gave an overall order to each operation purely in terms of the positive and negative non-technical behaviour observed.

In paediatric cardiac surgery this simple approach proved effective, useful and informative, and helped to establish a methodology and a substantive link between non-technical skills, process and, by implication with previous work (de Leval et al. 2000), outcome. There was a moderately close relationship between the number of minor process problems and the ranked Surgical NOTECHS score (Figure 7.2), since this type of surgery requires considerable use of these types of skills, particularly in the management of blood circulation between anaesthetist, perfusionist and surgeon. Moreover, because this type of surgery involved large teams, and is amongst the most complex, technically demanding, and potentially risky of any surgery, the surgical process can quickly fall apart if the operating team do not work together effectively. Combined with previous observations regarding operative risk and operative type, the Great Ormond Street team found that escalation from small problems to bigger

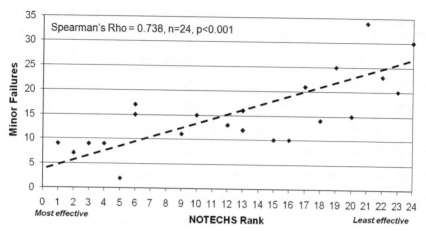

Figure 7.2   Relationship between minor failures and ranked non-technical skills performance in paediatric cardiac surgery

Source: Catchpole et al. 2005

problems was partially mitigated in teams with higher non-technical skills ratings (Catchpole et al. 2007). Thus, it was possible to describe a mechanism for surgical failure, which suggested direct methods for improvements in surgical performance and safety, one of which was the explicit training of non-technical skills.

Though the model also fitted orthopaedic surgery, it was clear that this simple method for scoring non-technical skills as a team did not fit as well when an operation had widely differing demands on individuals. Knee replacement operations are demanding of some members of the team, with success relying heavily on the relationship between the scrub nurse and the surgeon, while the anaesthetist was rarely involved directly with the surgical procedure, and had little interaction with the team, even though, for example, patients can have rare but extreme reactions to the surgical treatment. Thus, with nurses and surgeons who worked well together, the course of the operation might be smooth, even though the anaesthetist might not be as situationally aware – or as safe – as might be desirable. The escalation from small problems to bigger ones, and the influence of risk, operative type and non-technical performance is illustrated in Figure 7.3.

To provide greater quality to the evaluation of non-technical skills in a wider range of operations, and to evaluate the success of an aviation-style non-technical skills training programme in more common types of surgery, the original method for non-technical skills measurement needed refinement. The key limitation was that the first iteration of the Surgical NOTECHS system could not account for different contributions of individuals or sub-teams to the success of the surgery. This might be particularly important where certain types of surgery did not usually demand the constant interaction with another team member or sub-team, encouraging a lack of awareness that could prove deleterious during the development of more acute events in the process of surgery. Moreover, it might also help to better understand

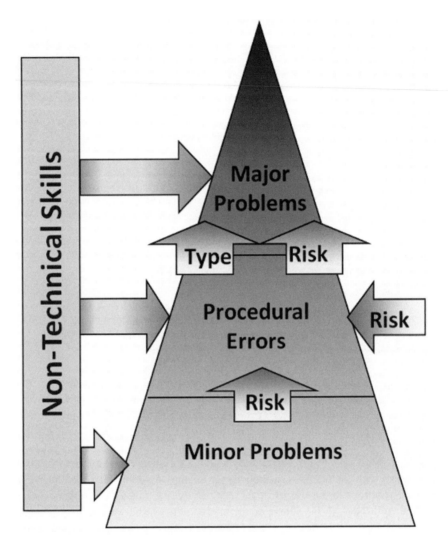

Figure 7.3   Mechanisms of surgical failure

the team dynamics, and the contribution of sub-teams to the overall success of an operation. In the remainder of this chapter, we describe the development and validation of this refined non-technical performance measurement methodology.

The Oxford NOTECHS System

The tool was developed by a consultant upper gastro-intestinal surgeon, a consultant vascular surgeon, a clinical research fellow, who was also a trainee surgeon, and the human factors researcher and aviation trainers involved in the first iteration. The most obvious change from the first iteration was the scoring of performance of each of the three sub-teams (surgeons, anaesthetists and nurses) in each dimension for every operation. Overall sub-team performance was taken as the sum of the dimension performances (out of 16). The overall team non-technical performance was calculated from the sum of the overall sub-team performance scores (out of 48). Each overall team dimension performance was scored as the sum of all the sub-team performances in that dimension (out of 12). Thus, a non-technical score was obtained in each dimension for the theatre team, and for each sub-team of surgeons, anaesthetists and nurses. Repeat scoring for three phases of the operation was abandoned to ease the burden on the observers, and because the operations were generally of shorter duration and without such clearly delineated phases as cardiac surgery.

As part of a larger study that sought to examine the value of multidisciplinary aviation-style teamwork training on performance in the operating theatre (McCulloch et al. 2009), we applied the Oxford NOTECHS scale to examine behavioural change. This provided the opportunity to examine a number of properties of the scale for validity and reliability purposes. We observed 65 laparoscopic cholecystectomies (LC) and 45 carotid endarterectomies (CEA) in the pre- and post-intervention phases of the study. For each case, a non-technical performance score was given using the Oxford NOTECHS system. We further evaluated relationships between technical errors, minor process problems and the sub-team non-technical scores, as well as the four dimensions. This allowed a more detailed analysis of the aspects of teamwork most closely associated with changes in these outcome measures. Technical errors were identified at the same time using the Observational Clinical Human Reliability Assessment (OCHRA) system (Tang et al. 2004), while minor process problems, were identified using the previous framework (Catchpole et al. 2006), and operative duration was also recorded. In 36 cases, the teams were assessed independently by the study's two principal observers, and in 14 other cases by a third independent observer. Five cases were also studied with one observer using Oxford NOTECHS, and the other using the Observational Teamwork Assessment for Surgery (OTAS) scale (Undre et al. 2007).

Reliability of the Oxford NOTECHS Tool

Inter-rater reliability was evaluated using the Rwg statistic for overall Oxford NOTECHS scores and component dimensions by parallel independent scoring of cases by two observers. Including all pre- and post-intervention cases, 24 LCs and 12 CEAs were independently dual observed. Reliability of Oxford NOTECHS scoring is reported for all 36 cases in Table 7.2, and in CEA operations only in Table 7.3. Results for the 24 LC operations on their own have been reported elsewhere (Mishra et al. 2009). In all cases, and for most sub-teams and dimensions, overall

Table 7.2   Reliability (R$_{wg}$) of Oxford NOTECHS tool for 36 dual observed LCs and CEAs

α	LM	TC	PD	SA	Total
Surgeons	0.89	0.89	0.91	0.86	0.96
Anaesthetists	0.94	0.91	0.93	0.93	0.97
Nurses	0.87	0.89	0.87	0.90	0.96
Total	0.94	0.93	0.96	0.96	0.98

Table 7.3   Reliability (R$_{wg}$) of Oxford NOTECHS for 12 dual observed CEAs

α	LM	TC	PD	SA	Total
Surgeons	0.87	0.90	0.83	0.83	0.96
Anaesthetists	0.90	0.97	0.83	0.93	0.97
Nurses	0.87	0.90	0.93	0.83	0.95
Total	0.91	0.94	0.96	0.93	0.98

reliability is high. In CEA reliability on the problem-solving and decision-making dimension was lower than might be desired for some teams, as were the ratings on the surgeons' cognitive dimensions. This reflects difficulties in scoring where observable behaviours may be limited.

For ten of the LCs and four of the CEAs, a third observer was invited to independently score the theatre teams on their non-technical performance. Overall reliability was good (Table 7.4) but again lowest reliability was noted in scoring of situation awareness (SA). This is perhaps because the third observer, from an aviation background, had a very basic understanding of the workings of an operating theatre.

Table 7.4   Reliability of Oxford NOTECHS in 14 cases observed independently with third observer

α	LM	TC	PD	SA	Total
Surgeons	1.00	0.89	0.91	0.83	0.98
Anaesthetists	0.94	0.94	0.94	0.97	0.98
Nurses	0.94	0.83	0.97	0.86	0.94
Total	0.98	0.91	0.96	0.93	0.98

We also examined the reliability of the non-technical skills ratings over time by dividing data in both pre- and post-intervention conditions into three, and comparing the performance in these one-third cohorts. In laparoscopic cholecystectomy, differences between the thirds of the cohorts were not significant using ANOVA either before (F=1.34, p=0.28) or after (F=1.03, p=0.34) the training intervention. Similarly in carotid endarterectomy, differences between the thirds of the cohorts were not significant before (F=1.93, p=0.17) or after (F=1.01, p=0.38). Though clearly, reliability over time needs to be studied in more detail, this at least suggested that when comparing between pre- and post-intervention data to examine the effect of the training programme, we could be more confident that the effect was not brought about by changes in scores over time.

Convergent Validity

Overall agreement between OTAS and Oxford NOTECHS was excellent (r= 0.88, n=5, p=0.04). The mean OTAS score for the five cases compared was 18.8 (range 14–22 out of a possible maximum of 30), and the mean Oxford NOTECHS score was 37.8 (range 33–45, out of a possible maximum of 48), also suggesting that data on both scales covered a similar range in relation to the overall scale maxima and minima (see Figure 7.4).

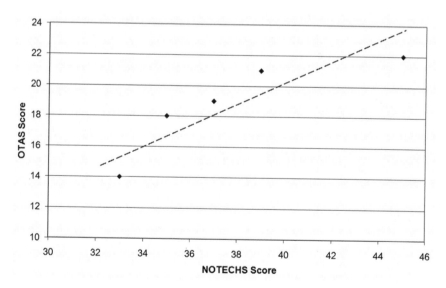

Figure 7.4   Oxford NOTECHS scores against OTAS scores for 5 LCs

Relationship between Oxford NOTECHS, Technical Errors and Minor Failures

We exploited our developing model of the relationship between non-technical skills and intra-operative performance to examine the relationship between the Oxford NOTECHS scores and technical errors and minor intra-operative problems. We observed 65 LCs and 45 CEAs, in which non-technical performance was evaluated using the Oxford NOTECHS scale, and technical errors noted using the OCHRA system. There were no associations between non-technical performances and technical errors of statistical significance in CEA, but in LC there was a strong association with surgeons' SA ($\rho = -0.54$, p<0.001). Linear regression analysis suggests that surgeons' SA and nurses' problem-solving and decision-making (PD) combined are responsible for 40.5 per cent of the variation in technical errors seen.

For carotid endarterectomy, significant relationships are between nurses' teamwork and cooperation (TC) and minor problems (ρ=–0.30, p=0.04) and between nurses' sub-team Oxford NOTECHS and minor problems, but there were no associations between non-technical skills performance and technical errors of statistical significance. As with LC, there is a suggestion of the number of technical errors being negatively related to the overall non-technical performance, but in this group the associations were not significant.

Examining operative duration, for LC, significant relationships were seen between anaesthetists' non-technical skills and operative duration (ρ=–0.25, p=0.041) and between team leadership and management (LM) and duration (ρ=–0.25, p=0.046). For CEA, correlations between surgeons' LM and non-technical skills (ρ=–0.31, p=0.037), and surgeons' SA and non-technical skills (ρ=–0.31, p=0.040) were significant.

Discussion

The Oxford NOTECHS tool has been found to be reliable and to relate in different ways, depending upon operative type, to other intra-operative performance measures. One finding was that greater surgical situation awareness may result in fewer technical errors for LC and CEA operations. Surgical SA is assessed by gauging the surgical team's awareness of the state of the patient, stage of the procedure and availability of theatre staff. It is unsurprising therefore that excellence in this dimension translates into technical outcome, and so perhaps disappointing that no relationship was found in the other type of operation (CEA). Laparoscopy is known to be cognitively demanding, which may explain the closer relationship with cognitive skills scores. Very few technical errors were recorded in CEA, and we did observe a trend toward the results in LC, so it may be that simply a greater sample of cases would be necessary to demonstrate the relationship. Clearly, we also need to be cautious with these results since SA can be difficult to observe.

Minor failures are a reflection of errors produced mainly outside the operating field, and it is therefore logical that better coordination amongst the nursing staff results in fewer problems. For example, where higher nursing teamwork scores were recorded, fewer psychomotor general errors (such as dropping instruments) were noted. Clearly, one criticism is that the Oxford NOTECHS and failure assessments were scored by the same observer and thus may be contaminating one another. However, this relationship was found to be consistent after analysis of scores performed by both observers, and the Oxford NOTECHS scores were further validated by comparison with scoring by an independent observer uninvolved in the recording of minor failures. So Oxford NOTECHS at least seems resistant to this contamination, even though the timing of the Oxford NOTECHS ratings at the end of the operation, after the recording of minor failures, means it would be the more likely measure to be contaminated.

In the UK, three groups working independently and more or less simultaneously have derived observational techniques of team performance in the operating theatre that have a great many resemblances. Indeed, we suspect that the differences largely relate to decisions made about the appropriate trade-offs between conflicting demands. The ANTS (Fletcher et al. 2003) and NOTSS (Yule et al. 2006) systems, for anaesthetists and surgeons respectively, have been developed at the University of Aberdeen to assess individuals, and primarily as training aids, and they are both extremely well designed for these purposes (see Chapters 2, 11 and 12 in this volume). The OTAS system (Undre et al. 2007), developed by the Clinical Safety Research Unit at Imperial College, London, has been developed to measure team behaviour in the operating theatre. It is prescriptive – so relatively easily trained – but requires the full attention of a single observer (see Chapter 6). Our Oxford NOTECHS tool has been developed to allow assessment of team performance simultaneously with other intra-operative parameters, and has evolved from assessing whole team performance to allow the rating of sub-teams. We have demonstrated here that, though it may require observational experience and some calibration, it can indeed be used reliably even by non-specialists and may relate to other aspects of intra-operative performance. We feel that establishing the relationship between teamwork and quality of care or operative duration may be one way to evaluate whether training for these skills in healthcare is valuable, and to engage front line staff in thinking differently about how they practice.

The complexity and difficulty of observing performance and behaviour in the operating theatre should not be underestimated. Meaningful, useful and reliable data are dependent upon the skills of the observer – who is the basic tool in the observation – and the design of the observational method to be appropriate for the type of operation, the parameters being studied, and the purpose of the observations. We have described the evolution and substantive affirmation of the value of the Oxford NOTECHS technique for evaluating non-technical skills in the operating theatre, and have demonstrated an iterative cycle that swings between measurement and theoretical development. Thus, by building on the excellent research work reported in this volume, we hope to work with others to develop better measurement methods, that require fewer trade-offs to be made, that examine these skills in more detail while being practical, inexpensive and easy to use, and that describe more closely the relationship between teamwork, performance, safety and quality.

Acknowledgements

This work was generously funded by the BUPA foundation, with our earlier reported work supported by the Patient Safety Research Programme. Thanks also to the rest of the Great Ormond Street project team, and especially Professor Marc de Leval and Mr Tony Giddings.

References

Avermaete, J.A.G. and van Kruijsen, E.A.C. (1998) *NOTECHS. The Evaluation of Non-technical Skills of Multi-pilot Aircrew in Relation to the JAR-FCL Requirements*. Amsterdam: EC NOTECHS Project final.

Catchpole, K., Godden, P.J., Giddings, A.E.B., Hirst, G., Dale, T., Utley, M., Gallivan, S. and de Leval, M. (2005) *Identifying and Reducing Errors in the Operating Theatre* (Rep. No. PS012). Patient Safety Research Programme. Available at <http://www.pcpoh.bham.ac.uk/publichealth/psrp/documents/PS012_Final_Report_DeLeval.pdf> [last accessed February 2009].

Catchpole, K.R., Giddings, A.E., de Leval, M.R., Peek, G.J., Godden, P.J., Utley, M., Gallivan, S., Hirst, G. and Dale, T. (2006) Identification of systems failures in successful paediatric cardiac surgery. *Ergonomics* 49, 567–88.

Catchpole, K., Giddings, A.E., Wilkinson, M., Dale, T., Hirst, G., and de Leval, M.R. (2007) Improving patient safety by identifying latent failures in successful operations. *Surgery* 142, 102–110.

de Leval, M.R., Carthey, J., Wright, D.J., and Reason, J.T. (2000) Human factors and cardiac surgery: A multicenter study. *Journal of Thoracic and Cardiovascular Surgery* 119, 661–72.

Fletcher, G.C.L., Flin, R.H., Glavin, R J., Maran, N.J. and Patey, R. (2004) Rating non-technical skills: Developing a behavioural marker system for use in anaesthesia. *Cognition, Technology and Work* 6, 165–71.

Fletcher, G.C.L., Flin, R.H., Glavin, R.J., Maran, N.J. and Patey, R. (2003) Anaesthetists' Non-Technical Skills (ANTS): Evaluation of a behavioural marker system. *British Journal of Anaesthesia* 90, 580–8.

Flin, R., Martin, L., Goeters, K., Hoermann, J., Amalberti, R., Valot, C. and Nijhuis, H. (2003) Development of the NOTECHS (Non-Technical Skills) system for assessing pilots' CRM skills. *Human Factors and Aerospace Safety* 3, 95–117.

Helmreich, R.L. and Musson, D.M. (2000) The University of Texas Threat and Error Management Model: Components and examples. *British Medical Journal* website. Available at: <http://homepage.psy.utexas.edu/homepage/

group/HelmreichLAB/Publications/pubfiles/Pub248.pdf> [last accessed February 2009].

Helmreich, R.L., Klinect, J.R. and Wilhelm, J.A. (1999) Models of threat, error, and CRM in flight operations. *Proceedings of the 10th International Symposium on Aviation Psychology* (pp. 667–82). Columbus, OH: The Ohio State University.

Lodge, M., Fletcher, G.C.L., Russell, S., Goeters, K.M., Hoermann, H., Nijhuis, H. et al. (2001) *Results of the Experiment*. JARTEL WP3 Final Report (Rep. No. JARTEL/BA/WP3/D5_20.). Brussels: The JARTEL Consortium, for the European Commission, DG TREN.

McCulloch, P., Mishra, A., Handa, A., Dale, T., Hirst, G. and Catchpole, K. (2009) The effects of aviation-style non-technical skills training on technical performance and outcome in the operating theatre. *Quality and Safety in Healthcare* 18, 109–115

Mishra, A., Catchpole, K., and McCulloch, P. (2009) The Oxford NOTECHS System: Reliability and validity of a tool for measuring teamwork behaviour in the operating theatre. *Quality and Safety in Healthcare* 18, 104–108.

O'Connor, P., Hormann, J., Flin, R.H., Lodge, M., Goeters, K.M. and The JARTEL Group (2002) Developing a method for evaluating Crew Resource Management skills: A European perspective. *International Journal of Aviation Psychology* 12, 263–85.

Tang, B., Hanna, G.B., Joice, P. and Cuschieri, A. (2004) Identification and categorization of technical errors by Observational Clinical Human Reliability Assessment (OCHRA) during laparoscopic cholecystectomy. *Archives of Surgery* 139, 1215–20.

Undre, S., Sevdalis, N., Healey, A.N., Darzi, A. and Vincent, C.A. (2007) Observational Teamwork Assessment for Surgery (OTAS): Refinement and application in urological surgery. *World Journal of Surgery* 31, 1373–81.

Yule, S., Flin, R., Paterson-Brown, S., Maran, N. and Rowley, D. (2006) Development of a rating system for surgeons' non-technical skills. *Medical Education* 40, 1098–104.

Chapter 8

RATE: A Customizable, Portable Hardware/ Software System for Analysing and Teaching Human Performance in the Operating Room

Stephanie Guerlain and J. Forrest Calland

Introduction

Researchers at the University of Virginia are studying human performance in the operating room in an effort to understand the factors that lead to or inhibit patient safety in this environment. In general, observation 'in the wild' is extremely difficult as there is no transcription or video recording upon which to base an analysis or to validate the result. Or, even with such recordings, the work to code and analyse these recordings is extremely labour intensive and thus may not be practical for 'real-world' projects that do not have enormous budgets (and time) to accommodate such analyses. We have developed and tested several methodologies that enable collecting team data 'on the fly', some of which are 'summative' evaluations and others that are more detailed process tracing of events and communications yielding directly usable data that can be analysed to characterize team behaviours immediately following the team process that was observed. We specifically report here on the design of a portable and customizable hardware/software system called Remote Analysis of Team Environments (RATE) that we have used to run two studies designed to improve team communication and coordination in the operating room (Guerlain et al. 2004, 2005, 2008), one handoff-of-care study for paediatric residents (Sledd et al. 2006) and one usability study (in progress). This chapter is based upon work supported by the National Science Foundation and describes how the system works; it has been used in our operating room studies. The hardware enables digitally recording up to four video feeds and eight audio feeds. The event-recording software enables observers to create a customized set of events of interest that can be logged into a time-stamped database when watching a case live. The playback software synchronizes the event-recording database with the audiovisual (AV) data for efficient review of the case.

Why Study Team Communication in the Operating Room?

In the United States, operating suites at academic medical centres do not have consistent standard procedures or protocols. Team members often rotate across different teams and techniques and procedures often vary depending on the staff and the technology available.

Research, though limited, has demonstrated that poor teamwork and communication exist during surgical procedures (Guerlain et al. 2008, Helmreich and Schaefer 1994, Sexton et al. 2002). Our pre-intervention observation studies showed that rarely is sufficient information shared between the surgeon and other team members from anaesthesia to nursing about the plan.

Researchers have begun to study team performance in the operating room, most often focusing on anaesthesiology. Gaba has studied the use of crew resource management (CRM) training for anaesthesiologists using an anaesthesia simulator (Gaba 1989). Xiao, McKenzie and the LOTAS group at the University of Maryland Shock Trauma Center have evaluated anaesthesiology performance on trauma teams (Xiao et al. 2000, Xiao and The LOTAS Group 2001), and have evaluated focused tasks, such as patient intubation. Little research, however, has been conducted evaluating team performance from the surgeon's perspective. This may be due to the difficulty of judging performance during long, complicated, primarily manual procedures (e.g., no computerized data are collected).

Evaluation of Teamwork

Because team members with distinct tasks must interact in order to achieve a shared goal, multiple factors play a role in determining the success of a team, such as organizational resource availability, team authority, team effort, leadership, task complexity and communication. These constructs cannot be measured in the same sense as temperature or pressure and may interact with each other in complex ways. Collecting behavioural data means that an observer needs to capture 'the moment-to-moment aspects of team behaviors'. 'While reliance on expert observer ratings may be a necessity, there is considerable discretion about what is measured', creating noise in the data as well as missing data points (Rouse et al. 1992, p. 1298). In crew resource management training and evaluation, trained raters judge the adequacy of communication overall on a rating scale, either periodically or at the end of a test (or live) situation. Thus, the team is given one or a few overall scores. It is difficult, however, to develop reliable, sensitive scoring metrics, although significant work has been done in this area (Flin and Maran 2004, Law and Sherman 1995). Others look at just performance metrics or knowledge of team members at particular points during a team activity or at the end (e.g., Endsley 1995) or count 'utterances' or communication 'vectors' (who is talking to whom) (e.g., Moorthy et al. 2005). If one has transcribed verbal data, then verbal protocol analysis (Simon and Ericsson 1993) or even automated linguistic analysis can be conducted. For example, in a study conducted by Sexton and Helmreich (2000), a computer-based linguistic tool was used to analyse how various language usages affect error rates by flight deck crew members. The study indicated that 'specific language variables are moderately to highly correlated with individual performance, individual error rates, and individual communication ratings' (p. 63). Thus, frequent usage of first person plural (we, our, us) tends to be correlated with a reduced occurrence of error. The study also pointed out the number of words used by the crew members increases in an abnormal hostile situation or during times when workload is increased. Such techniques, however, first require that all communications are transcribed, an extremely labour-intensive, time-consuming and tedious task.

Our approach was to have a 'happy medium' that provides a fairly detailed process tracing of events and communications that goes beyond just utterances but does not require transcription of verbal data. RATE enables trained observers to mark events of interest 'on the fly' while watching the team process, knowing that the resultant data set may not be 100 per cent accurate, but benefiting from the fact that the data are immediately available for summarization of events (e.g., number of observed contaminations, or amount of communication that was focused on teaching vs. coordination) with the ability to immediately jump the AV record to a few seconds before any event that was marked, either for teaching or review purposes or to further validate the data. Thus, we end up with a human-indexed summarization of events with an ability to play back those events of interest without having to search through a long AV record.

The methods reported here were developed to support observation and scoring of teams performing laparoscopic cholecystectomy, a surgical procedure to remove the gallbladder. The procedure created an ideal situation due to its frequency of performance and relatively short time length of procedure (1–1.5 hours from patient entering to patient leaving the room). The challenges include the fact that a standard team is made up of at least five people: anaesthesiologist, attending surgeon, resident surgeon, scrub tech, circulating nurse; in our institution, a medical student who acts as the laparoscopic camera operator and an anaesthetist is most often included too. Others such as technicians and nurses-in-training may also be present. Reliability of the data becomes an issue when the observer is confronted with tracking multiple events by multiple test subjects when evaluating a team (Simon and Ericsson 1993).

One of the biggest problems in collecting such data is determining how much individual interpretation by an observer affects the make-up of the data. If the purpose of the data collection tool is to produce consistent and valid data, then the data collection tool/methodology should also produce data that has high inter-rater agreement between multiple observers. A data collection tool that can minimize the effects of individual interpretation may result in a data set that has high degree of inter-rater agreement. This can be aided with a computerized system that helps standardize the data collection options. In our system, we agreed ahead of time on the types of events we wanted to track, and the event-marking software aids in this process. Events can be 'one-time' checkboxes, such as 'Patient enters room', 'Antibiotics given', 'First skin incision', etc., 'countable' list items, such as 'Dropped the gallbladder', 'Contamination', 'Distraction', etc. or a series of pick lists that enable the observer to quickly summarize a communication event, such as 'Surgery Attending → Scrub Tech → Requesting → Tools', 'Surgery Resident → Medical Student → Teaching → Camera', etc. The observer also has the ability to type in free-hand notes at any time. All of these events are time-stamped and synchronized with the AV recordings (if any) using a method described further below. We have also experimented with creating a 'union' of the two scorers' data files, such that if one observer marked communication events that the other did not or vice versa, a more complete data set would result by joining the two data files and eliminating any that are the 'same', with the ability to also measure inter-rater agreement on those that were an interpretation of the 'same' communication event (Shin 2003). In other words, the moving window alignment algorithm automatically detects the 'same' conversations that were encoded so that a union of the two data sets can be made, and inter-rater agreement can be measured on just the intersection.

Interestingly, in our second operating room study, RATE was used as part of the *Independent* variable, which was the training of crew resource management skills. Thus, RATE was used to help train surgeons on their team communication and coordination skills. In this longitudinal study, the dependent variables were composed of answers to a questionnaire distributed to all team members immediately following each case. Improvements over time in questionnaire scores was the method for measuring impact (Guerlain et al. 2008). This method of measuring team performance has several advantages, including ease of collection, increased power (due to all team members rating the team performance, one case gets seven or so ratings) and no need to train observers on a team scoring metric.

Data Collection System

We list here the set of equipment used for the operating room studies along with some details about how and when it is used. Researchers can choose to use less recording equipment, depending on their methodological needs.

- *Rolling cart.* This cart stores all of the equipment listed below (except the two scoring laptops). It is rolled into the operating room, placed in the corner of the room to the left of the anaesthesia monitor to be most out of the way, the AV equipment is set up and recording is started prior to the patient's arrival. After the patient leaves, recording is stopped, the AV equipment is taken down and the cart is rolled out.
- *Four Pentium III computers*, each with a video capture card, corresponding video compression software and a large hard drive. These computers are placed on the bottom half of the cart. Each video card and corresponding

software automatically compresses one video feed (laparoscopic image view, table view, anaesthesia monitor view or room view) and two audio feeds. Upon playback, we can thus view all four videos and hear all conversations, or selectively mute any of the four pairs of audio feeds.

- *One LCD monitor, mouse, keyboard and switcher.* These are placed on the top half of the cart. The switcher enables switching the control of the monitor, keyboard and mouse among the four computers.
- *Eight Shure wireless microphones* (each on a different frequency). The receivers are placed on the top of the cart, to the right and left of the LCD monitor, with each audio feed going into one of the stereo (left/right) audio input lines of the video capture cards on the four computers. The lapel microphones are placed on staff as they arrive. For the surgeons, the lapel receiver is clipped onto the front of the scrub top, with the wire running over the shoulder, taped to the back of the scrub top, and the microphone itself is turned on and placed into the pocket of the scrub bottom. This is done before the surgeon scrubs and has a gown put on.
- A *video cable* is directly connected from the output jack on the back of the laparoscopic monitor to the laparoscopic view recording computer, thus enabling video capture of the laparoscopic image.
- *One high definition digital camera* (requires running cabling to it), which has remote pan/tilt/zoom capabilities and can handle the bright lights vs. dark room changes that occur during surgery is installed on one of the booms over the operating table to get a 'table' (operating area) view. Each boom in our operating rooms now has Velcro placed in the correct spot, as does the back of the camera. Due to the camera's weight, we also use surgical tape to secure the camera in place prior to each surgery. The camera is adjusted using the remote pan/tilt/zoom capability such that just the abdominal area is in view and the cable is secured out of the way using surgical tape along the boom and runs under the anaesthesia monitor etc. to get to our cart, and is plugged into the video capture card of the table view recording computer.
- A *digital-to-analogue scan converter.* This is an off-the-shelf product that can be used to 'split' the video feed of any computer monitor. We use it to get a video capture of the anaesthesiologist's computer screen, the analogue output of which is connected to the anaesthesia view recording computer (which then digitizes the analogue input).
- *One wireless video camera* (low resolution but extremely small and portable, we use this to get a 'room view' of the operating room). All of our operating suites now have Velcro on the upper corner of the wall, and we have Velcro on the back of the wireless video camera such that we can quickly place this camera prior to a surgery. The receiver is on the top of the cart. One person climbs onto a stool to place the video camera and a second person looks at the output on the room view recording computer so that the person placing the camera knows at what angle to point the camera (as it has no remote pan/tilt features).

- *Two laptop computers*, each running the RATE event-marking software. We have two people observe each case live and manually 'mark' events of interest using predefined categories of information described further in the next section. The observers stand on one or two steps to get a better view, and are behind the attending, on the surgeon's left side.
- *Two headsets*. These are worn by the observers to enable hearing all conversations.
- *One eight-jack local area network* (LAN) hub, which enables all four computers to have internet access through one ethernet cable. We also use this hub to connect external computers (e.g., the laptops we use to manually mark events of interest when observing the case) to the four recording computers.

Thus, to summarize, we designate the audio-video input to the four computers as follows:

- For the laparoscopic image computer, we capture the image coming off the laparoscopic camera (using a video cable), along with the surgery attending's and surgery resident's voices (using one pair of Shure wireless microphones).
- For the table view computer, we capture video taken from just above the operating table (using a high-definition video camera). On this view, we capture the voices of the scrub tech and camera operator using a second pair of Shure wireless microphones.
- For the anaesthesia monitor computer, we capture the video from the anaesthesiologist's monitor (using a scan converter) along with the voices of the anaesthetist(s) using a third pair of Shure wireless microphones.
- For the room view computer, we capture an overall room video, taken from high up in the corner of the OR (using a wireless video camera) and, on this view, we capture the circulating nurse's voice along with any 'extra' person in the room using the final pair of Shure wireless microphones.
- The observers set up and take down all equipment, and then make live observations using the RATE event-marking software.

General Setup Procedure

Our method of synchronizing the four audio-video files and the observers' event database file require that four activities take place. First, we manually synchronize the four Pentium III computers' clocks prior to each recording session (e.g., the morning before a case), to an external time server, which we do by using a software tool, available for free download from <www.arachnoid.com/abouttime/>.

Second, once all equipment is set up, we start compressing/recording the laparoscopic view first, as this is the reference recording time from which the other three computers' recording times are offset upon playback.

Third, once the four audio-video feeds are up and running (e.g., all the above equipment is set up and each computer is recording/compressing their respective audio-video inputs), we start the RATE event-marking software, set the 'start time' to approximately 30 seconds ahead of the currently counting up recording time on the laparoscopic view, and then hit 'Start' on the RATE event-marking software just as the recording time on the laparoscopic view reaches the just-entered start time. The RATE event-marking software will then 'count up' from the start time; this counting up time remains approximately in sync with the counting up time of the laparoscopic view. This enables the time stamps captured with the RATE event-marking software to be synchronized with the four video feeds upon playback (all computers' clocks are slightly different, so the two recording laptops and laparoscopic video capture time will eventually go out of sync, but not by more than a few seconds by the end of the case).

Finally, all software files are named with a unique ID for that case, followed by a description of the file (e.g., 6134_LapView.mpg, 6134_TableView.mpg, 6134_AnesthView.mpg and 6134_RoomView.mpg for the four AV files and 6134_Observer1.mdb, 6134_Observer2.mdb for the two observers' database files). Thus, when running the playback software, one can select the appropriate observer data file (e.g., 6134_Observer1.mdb) and know which four video files to load along with that file (e.g., 6134_LapView.mpg, 6134_TableView.mpg, 6134_AnesthView.mpg, and 6134_RoomView.mpg). In our studies, we had two observers recording but designated one as the 'primary' observer, and used this person's log file for debriefing purposes immediately following the case. Some work was done later to measure inter-rater agreement of the two observers etc. as described above.

Of note, upon playback, we run the four video using the LAN hub. The playback software just opens and plays the videos directly from their location on the recording computers. In other words, we avoid the extensive time it would take to copy the videos to a single computer. Thus, we can review the case immediately, which is how we are able to debrief the surgeons on their crew resource management and/or non-technical skills in a breakout room during the time between cases (see Figure 8.1). We tear down the equipment as soon as the patient is wheeled out of the room, store it on the cart, wheel the cart to the break-out room and meet the surgeons there once they are finished dictating the case. (In our studies, the surgery attending always attended the debriefs and sometimes the surgery resident joined as well. The other team members are busy during this change-over time).

The RATE Playback Software

Both the 'event marking' and 'playback' components of RATE are programmed using Visual Basic 6.0 (VB). The time-stamped events are stored in an Access database.

RATE playback is used to synchronize the four video feeds upon playback by offsetting the start of each video based on the time the videos were encoded.

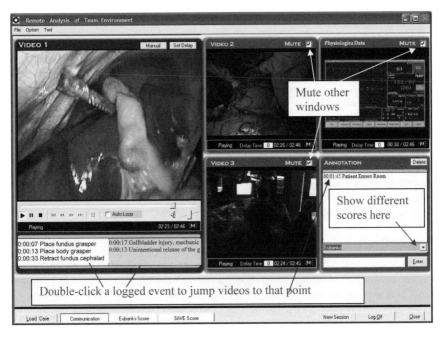

Figure 8.1   The RATE software

Thus, the playback software allows the observer to watch all four video feeds simultaneously and to jump all the videos instantly to a different point based on any marked event (that was marked by the observer watching the case using the RATE event-marking software) (see Figure 8.2).

The RATE Event-Marking Software

Figure 8.2 shows a screen shot of the RATE event-marking software just after a case has started. The left half of the screen is for conversation tracking and the right half of the screen is for event tracking. In particular, the upper portion of the left half of the screen allows observers to manually track conversations between members of the team by marking who is talking to whom, using what type of communication (e.g., joking, requesting, coaching) and about what topic (e.g., the patient, the room, the surgical tools, other cases). The observer clicks four times in the four columns, or can use 'type-ahead' and the 'Tab' key to mark a communication event. The summary is placed in the box to the right of these pick lists and is double-clicked by the observer when the communication event is finished. One can also single click on one of these conversations and click 'Answer Back' (below the 'Talk' button) and this will cause the 'From' and 'To' columns to automatically switch (e.g., 'Surgery Attending (SA) → Other → Discussing → Other Cases' automatically gets selected in the four boxes as 'Other → SA → Reply → Other Cases') and then the observer

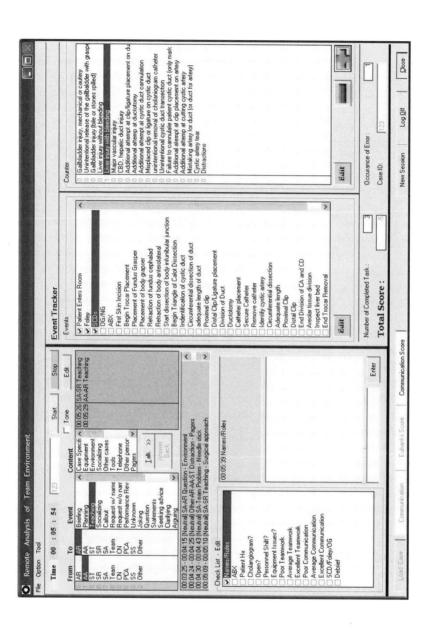

Figure 8.2   The RATE event-marking software

hits the 'Talk' button or edits one of these entries first if desired. The software user interface enables keeping up with conversations fairly well so long as the observer does not spend too much time typing in free-text comments (possible using the text entry box on the bottom left of the screen).

Based on these conversation traces, RATE tracks communication counts of each individual and each pair of individuals, by communication type and by categorized communication content (as judged by the observer when tracking the conversations live during the case). This enables summary analyses such as determining the (surprisingly large) percentage of time spent directing a medical student on how to operate the camera effectively during a case.

In the bottom half of the left side of the screen, we put in a few entries that we specifically wanted to track regarding communication during the case, e.g., we checked off these boxes if the following aspects were specifically *discussed* by the surgeon during a pre-operative briefing prior to first skin incision: introductions of people by name and their roles during the case, confirmation of antibiotics dosed, patient history, whether a cholangiogram procedure was planned, the likelihood the case might convert to an open procedure, any planned turnovers of personnel during the case, and confirming that all equipment and appliances were set up and ready for case start. These events could likely have been inferred from our more generic conversation tracker above, but they were important enough for our study to warrant a separate checkbox just for those events. We also placed here the ability to give an 'overall' communication score to the team at the end of the case, but found it was impossible to judge this and we thus quickly gave up using this feature.

The right half of the screen enables marking one time events that should/could occur for every case (left column) and things that could happen more than once (right column). The former are very useful for jumping to a particular part of the surgery later, and the latter are counts of errors with the added ability to jump the case to just prior to any of these upon review.

Determine Coding Scheme between Observers for Communication

In general, the software is designed to be customizable. All fields and events are editable, either directly through the Access back end, or by using the 'Edit' buttons that are placed around the screen. The observers need to define the codes and rules to follow when encoding data. The three communication categories that we used are team members, communication type (event), and the content as shown in Figure 8.2 (with an option to type in a free-text keyword, comment or summary of what was said). The team members and communication content are domain specific and can be changed depending on the process being observed, but we hypothesize (but have not tested) that the communication types, such as coaching, empowering and greeting, are generic.

Conclusion

This chapter described a hardware/software system called RATE that was developed to integrate data collection, processing and analysis for monitoring and training team performance. RATE allows observers to code real-time events with time codes, align and combine multiple codes, and compare for inter-rater agreement. Because RATE is a multimedia system, the time-stamps can be used to replay back the video segments of marked events immediately. A complete user's manual with screen shots of RATE, along with the executable software, is free to download for non-profit use from <http://www.sys.virginia.edu/hci/hcilab.asp>.

References

Endsley, M. (1995) Measurement of situation awareness in dynamic systems. *Human Factors* 37(1), 65–84.

Flin, R. and Maran, N. (2004) Identifying and training non-technical skills for teams in acute medicine. *Quality and Safety in Healthcare* 13, i80–i84.

Gaba, D. (1989) Human error in anesthetic mishaps. *International Anesthesiology Clinics* 27(3), 137–47.

Guerlain, S., Turrentine, B., Calland, J.F., and Adams R. (2004) Using video data for analysis and training of medical personnel. *Cognition Technology and Work* 6, 131–8.

Guerlain S., Adams R.B., Turrentine F.B., Shin T., Guo H., Collins S.R. and Calland J.F. (2005) Assessing team performance in the operating room: Development and use of a 'black-box' recorder and other tools for the intraoperative environment. *Journal of the American College of Surgeons* 200(1), 29–37.

Guerlain, S. Turrentine, F. Collins, S., Calland, J.F. and Adams, R. (2008) Crew resource management for surgeons: Feasibility and impact. *Cognition, Technology and Work* 10(4), 255–64.

Helmreich, R. and Schaefer, H. (1994) Team performance in the operating room. In M. Bogner (ed.), *Human Error in Medicine* (pp. 225–53). Hillsdale, NJ: Lawrence Erlbaum.

Law, J. and Sherman, P. (1995) Do raters agree? Assessing inter-rater agreement in the evaluation of air crew resource management skills. In R. Jensen (ed.), *Proceedings of the 8th Symposium of Aviation Psychology* 608–12.

Moorthy, K., Munz, Y., Adams, S., Pandey, V. and Darzi, A. (2005) A human factors analysis of technical and team skills among surgical trainees during procedural simulations in a simulated operating theatre. *Annals of Surgery* 242(5), 631–9.

Rouse, W., Cannon-Bowers, J. and Salas, E. (1992) The role of mental models in team performance in complex system. *Institute of Electrical and Electronics Engineers* 22(6), 1296–308.

Sexton, J. and Helmreich, R. (2000) Analyzing cockpit communication: The links between language, performance, error, and workload. *Human Performance in Extreme Environments* 5(1), 63–8.

Sexton, J., Marsch, S., Helmreich, R., Betzendoerfer, D., Kochre, T. and Scheidegger, D. (2002) Jumpseating in the operating room. In L. Henson, A. Lee and A. Basford (eds), *Simulators in Anesthesiology Education* (pp. 107–108). New York: Plenum.

Shin, T. (2003) Team Performance Measurement: Measuring Inter-Rater Reliability/Agreement of Independent Team Scores. University of Virginia Masters thesis.

Simon, H., and Ericsson, K. (1993) *Protocol Analysis: Verbal Reports as Data.* Cambridge, Mass: Massachusetts Institute of Technology Press.

Sledd, R. Bass, E. Borowitz, S. and Waggoner-Fountain, L. (2006) Supporting the characterization of sign-out in acute care wards. In *Proceedings of the 2006 IEEE Conference on Systems, Man, and Cybernetics*, 5215–20.

Xiao, Y., Mackenzie, C., Seagull, F., and Jaberi, M. (2000) Managing the monitors. An analysis of alarm silencing activities during an anesthetic procedure. *Proceedings of International Ergonomics Association 2000 Human Factors and Ergonomics Society 2000 Congress* 4, 250–3.

Xiao, Y. and The LOTAS Group (2001) Understanding coordination in a dynamic medical environment. Methods and results. In M. McNeese, E. Salas and M. Endsley (eds), *New Trends in Cooperative Activities* (pp. 242–58). Santa Monica, CA: Human Factors and Ergonomics Society.

Chapter 9

A-TEAM: Targets for Training, Feedback and Assessment of all OR Members' Teamwork

Carl-Johan Wallin, Leif Hedman, Lisbet Meurling and Li Fellländer-Tsai

Background

The objective for our research is to increase our knowledge about the teamwork training process that helps account for improving teamwork outcome and patient safety. In this chapter we will focus on the development of a new instrument to assist team performance assessment in a variety of real and simulated clinical events in the operating theatre. This tool could be used in the study of the relationship between the teamwork process and teamwork outcome, as well as for feedback during training. Laborious work has been done earlier in this field and we want to further explore whether refinements of existing behaviour scales will add to our understanding of teamwork in general and to understanding of the team training process in particular (for reviews see Baker et al. 2005b, Rosen et al. 2008).

The process of providing healthcare is inherently interdisciplinary, requiring physicians, nurses and allied health professionals from different specialties to work in teams. Compared to teams in other industries, medical teams work under conditions that change frequently, may be assembled ad hoc, have a dynamically changing team membership, often work together for a short period of time, consist of different specialists and have to integrate different professional cultures (Manser 2009). In order to effectively train teamwork, it is necessary to reliably assess behaviours associated with effective teamwork and their interplay in relation to clinical performance ratings and ultimately to patient outcome (Baker et al. 2005a, Rosen et al. 2008).

There are three parts in this chapter: (i) rationale for developing the all team members' behaviour scale (A-TEAM), (ii) presentation of A-TEAM, and (iii) application of A-TEAM in an operating theatre setting.

Rationale for Developing the A-TEAM Scale

A Generic Behavioural Scale for Teamwork in Healthcare

In the operating theatre, failures in communication and ineffective teamwork during surgical procedures have observable consequences such as delay, tension among team members, or procedural errors (Catchpole et al. 2007, Lingard et al. 2004a, Wiegmann et al. 2007). Although it is often claimed that many adverse events could have been prevented by improved teamwork, most studies do not make explicit exactly which aspects of teamwork that have to be improved (Baker et al. 2005b, Manser 2009). To exactly identify the demands in each particular setting in the operating theatre is a prerequisite for efficient training, although research in this field has just started (Rosen et al. 2008). However, when looking at the coordination problems that occur in healthcare, it is obvious that generic well-known coordination behaviours are not always applied and providers have not received formalized training in how to interact with one another. Therefore health care authorities recommend implementation of team training to improve teamwork (Agency for Healthcare Research and Quality 2006, Burke et al. 2006, Kohn et al. 2000, Veterans Affairs National Center for Patient Safety 2004). Murray and Foster (2000) recommended bringing together individuals from different healthcare professions and specialties to take part as 'strangers' in team training using generic team behaviours as targets for training. Ostergaard et al. (2004) have also argued for multidisciplinary team training in medicine aiming at improving team skills in order to increase patient safety. Frankel and collaborators (2007) argued for teamwork skills that are widely applicable and reflect good practice for a wide variety of healthcare professions. Applying generic coordination principles in team training of the operating theatre staff would be an advantage also for the safety of the surgical patient. For this purpose, a generic behaviour scale as target for team training in medicine is needed. This should also be applicable in the operating theatre. Refining the training programme in future by applying specific behaviours revealed by research would add to this advantage.

A Scale Feasible to use as a Target for Training, Formative Assessment and Feedback

Applying cognitive behaviour principles (for review see McGuire 2000) in industrial and organizational training settings (Cannon-Bowers and Salas 1997, Salas et al. 1999) aligns target for training with formative assessment for feedback, 'assessment is the tail that wags the dog' as someone said. In order not to tax trainees' limited working memory (Baddley and Logie 1999, Cowan 2005, Miyake et al. 2001) during training, targets for training should be limited. Social psychology has made considerable progress over the last few decades regarding the development of observational methods. Despite this headway, there still remains a number of methodological issues about which little can be said. One such issue is how to consider findings of human working memory when developing observational methods and protocols. Tools for observation and rating of behaviour should be very easy to understand and use, since observational methods are vulnerable to limitations of human perceivers. Weick (1968, p. 433) also advocated the use of:

> simple, unequivocal behavioural indices [i.e., checklists] ... [which] are easy to grasp [i.e., easy to train to a high degree of interjudge agreement], and do not impose excessive demands on the observer.

Working memory, previously termed short-term memory, is a theoretical construct studied within cognitive psychology which has been applied to image guided surgical simulation (Hedman et al. 2007). It refers to the mental structures and processes used for temporarily storing and elaborating information. Working memory is generally considered to have limited capacity. We cannot focus on everything at once. We quickly become overburdened. In his classical article in the history of psychology, Miller (1956) was the first cognitive psychologist who introduced the 'magical number seven' as a quantification of the capacity limit associated with short-term memory. The memory span of young adults was around seven elements (chunks), regardless whether the elements were letters, words, digits or other units. However, more recent research has shown that many different factors affect a person's measured span. It is therefore generally difficult to state that the capacity of short-term or working memory is an absolute number of chunks. Nonetheless, Cowan (2005) suggested that working memory may have a capacity of about four chunks in young adults, and fewer in children and old adults.

Numerous theories of working memory exist. For example, according to Baddeley and Logie (1999), working memory is the information we are actively thinking about and processing at any given moment, and working memory is consequently closely related to the allocation of our attention to the most important events in a situation. Baddeley and Hitch (1974) introduced their multi-component model of working memory, which proposes that two *slave systems* are responsible for short-term maintenance of information, and a *central executive* is responsible for coordinating the *slave systems* as well as for the supervision of information integration. For Cowan (2005) working memory is not as a separate theoretical system, but a part of long-term memory. The hypothesis that working memory is crucial for reducing distraction by maintaining the prioritization of relevant information was tested by de Fockert and collaborators (2001) by functional magnetic resonance imaging (fMRI) and psychological experiments in humans. The researchers demonstrated that when a person's working memory is occupied his or her brain cannot filter out distracting sights in a separate attention task. Hence, working memory is crucial for reducing distraction by maintaining the prioritization of relevant information. It therefore became very important for us to select as few behavioural categories and descriptions of poor to proficient behaviours as possible for a behaviour observation tool, in order not to tax the observer's limited working memory.

Taking into consideration findings on working memory, we designed the A-TEAM scale with only a few and distinct categories of behaviour to be identified. The scale should be exceedingly simple since the task for the observers is to simultaneously observe the behaviours of both leaders and followers. Moreover, an easy way to align targets and assessment is to use the same scale for both purposes. For training teamwork in medicine, we need a scale that has a limited number of behaviour items, easily understood by trainees and feasible to use for formative feedback. In order to evaluate the training per se the scale must also be feasible to use for summative assessment, i.e., provide pseudo-quantitative data to measure progress in teamwork after training. Most of the available behaviour rating instruments for healthcare settings, such as ACRM (Anesthesia Crisis Resource Management; Howard et al. 1992), revised teamwork behaviour matrix (Small et al. 1999), Team Dimensions Rating Form (Morey et al. 2002), OTAS (Observational Teamwork Assessment for Surgery; Carthey et al. 2003, Healey et al. 2004), ANTS (Anaesthetists' Non-Technical Skills; Fletcher et al. 2003, Flin et al. 2004), EMCRM (Emergency Medicine Crisis Resource Management Behavioural Performance Evaluation; Reznek et al. 2003, Wallin et al. 2007), BARS (Behaviourally Anchored Rating Scales, Shapiro et al. 2004), NOTSS (Surgeons' Non-Technical skills in the operating theatre; Flin et al. 2006, Yule et al. 2008), Ottawa GRS (Ottawa Crisis Resource Management Global Rating Scale, Kim et al. 2006), CATS (Communication and Teamwork Skills; Frankel et al. 2007), are designed for summative use, and as such too overburdened with elements to be used effectively in training.

A Behaviour Scale for Recognition of all Individuals in the Team

The core feature of teamwork is coordination of task execution to achieve a specified and shared goal. Timely and correct execution of tasks is coordinated through collaborative information sampling to build a shared mental model of the situation, collaborative decision-making, prioritizing and delegating tasks. The process can be described with help of a straightforward decision-making strategy as presented by St. Pierre et al. for individuals (2008, p. 122) applied to a team (see Figure 9.1).

They emphasize that all strategies and decisional aids in the literature of decision-making in high stake environments (e.g., Gaba 1992, Murray and Foster 2000) contain at least the following five steps of a good strategy:

1. preparedness;
2. analysis of the situation (gathering of information, building mental models);
3. planning of actions (formulating of goals, risk assessment, planning, decision-making);
4. execution of action;
5. review of effects (review of actions, revision of strategy, self-reflection).

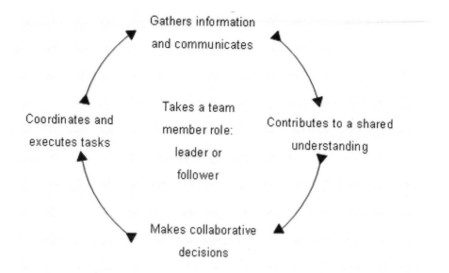

Figure 9.1 **A schematic presentation of a structured team decision-making process**

Team members are delegated different tasks while working together; task functions are not interchangeable, although change of the distribution of tasks between members may vary over time. In order to collaborate, a team member must adjust his/her behaviour to other members', quoting Brannick and Prince (1997, p. 10):

> The interpersonal part of the process can thus be thought of as providing the grease that keeps the part of the team working together smoothly. On the other hand, difficulties in individual member performance can act like sand in creating friction within a team, thus interfering with interpersonal harmony.

Leading and following are significant collaborative adjustment behaviours; an evolutionary strategy for solving social coordination problems (Van Vugt et al. 2008).

All individuals in healthcare are involved in teamwork, most often in the follower position; some individuals also regularly take a leader position. No single individual has the privilege to always be the leader, more likely he/she will work together with others in a team where somebody else holds the leader position. The situation during work may also demand a quick change in roles between a leader and one of the followers in the team. All healthcare personnel must thus be able to function as both a follower and a leader in a team and to quickly change position without prestige. The relationship is symbiotic; no one can lead without followers. Leader and follower are distinct entities but of equal value to team collaboration and both are partners in the team. Both leader and follower need to support the mutual role assignment to support the integrity of team structure and process. Some attributes and characteristics associated with leaders are requisites of followers as well, referred to as good leadership or as good followership. Van Vugt (2006), who evaluated vast psychological literature on leadership as a database to test several evolutionary hypotheses about the leadership and followership in humans, found that leadership correlates well with initiative taking, trait measures of intelligence, specific task competencies, and several indicators of generosity, but he found no link between leadership and dominance. Burke and co-workers (2006, p. 302), who conducted a meta-analysis to examine the relationship between leadership behaviour in teams and behaviourally based team performance outcomes found that:

> Surprisingly, the results of the current literature review indicate the preponderance of empirical research conducted to date to examine team leadership has largely been grounded in traditional leadership theory. In other words, researchers are just transporting traditional theories of leadership to team settings. This is a concern because classical leadership theories have often been criticized for failing to fully appreciate and model the dynamism and complexities of team leadership (Kozlowski and Bell, 2002, Salas, Stagl and Burke, 2004, Ziegert 2004). In fact, most existing leadership theories are advanced as if 'leader–follower relationships exist in a vacuum'. (House and Aditya 1997, p. 445)

As current leadership theory and research predominantly refers to leader style, Avolio (2007) argues that future work needs to consider the dynamic interplay between leaders and followers. Presumptions about leadership and followership – such as leaders are more important than followers, followers are only doing what they are told, followers get their energy and aims from the leader – should be challenged also in theory and research regarding medical teams.

Our general working hypothesis is that all team members are important for successful goal achievement and that the roles and interaction between sub-teams, professions, specialities, leader and followers have to be further explored in relation to patient outcome. Our specific working hypothesis is that training effectiveness will be better when these roles and interactions are identified for each sub-team, profession, speciality, leader and follower and used as targets in team training. In order to further elucidate the individual team members' contribution to the collaborative teamwork and the interpersonal interaction between team members, we need an observational behaviour instrument that allows for rating all team members' team skills.

Leadership and Followership; Attitudes in Teamwork

We consider leadership/followership, to be a significant element of teamwork, in two aspects: attitudes and behaviours. Dickinson and McIntyre (1997, p. 25) explain team leadership:

> Involves providing direction, structure, and support for other team members. It does not necessarily refer to a single individual with formal authority over

others. Team leadership can be shown by several team members: explains to other team members exactly what is needed from them during assignment, listens to the concerns of other team member.

Thomas et al. (2004, p. 160) comment, regarding observation of neonatal resuscitation, that:

> Leadership activities may include sharing of a mental model, assigning tasks, and sharing of information and opinion. This may be rated for any provider at the resuscitation. There is usually not a clear leader (either in deed or word), so the observability rating is often 0. Lack of leadership was not obviously detrimental to the process of care.

Thus in a successful team, all team members, not only the formal leader but also the followers, embrace positive team attitudes such as team orientation, conflict efficacy, shared vision, team cohesion, interpersonal relations, mutual trust, task-specific teamwork attitudes, collective orientation and importance of teamwork. Such leadership or followership attitudes facilitate a culture of non-negotiable mutual respect and trust so that effective teamwork can flourish.

Leader Behaviour and Follower Behaviour

The reasoning regarding leader and follower attitudes does not apply to the issue of leader behaviour and follower behaviour. In contrast to attitudes, if several members of a team simultaneously apply some of the identified 'leadership' behaviours, there is an obvious risk of confusion and conflict in the team, which jeopardizes team structure and process. A leader is recognized by his/her leader behaviour which might include taking the initiative to prompt discussions, making decisions, verbalizing plans and having the 'last word'. A situation when a follower simultaneously behaves in that manner, or shows other leader behaviours, will confuse other members as to who is the leader. Tension arises and a prestige conflict between team members might result which undermines, rather than enhances, the leader's position, and demoralizes the team. Obviously, regarding certain behavioural elements there is a reciprocal relationship between leader behaviour and follower behaviour. Another recognized behavioural element, such as good communication, is identical for all team members. In agreement with Thomas et al. (2004), we seek behavioural markers that allow the rating of any team member's team skills, whether as leader or as follower, or just as a good team member. Accordingly, in agreement with Murray and Foster (2000) and Ostergaard et al. (2004), we advocate using specified leader behaviours, follower behaviours and member behaviours as targets for team training to emphasize the complementary behaviours and to facilitate individual feedback to each individual team member.

Behaviour markers for healthcare, many of them based on crew resource management (CRM) used in aviation (Gaba et al. 1994, Flin et al. 2003, Helmreich et al. 1999) and adapted to medical settings, such as ACRM (Anesthesia Crisis Resource Management; Howard et al. 1992), Revised teamwork behaviour matrix (Small et al. 1999), Team Dimensions Rating Form (Morey et al. 2002), OTAS (Observational Teamwork Assessment for Surgery; Carthey et al. 2003, Healey et al. 2004), ANTS (Anaesthetists' Non-technical Skills; Fletcher et al. 2003, Flin et al. 2004a), EMCRM (Emergency Medicine Crisis Resource Management Behavioural Performance Evaluation; Reznek et al. 2003, Wallin et al. 2007), CARMA (Crisis Avoidance Resource Management for Anaesthetists; Flin et al. 2004b), BARS (Behaviourally Anchored Rating Scales; Shapiro et al. 2004), NOTSS (Surgeons' Non-Technical skills in the operating theatre; Flin et al. 2006, Yule et al. 2008), Ottawa GRS (Ottawa Crisis Resource Management Global Rating Scale; Kim et al. 2006), CATS (Communication and Teamwork Skills; Frankel et al. 2007), are focused on the team leader alone (i.e., the anaesthetist or the surgeon) and/or the team (e.g., the crew). Only the instrument designed by Thomas et al. (2004) – University of Texas behavioural markers for neonatal resuscitation (UTBMNR) – is explicitly constructed for summative assessment of any team member's team skills.

In summary, we need a behaviour-based assessment instrument suitable for gauging all team members' teamwork skills on an individual basis that is widely applicable and reflects good practice across the healthcare professions, disciplines and medical environments, and that can be used as target for training, formative assessment for feedback and for summative evaluation of training.

Description of the A-TEAM Scale

Development of the A-TEAM Scale

We used the decision loop (Figure 9.1) as a template for four behavioural categories: 'Gathers information and communicates', 'Contributes to shared understanding', 'Makes collaborative decisions', 'Coordinates and executes tasks', and added a fifth category, 'Takes a team member role', which has three subcategories: 'All members' behaviour', 'Leader behaviour' and 'Follower behaviour'. From our experience these categories are easy for trainees to comprehend. We scanned the literature and sampled verbally defined behavioural elements from other scales and CRM programmes as generic behaviours of effective collaboration (Burke et al. 2004, Carthey et al. 2003, Dickinson and McIntyre 1997, Fletcher et al. 2003, Flin et al. 2004a, Flin and Maran 2004, Flin et al. 2006, Frankel et al. 2007, Healey et al. 2004, Howard et al. 1992, Kim et al. 2006, Moorthy et al. 2006, Morey et al. 2002, Morgan et al. 2007, Murray and Foster 2000, Ostergaard et al. 2004, Ottestad et al. 2007, Reznek et al. 2003, Shapiro et al. 2004, Small et al. 1999, Thomas et al. 2004, Wallin et al. 2007, Undre et al. 2007). We selected behavioural elements meeting two criteria: a trainee should, voluntarily, be able to display the behaviour at work, and the behaviour should be observable for trainees. Behavioural elements related to the four categories – 'Gathers information and communicates', 'Contributes to shared understanding', 'Makes collaborative decisions', 'Coordinates and executes tasks' – were sorted to respective categories. In order to sort behavioural elements into the leader, follower and member sub-categories, we used our clinical experience of working in anaesthesia, intensive care and emergency medicine, and experience from acting as 'consultant on call' in hundreds of simulator scenarios with younger medical colleagues and nurses. The intention was that a senior consultant would stay in a follower position to give a second opinion and support to a younger, less experienced colleague. Behaviours by the consultant that immediately would dislodge this balance were categorized as leader behaviour. Examples of these behaviours were taking initiative to provide briefings, decision-making, confirming and verbalizing plans, and 'having the last word'. Behaviours that stabilized the relationship, yet allowed use of all expertise available, were categorized as follower behaviours. These behaviours were such as giving the junior colleague suggestions to take initiative for briefings and decision-making, suggesting that he/she verbalize plans and let him/her 'have the last word' in order to support him/her as leader. The vast majority of behaviours sampled were both leader and follower behaviours and as such categorized as team member behaviours.

For each category, we condensed the vast number of sampled behavioural elements so that the sum of them would be limited and not tax the observer's, trainee's or trainer's, limited working memory, and hence easy to use as target for training, formative assessment and feedback.

Using A-TEAM as Target for Training, Formative Assessment and Feedback

The A-TEAM form should be presented and discussed with trainees and demonstrated by trainers before practice. During practice, non-active trainees can observe and grade active participants using an A-TEAM protocol, which enhances learning. All elements are directly observable; the text is short and in simple language. During feedback, trainers have the opportunity to further elucidate behaviour issues related to coordination using A-TEAM. During training, observers and trainers use the following four grades for classifying team member behaviours:

- *Poor*: Behaviour that intentionally counteracts desirable team behaviour.
- *In need of considerable improvement*: Behaviour that neither counteracts nor fully contributes to desirable team behaviour.
- *Good*: Behaviour that really helps in solving the task and strives towards desirable team behaviour, but is not excellent.
- *Proficient*: Proficient behaviour, role model.

The result of the development process is presented in Table 9.1. There are five main categories of behaviours, and the first, 'Takes a membership role', is divided into three subcategories. Each category and subcategory is defined separately. Examples of behavioural elements representative for each category are given for four grades in columns, read from left to right with increasing proficiency. The grades 'Good' and 'Proficient' are used as targets for training, while all grades are used for feedback and assessment of training outcome.

During debriefing, advantages and disadvantages of using leader and follower behaviours can be discussed in relation to conflicts and outcome for the (simulated) patient. Future research may elucidate in which situations leader behaviour, follower behaviour and member behaviour are of particular importance for patient outcome and integrated in training.

Using A-TEAM for Summative Assessment

All elements to be assessed for each category are directly observable, so no further assumptions/interpretations have to be made by the observers. Active verbs are used for describing observable behaviours. Global rating of an individual's team skills and/or global rating of the complete team performance can also be registered if needed.

Scoring Method in Summative Assessment

For feedback during training, it is easier to 'pinpoint' the most important behaviours observed using four grades. However, for evaluation of training and for research purposes, it is statistically correct to handle these ordinal data as binary data. All raw data are converged into the following two stages:

> 0 = Poor and in need of considerable improvement.
> 1 = Good and proficient.

In summary, the A-TEAM instrument is designed for both training and research purposes. All team members are scored in terms of the occurrence and quality of certain behaviours. Hence, it will assist team performance assessment in a variety of real and simulated clinical events and can be used in the study of the relationship between the teamwork process and teamwork outcome, as well as for feedback during training of instructors and trainees. People with quite different educational backgrounds should be able to use the scale. Lipshitz (2005, p. 370) argued that pure factual reports: 'without interpretation are either impossible or not meaningful'.

Human beings do not simply perceive, but elaborate and interpret information and reflect upon it (cognition) and so the observer is an interpreter of raw data. By using video recordings, good observational data can be obtained and the observer takes advantage of the serendipity. Discrepant observations are not

Table 9.1   The A-TEAM scale for assessment of individual team behaviour

1. Takes a team member role

All members' behaviour

A team member participates actively in all relevant aspects of teamwork and task work, observes other team members' performance and activities, and provides and accepts feedback and assistance.

Poor	In need of improvement	Good	Proficient
Does not give or welcome any support. Does not acknowledge other members. Work on his/her own. Does not give or take advice gracefully.	Support others only if challenged, not spontaneously. Supports in a reluctant way.	Supports others, e.g., by helping when obviously needed.	Accepts and gives support directly. Acknowledges and involves others frequently. Asks quickly for help when needed. Protests clearly against inaccuracies.

Leader behaviour

A team leader takes initiative to provide structure and direct team- and task work.

Poor	In need of improvement	Good	Proficient
Does not identify himself/herself as person in charge of the situation. Makes no final decisions. Tries to 'do it all'. Does not take initiatives.	Tries to make decisions and give orders but very unclear and vague. Takes initiative, but not in time when needed.	Makes decisions, but not clear enough. Gives orders, but not directed.	Makes final decisions. Gives clear orders. Takes initiatives to e.g., short briefings; confirms and verbalizes decisions. Accepts a non-leading role when appropriate.

Follower behaviour

A team follower supports the leader's initiatives, and assumes assigned responsibilities and directives.

Poor	In need of improvement	Good	Proficient
Challenges the leader in an obstructive way. Stands back, takes a 'hands-off approach'. Demonstratively does not participate in briefings.	Performs task duties, but only on demand. Does not support the leader verbally or in other ways.	Supports the leader both verbally and in other ways. Takes a 'hands-on approach'.	Supports the leader. Takes a 'hands on' approach. Challenges constructively. Requests and participates actively in briefings. Takes over leadership if required.

Table 9.1　Continued

2. Gathers information and communicates

All team members actively gather and exchange information.

Poor	In need of improvement	Good	Proficient
Does not communicate at all. Masters through oral or body language. Engages in unnecessary conversation. Makes inappropriate comments.	Communicates vaguely, quietly or continuously without pause.	Communicates in round terms, but not aimed at a team member. Does not give feedback.	Communicates in round terms. Uses closed-loop communication. Uses SBAR format for briefings. Calls out critical information during emergent events. Makes good eye contact. Uses team members' names.

3. Contributes to a shared understanding of the situation

In collaboration, all team members develop and maintain a common understanding of the situation, and have team situational awareness.

Poor	In need of improvement	Good	Proficient
Does not share any information. Demonstratively does not contribute.	Reports findings unclearly. Gets distracted by non-essentials. Acts independently on symptoms without confirming with others.	Reports findings (positive and negative) in a clear and concise way. Does not try to explain things to others when obviously needed to.	Interprets information in a timely manner. Shares information and explains core events, thus making them understandable to the whole team.

4. Makes collaborative decisions

In collaboration, all team members consider options, resources and risks to be able to take decisions.

Poor	In need of improvement	Good	Proficient
Defies any attempts to decision and does not state an alternative. Demonstratively does not take part.	Makes decision right away without discussing alternatives with the team though time and opportunity exists.	Contributes with ideas, but does not state any own opinion.	Re-evaluates, discusses and takes other alternatives in consideration with other team members before reaching a conclusion. Actively drives the decision process forward.

Table 9.1 *Concluded*

5. Coordinates and executes tasks

A team member coordinates his/her tasks in a timely and integrated manner with other team members' activities, facilitating the performance of other members' jobs.

Poor	In need of improvement	Good	Proficient
Does not coordinate at all. Acts on his/her own. Stops others. Carries out inappropriate courses of action. Does not adhere to guidelines.	Obstructs but does not stop. Does not change plans despite new information.	Coordinates, but not for the whole team. Keep things progressing, but not in a clear and efficient way.	Coordinates his/her activities with others. Adapts to any changes in the present situation. Prioritizes tasks. Tells others of plan for further care. Adheres to guidelines.

always unreliable observations reducing the validity and reliability of findings, but could be signs of originality and perceptiveness of the observer. As in most true discoveries, the observer can shift his/her focus from originally defined data collection to also include observation of new phenomena. Since the locus of exploratory observational studies is on discovery, several techniques should be used to broaden the set of observations and maximize the observers' opportunity for uncovering interesting data. Roth and Patterson (2005, p. 382) have exemplified some good techniques: (i) broadly sampling domain practice (e.g., multiple trainees at several different levels of experience, many test sites), (ii) using multiple converging techniques (e.g., field observations, interviews, questionnaires), and (iii) using several observers (who bring different conceptual frameworks for observation and interpretation).

In future studies, A-TEAM could also be used in exploratory observational studies as contrasted with studies designed to test specific research hypotheses on human decision-making in complex medical domains.

Application in the Operating Theatre

Optimal surgical performance includes both technical and non-technical aspects. Regarding the latter, the equal importance of leadership and followership challenges the current dogma with respect to leadership. We outline a new hypothesis regarding the teamwork process in the operating theatre and identify the equal importance of leadership and followership, as well as the ability to engage in reciprocal rotation of these functions depending on the situation. There is a clear need for more awareness of these metacognitive aspects in the surgical community. Patient safety on the agenda facilitates this evolution.

The A-TEAM instrument could be applicable in many different surgical challenges from simple surgical procedures to demanding and complex tasks such as liver transplantation, cardiothoracic surgery and spinal surgery where system failure is deleterious. The results should also be coupled to traditional performance variables and patient outcome. Regarding inability or failure of followership in the operating room (OR), Lingard et al. (2004a), for example, observed a failure in 30 per cent of communication events during surgical procedures. Of these failures, 36 per cent had observable consequences such as delay, tension among team members or procedural error. These results are supported by another observational study (Wiegmann et al. 2007) focusing on the effects of disruptions of the surgical process (e.g., communication failures, equipment problems). Their study found that surgical errors increased significantly with increased disruptions and that teamwork and communication problems were the strongest predictors of surgical errors. Communication is a very important causal factor in errors made in surgery (Gawande et al. 2003). An observational study in paediatric cardiac and orthopaedic surgery found that effective teamwork was associated with fewer minor problems per operation (i.e., negative events that were seemingly innocuous but many of which contributed to major problems), higher intra-operative performance (i.e., fewer key operating tasks were disrupted) and shorter operating times (Catchpole et al. 2007).

Achievement of medical goals and patient safety are the main objectives for teamwork in medicine. In the operating theatre patient outcome can be quantified in mortality, morbidity, time to recovery, absence of iatrogenic injury i.e., a technically successful surgical procedure, time of low oxygen saturation etc. The team's task work gives information whether the team has executed procedures, algorithms and routines as planned and expected. Task work can be related to patient outcome to provide information whether team performance is effective. The individual, interpersonal teamwork behaviour gives information on how a team member contributes to coordination of task work and to internal team structure and process. Assessment of team skills is necessary for feedback during training and as such a formative assessment.

The aggregate of all team members' behaviour gives information on the teams' internal effectiveness and can be related to task execution (Lingard et al. 2004a, Catchpole et al. 2007, Ottestad et al. 2007) and to patient outcome (Catchpole et al. 2007, Wiegmann et al. 2007). Further analysis of the individual, interpersonal teamwork behaviour can provide information whether a certain subteam of members, such as surgical (Moorthy et al. 2005, Undre et al. 2007), anaesthetic (Undre et al. 2007), nursing (Undre et al. 2007), leader or followers, or a specific leadership style (Cooper and Wakelam 1999, Entin and Serfaty 1999, Klein et al. 2006, Marsch et al. 2005, Tschan et al. 2006), have favourable impact on task execution and patient outcome. Although team performance is a collective effort, there is lack of information on the impact of the quality of followers' behaviour on teamwork, team performance and patient outcome. Observational studies of teamwork have identified patterns of communication, coordination and leadership that support effective teamwork. However, only a few studies could establish a direct link between specific teamwork behaviours and clinical performance or patient outcome.

Communication Patterns Supporting Effective Teamwork

Among the most prominent themes in communication research in healthcare are the effects of interruptions and tensions on effective team functioning. For example, ethnographic studies showed that tensions in team communications in the operating room often evolve around the issues of time, safety and sterility, resources and work roles (Lingard et al. 2002 and 2004b). In medicine, CRM and simulation traditionally emerged within anaesthesia and intensive care. Human reliability from a team perspective is the focus. Within the different fields of surgical intervention, until recently, simulation was most commonly focused on technical skills i.e., manual dexterity of the operating surgeon. High fidelity and full procedural simulation in image guided surgery have clearly emerged as contemporary state-of-the-art training tools which are being embedded into curricula and as part of certification procedures in surgical education and training. Since metrics are inherent in image guided surgical simulators, the trainee gets evidence-based feedback and learning curves as well as proficiency gains can easily be monitored. Extensive validation studies are convincing and demonstrate transfer of skills acquired in surgical simulators to real surgery performed on patients (Ahlberg et al. 2007, Seymour et al. 2002, Grantcharov et al. 2004). Factors underpinning technical performance such as visual spatial abilities, working memory and computer game experience have also been demonstrated (Enochsson et al. 2004, Hedman et al. 2006 and 2007, Kolga Schlickum et al. 2008). However, several initiatives now also focus on non-technical OR skills of surgeons and the whole surgical team (e.g., Moorthy et al. 2006). This evolution transforms simulation towards systems orientation and points out that the result of surgery is neither related to patient pathophysiology nor the surgeons' technical skills alone but rather to the competence of the whole perioperative team.

Traditionally, the OR team consists of the surgeons (attending staff and residents), the scrub nurse, the anaesthetist, the anaesthesia nurse and nurse assistants. As in all high hazard fields, it is clear and evident that communication skills are crucial for outcome. Increasing clinical complexity requires a reciprocal increase in communication skills not only within professions and disciplines, but also across professional culture barriers. A multidisciplinary and transprofessional approach is needed. As in other high risk industries, surgery requires a minimum amount of system redundancy. One major challenge is the unpredictable nature of surgery and the ability of the whole team to be able to shift from working in a routine mode to a state of emergency accommodating rapid and efficient coordination. Verbal communication and feedback has been shown to improve team performance in image guided surgical teams (Shiliang Chang et al. 2008).

Bearing the recent evolution in medical simulation in mind, it is now prime time to take one step further, looking at the whole perioperative team, the OR team and not only the patient's pathophysiology and the surgeon. The A-TEAM scale which rates all team members enables this step towards increased team coordination. As shown in Table 9.1 it assesses behaviours. It is important to keep in mind the impact of patient outcome variables, clinical performance and team members' subjective experiences of the process of teamworking. Consequently, such additional assessments also have to be addressed by other scales in order to yield a more fine-grained analysis. True mastery of intra-operative skills transcends from teamwork in harmony with manual dexterity. It stems from mastery of oneself, being fully aware and in tune with the rest of the team, despite leadership or followership and irrespective of the current context. The traditional focus being mainly on the leader deserves challenge and a new hypothesis needs to be outlined; the equal importance of followership for successful surgery. This evolution can be considered as sluggish within the field of perioperative care. According to empirical evidence, one reason could be the inherent promotion of vertical climbing of the pyramid of hierarchy within surgery, rather than a horizontal process-oriented approach. Intimidation and harassment have been described as functional educational tools in surgical education (Musselman et al. 2005). The authors found that intimidation was sustained in the surgical education by encapsulation and rationalizing the behaviour to 'good' or 'beneficial' intimidation. These fundamental values in the surgical community towards education have no doubt served as conservers of the old system.

This mastery of teamwork can be developed and trained by a systematic approach and requires the attempt to assess all team members' performance, since it is the combined effort of the team that yields the net result for the ones we are set to treat and help – the patients.

In summary, the A-TEAM scale could be a suitable tool for elucidating the complex interaction between leaders and followers. Further, it could be used in the study of the relationship between the teamwork process and teamwork outcome, as well as for feedback during training. We propose further validation of the A-TEAM scale with the ultimate goal to enhance teamwork output for optimal perioperative care.

References

Agency for Healthcare Research and Quality (2006) *TeamSTEPPS™: Strategies and Tools to Enhance Performance and Patient Safety.* Available from: <http://teamstepps.ahrq.gov/abouttoolsmaterials.htm> [last accessed September 2008].

Ahlberg, G., Enochsson, L., Gallagher, A.G., Hedman, L., Hogman, C., McClusky, D.A. 3rd, Ramel, S., Smith, C.D.and Arvidsson, D. (2007) Proficiency-based virtual reality training significantly reduces the error rate for residents during their first 10 laparoscopic cholecystectomies. *American Journal of Surgery* 193 (6), 797–804.

Avolio, B.J. (2007) Promoting more integrative strategies for leadership theory-building. *American Psychologist* 62 (1), 25–33.

Baddeley, A.D. and Hitch, G.J. (1974) Working memory. In G.A. Bower (ed.), *Recent Advances in Learning and Motivation* (pp. 47–90). New York: Academic Press.

Baddeley, A.D. and Logie, R.H. (1999) Working memory: The multicomponent model. In A. Miyake and P. Shah (eds) *Models of Working Memory: Mechanisms of Active Maintenance and Executive Control* (pp. 22–61). New York: Cambridge University Press.

Baker, D.P., Gustafson, S., Beaubien, J., Salas, E. and Barach, P. (2005a) Medical team training programs in health care. *Advances in Patient Safety* vol. 4, Agency for Healthcare Research and Quality, Rockville, MD. Available from: <http://www.ahrq.gov/downloads/pub/advances/vol4/Baker.pdf> [accessed September 2008].

Baker, D.P., Gustafson, S., Beaubien, J., Salas, E. and Barach, P. (2005b) Medical teamwork and patient safety: The evidence-based relation. *Literature Review. AHRQ Publication No. 05-0053, April 2005*. Agency for Healthcare Research and Quality, Rockville, MD. Available from: <http://www.ahrq.gov/qual/medteam/> [accessed September 2008].

Brannick, M.T. and Prince, C. (1997) An overview of team performance measurement. In M.T. Brannick, E. Salas and C. Prince (eds) *Team Performance Assessment and Measurement* (pp. 3–16). Mahwah: Lawrence Erlbaum Associates.

Burke, C.S., Salas, E., Wilson-Donnelly, K. and Priest, H. (2004) How to turn a team of experts into an expert medical team: Guidance from the aviation and military communities. *Quality and Safety in Health Care* 13 (Suppl. 1), i96–104.

Burke, C.S., Stagl, K.C., Klein, C., Goodwin, G.F., Salas, E. and Halpin, S.M. (2006) What type of leadership behaviors are functional in teams? A meta-analysis. *The Leadership Quarterly* 17, 288–307.

Cannon-Bowers, J. and Salas, E. (1997) A framework for developing team performance measures in training. In M.T. Brannick, E. Salas, C. Prince (eds) *Team Performance Assessment and Measurement* (pp. 45–62). Mahwah, NJ: Lawrence Erlbaum Associates.

Carthey, J., de Leval, M.R., Wright, D.J., Farewell, V.T., Reason, J.T. and all UK paediatric cardiac centres (2003) Behavioural markers of surgical excellence. *Safety Science* 41 (5), 409–25.

Catchpole, K.R., Giddings, A.E., Wilkinson, M., Hirst, G., Dale, T. and de Leval, M.R. (2007) Improving patient safety by identifying latent failures in successful operations. *Surgery* 142 (1), 102–10.

Cooper, S. and Wakelam, A. (1999) Leadership of resuscitation teams: 'Lighthouse Leadership'. *Resuscitation* 42 (1), 27–45.

Cowan, N. (2005) *Working Memory Capacity.* New York, NY: Psychology Press.

de Fockert, J.W., Rees. G., Frith, C.D. and Lavie. N. (2001) The role of working memory in visual selective attention. *Science* 291, 1803–806.

Dickinson, T.L. and McIntyre, R.M. (1997) A conceptual framework for teamwork measurement. In M.T. Brannick, E. Salas and C. Prince (eds) *Team Performance Assessment and Measurement*, (pp. 19–43). Mahwah: Lawrence Erlbaum Associates.

Enochsson, L., Isaksson, B., Tour, R., Kjellin, A., Hedman, L., Wredmark, T. and Tsai-Felländer, L. (2004) Visuospatial skills and computer game experience influence the performance of virtual endoscopy. *Journal of Gastrointestinal Surgery* 8 (7), 876–82; discussion 882.

Entin, E.E. and Serfaty, D. (1999) Adaptive team coordination. *Human Factors* 41, 312–25.

Fletcher, G., Flin, R. McGeorge, P., Glavin, R., Maran, N. and Patey, R. (2003) Anaesthetists' Non-Technical Skills (ANTS): Evaluation of a behavioural marker system. *British Journal of Anaesthesia* 90 (5), 580–8.

Flin, R., Martin, L., Goeters, K.M., Hormann, H.J., Amalberti, R., Valot, C. and Nijhuis, H. (2003) Development of the NOTECHS (non-technical skills) system for assessing pilots' CRM skills. *Human Factors and Aerospace Safety* 3 (2), 97–119.

Flin, R., Glavin, R., Maran, N. and Patey, R. (2004a) *Anaesthetists' Non-technical Skills (ANTS) System Handbook v1.0.* Available from: < http://www.abdn.ac.uk/iprc/ants/> [accessed March 2009].

Flin, R. and Maran, N. (2004b) Identifying and training non-technical skills for teams in acute medicine. *Quality and Safety in Health Care* 13 (Suppl. 1), i80–4.

Flin, R., Rowley, D., Paterson-Brown, S. and Maran, N. (2006) *The Non-technical Skills for Surgeons (NOTSS) System Handbook v1.2.* Available from: <http://www.abdn.ac.uk/iprc/notss [accessed March 2009].

Frankel, A., Gardner, R., Maynard, L. and Kelly, A. (2007) Using the Communication and Teamwork Skills (CATS) Assessment to measure health care team performance teamwork and communication. *The Joint Commission Journal on Quality and Patient Safety* 33 (9), 549–58.

Gaba, D.M. (1992) Dynamic decision-making in anaesthesiology: Cognitive models and training approaches. In D.A. Evans and V.L. Patel (eds) *Advanced Models of Cognition for Medical Training and Practice.* Berlin: Springer.

Gaba, D.M., Fish, K.J. and Howard, S.K. (1994) *Crisis Resource Management in Anesthesia.* New York: Churchill Livingstone.

Gawande, A.A., Zinner, M.J., Studdert, D.M. and Brennan, T.A. (2003) Analysis of errors reported by surgeons at three teaching hospitals. *Surgery* 133 (6), 614–21.

Grantcharov, T.P., Kristiansen, V.B., Bendix, J., Bardram, L., Rosenberg, J. and Funch-Jensen, P. (2004) Randomized clinical trial of virtual reality simulation for laparoscopic skills training. *British Journal of Surgery* 91 (2), 146–50.

Healey, A.N., Undre, S. and Vincent, C.A. (2004) Developing observational measures of performance in surgical teams. *Quality and Safety in Health Care* 13 (Suppl. 1), i33–40.

Hedman, L., Ström, P., Andersson, P., Kjellin, A., Wredmark, T. and Felländer-Tsai, L. (2006) High-level visual-spatial ability for novices correlates with performance in a visual-spatial complex surgical simulator task. *Surgical Endoscopy* 20 (8), 1275–80.

Hedman. L., Klingberg, T., Enochsson, L., Kjellin, A. and Felländer-Tsai, L. (2007) Visual working memory influences the performance in virtual image-guided surgical intervention. *Surgical Endoscopy* 21 (11), 2044–50.

Helmreich, R.L., Merritt, A.C. and Wilhelm, J.A. (1999) The evolution of Crew Resource Management training in commercial aviation. *International Journal of Aviation Psychology* 9 (1), 19–32.

House, R.J. and Aditya, R.N. (1997) The social scientific study of leadership: Quo vadis? *Journal of Management* 23 (3), 409–73.

Howard, S.K., Gaba, D.M., Fish, K.J., Yang, G. and Sarnquist, F.H. (1992) Anesthesia crisis resource management training: Teaching anesthesiologists to handle critical incidents. *Aviation, Space & Environmental Medicine* 63 (9), 763–70.

Kim, J., Neilipovitz. D., Cardinal P., Chiu, M. and Clinch, J. (2006) A pilot study using high-fidelity simulation to formally evaluate performance in the resuscitation of critically ill patients: The University of Ottawa critical care medicine, high-fidelity simulation, and crisis resource management I study. *Critical Care Medicine* 35 (8), 2167–74.

Klein, K.J., Ziegert, J.C., Knight, A.P. and Xiao, Y. (2006) Dynamic delegation: Hierarchical, shared and deindividualized leadership in extreme action teams. *Administrative Science Quarterly* 51, 590–621.

Kohn, L.T., Corrigan, J.M. and Donaldson, M.S. (eds) (2000) *To Err is Human; Building a Safer Health System.* Washington DC: National Academy Press.

Kolga Schlickum, M., Hedman, L., Enochsson, L., Kjellin, A. and Felländer-Tsai, L. (2008) Transfer of systematic computer game training in surgical novices on performance in virtual reality image guided surgical simulators. *Studies in Health Technology and Informatics* 132, 210–15.

Kozlowski, S.W.J. and Bell, B.S. (2002) Work groups and teams in organizations. In W.C. Borman, D.G. Ilgen and R.J. Klimoski (eds) *Comprehensive Handbook of Psychology vol. 12: Industrial and Organizational Psychology* (pp. 333–75). New York: Wiley.

Lingard, L,. Reznick, R., Espin, S., Regehr, G. and DeVito, I. (2002) Team communications in the operating room: Talk patterns, sites of tension, and implications for novices. *Academic Medicine* 77 (3), 232–7.

Lingard, L., Espin S., Whyte, S., Regehr, G., Baker, G.R., Reznick, R., Bohnen, J., Orser, B., Doran, D. and Grober, E. (2004a) Communication failures in the operating room: An observational classification of recurrent types and effects. *Quality and Safety in Health Care* 13, 330–4.

Lingard, L., Garwood, S. and Poenaru, D. (2004b) Tensions influencing operating room team function: Does institutional context make a difference? *Medical Education* 38 (7), 691–9.

Lipshitz, R. (2005) There is more to seeing than meets the eyeball: The art of science and observation. In H. Montgomery, R. Lipshitz, B. Brehmer (eds) *How Professionals make Decisions* (pp. 365–78). Mahwah, NJ: Lawrence Erlbaum Associates.

Manser, T. (2009) Teamwork and patient safety in dynamic domains of healthcare: A review of the literature. *Acta Anaesth Scand* 53 (2), 143–51.

Marsch, S.C., Tschan, F., Semmer, N., Spychiger, M., Breuer, M. and Hunziker, P.R. (2005) Performance of first responders in simulated cardiac arrests. *Critical Care Medicine* 33 (5), 963–7.

McGuire, J. (2000) *Cognitive–Behavioural Approaches. An Introduction to Theory and Research.* Available from: <http://inspectorates.homeoffice.gov.uk/hmiprobation/docs/cogbeh1.pdf> [accessed September 2008].

Miyake, A., Friedman, N.P., Rettinger, D.A., Shah, P. and Hegarty, M. (2001) How are visuospatial working memory, executive functioning, and spatial abilities related? A latent variable analysis. *Journal of Experimental Psychology: General* 130, 621–40.

Miller, G.A. (1956) The magical number seven, plus or minus two: Some limits on our capacity for processing information. *Psychological Review* 63, 81–97.

Moorthy, K., Munz, Y., Adams, S., Pandey, V. and Darzi, A. (2005) A human factors analysis of technical and team skills among surgical trainees during procedural simulations in a simulated operating theatre. *Annals of Surgery* 242 (5), 631–9.

Moorthy, K., Munz, Y., Forrest, D., Pandey, V., Undre, S., Vincent, C. and Darzi, A. (2006) Surgical crisis management skills training and assessment: A simulation-based approach to enhancing operating room performance. *Annals of Surgery* 244 (1), 139–47.

Morey, J.C., Simon, R., Jay, G.D., Wears, R.L., Salisbury, M., Dukes, K.A. and Berns, S.D. (2002) Error reduction and performance improvement in the emergency department through formal teamwork training: Evaluation results of the MedTeams project. *Health Services Research* 37 (6), 1553–81.

Morgan, P. J., Pittini, R., Regehr, G., Marrs, C. and Haley, M.F. (2007) Evaluating team work in a simulated obstetric environment. *Anesthesiology* 106 (5), 907–15.

Murray, W.B. and Foster, P.A. (2000) Crisis resource management among strangers: Principles of organizing a multidisciplinary group for crisis resource management. *Journal of Clinical Anesthesia* 12 (8), 633–8.

Musselman, L.J., MacRae, H.M., Reznick, R.K. and Lingard, L.A. (2005) You learn better under the gun': Intimidation and harassment in surgical education. *Medical Education* 39 (9), 926–34.

Ostergaard, H.T., Ostergaard, D. and Lippert, A. (2004) Implementation of team training in medical education in Denmark. *Quality and Safety in Health Care* 13 (Suppl 1), i91–5.

Ottestad, E., Boulet, J.R. and Lighthall, G.K. (2007) Evaluating the management of septic shock using patient simulation. *Critical Care Medicine* 35 (3), 769–75.

Reznek, M., Smith-Coggins, R., Howard, S., Kiran, K., Harter, P., Sowb, Y., Gaba, D. and Krummel, T. (2003) Emergency medicine crisis resource management (EMCRM): Pilot study of a simulation-based crisis management course for emergency medicine. *Academic Emergency Medicine* 10 (4), 386–9.

Rosen, M.A., Salas, E., Wilson, K.A., King, H.B., Salisbury, M., Augenstein J.S., Robinson, D.W. and Birnbach, D.J. (2008) Measuring team performance in simulation-based training: Adopting best practices for healthcare. *Simulation in Healthcare* 3 (1), 33–41.

Roth, E.M. and Patterson, E.S. (2005) Using observational study as a tool for discovery: Uncovering cognitive and collaborative demands and adaptive strategies. In H. Montgomery, R. Lipshitz and B. Brehmer (eds) *How Professionals make Decisions* (pp. 379–93). Mahwah, NJ: Lawrence Erlbaum Associates.

Salas, E., Prince, C., Bowers C.A., Stout, R.J., Oser, L. and Cannon-Bowers, J.A. (1999) A methodology for enhancing crew resource management training. *Human Factors* 41 (1), 161–72.

Salas, E., Stagl, K.C. and Burke, C.S. (2004) 25 years of team effectiveness in organizations: Research themes and emerging needs. In C.L. Cooper and I.T. Robertson (eds) *International Review of Industrial and Organizational Psychology* (pp. 47–91). New York: John Wiley & Sons.

Seymour, N.E., Gallagher, A.G., Roman, S.A., O'Brien, M.K., Bansal, V.K., Andersen, D.K. and Satava, R.M. (2002) Virtual reality training improves operating room performance: Results of a randomized, double-blinded study. *Annals of Surgery* 236 (4), 458–63.

Shapiro, M.J., Morey, J.C., Small, S.D., Langford, V., Kaylor, C.J., Jagminas, L., Suner, S., Salisbury, M.L. and Simon, R., Jay, G.D. (2004) Simulation based teamwork training for emergency department staff: Does it improve clinical team performance when added to an existing didactic teamwork curriculum? *Quality and Safety in Health Care* 13 (6), 417–21.

Shiliang Chang, Waid, E., Martinec, D.V., Zheng, B., Swanstrom, L.L. (2008) Verbal communication improves laparoscopic team performance. *Surgical Innovation* 15 (2), 143–7.

Small, S.D., Wuerz, R.C., Simon, R., Shapiro, N., Conn, A. and Setnik, G. (1999) Demonstration of high-fidelity simulation team training for emergency medicine. *Academic Emergency Medicine* 6(4), 312–23.

St. Pierre, M., Hofinger, G. and Buerschaper, C. (2008) *Crisis Management in Acute Care Settings: Human Factors and Team Psychology in a High Stakes Environment.* Berlin: Springer.

Thomas, E.J., Sexton, J.B. and Helmreich, R.L. (2004) Translating teamwork behaviours from aviation to healthcare: Development of behavioural markers for neonatal resuscitation. *Quality and Safety in Health Care* 13 (Suppl 1), i57–64.

Tschan, F., Semmer, N.K., Gautschi, D., Hunziker, P., Spychiger, M. and Marsch, S. (2006) Leading to recovery: Group performance and coordinative activities in medical emergency driven groups. *Human Performance* 19 (3), 277–304.

Undre, S., Sevdalis, N., Healey, A.N., Darzi, A. and Vincent, C.A. (2007) Observational teamwork assessment for surgery (OTAS): Refinement and application in urological surgery. *World Journal of Surgery* 31 (7), 1373–81.

Van Vugt, M. (2006) Evolutionary origins of leadership and followership. *Personality and Social Psychology Review* 10 (4), 354–71.

Van Vugt, M., Hogan, R. and Kaiser, R.B. (2008) Leadership, followership, and evolution: Some lessons from the past. *American Psychologist* 63 (3), 182–96.

Veterans Affairs National Center for Patient Safety (2004) *Medical Team Training.* Available from: <http://www.patientsafety.gov/mtt> [accessed September 2008].

Wallin, C.J., Meurling, L., Hedman, L., Hedegård, J. and Felländer-Tsai, L. (2007) Target-focused medical emergency team training using a human patient simulator: Effects on behaviour and attitude. *Medical Education* 41 (2), 173–80.

Weick, K.E. (1968) Systematic observational methods. In G. Lindzey and E. Aronson (eds), *Handbook of Social Psychology*, Vol. 2, 2nd edition (pp. 357–451). Reading, MA: Addison Wesley.

Wiegmann, D.A., ElBardissi, A.W., Dearani, J.A., Daly, R.C., Sundt, T.M. 3rd (2007) Disruptions in surgical flow and their relationship to surgical errors: An exploratory investigation. *Surgery* 142 (5), 658–65.

Yule, S. Flin. R., Maran. N., Rowley. D., Youngson. G., Paterson-Brown. S. (2008) Surgeon's non-technical skills in the operating room: Reliability testing of the NOTSS behaviour rating system. *World Journal of Surgery*, 32 (4), 548–56.

Ziegert, J.C. (2004) A unified theory of team leadership: Towards a comprehensive understanding of leading teams. Paper presented at the 19th Annual Conference of the Society for Industrial and Organizational Psychology, Chicago, IL.

Chapter 10
Introducing TOP*plus* in the Operating Theatre

Connie Dekker-van Doorn, Linda Wauben, Benno Bonke,
Geert Kazemier, Jan Klein, Bianca Balvert, Bart Vrouenraets,
Robbert Huijsman and Johan Lange

Introduction

The focus in healthcare is changing from cost-effective ways of delivering care to delivering care that is safe, has a high standard of quality and improves patient outcomes like a shorter hospital stay and less complications. In this respect, concerns about patient safety are rising worldwide. Different studies suggest that 30–40 per cent of patients do not receive care in compliance with current scientific evidence and, possibly even worse, 20–25 per cent of the care provided is not needed or potentially harmful (Grol 2001, Schuster et al. 1998). Although surgical safety knowledge has improved substantially, it is estimated that 3–16 per cent of all hospitalized patients are affected by adverse events and almost 50 per cent of these events occur during surgical care, involving all surgical disciplines (Cuschieri 2006, World Health Organization 2008). The replication of the Harvard Medical Study in the Netherlands showed that 5.7 per cent of all patients hospitalized suffered from adverse events causing temporary or permanent disabilities, and 4.1 per cent of all patients who die during hospitalization die because of these probably preventable incidents (de Bruijne 2007, Wagner and de Bruijne 2007). Inadequate anaesthetic safety practices, avoidable surgical infection and poor communication among team members are issues that are common, deadly and preventable problems in all countries and all settings (World Health Organization 2008).

It is suggested that half of adverse events can be prevented, provided professionals in healthcare accept that human error is inevitable, teams are willing to learn from mistakes and organizations are looked at from a systems perspective. In this context the team is a small separate unit of a larger organizational system in which management decisions and organizational processes are important factors in relation to patient safety. The lack of support (managerial as well as financial), inadequate training and staff or the absence of reliable management information systems can all be causes for latent failures that eventually lead to adverse events (see Figure 10.1).

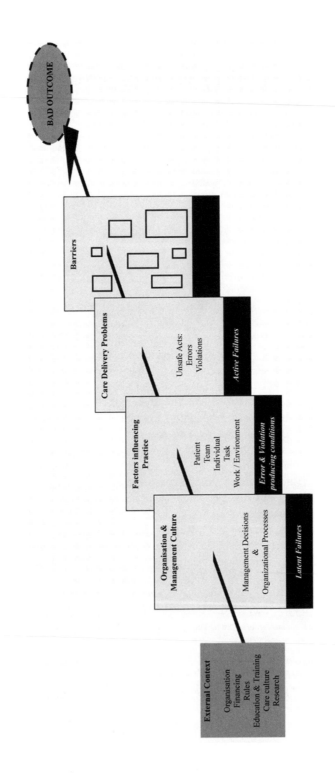

Figure 10.1   Causes for latent failures leading to adverse events (adapted from Reason 2005)

If a team works together effectively in the right working environment, it can avert a considerable proportion of life-threatening complications. 'Cooperation among team members' and 'Promote effective team functioning' are two recommendations of the Institute of Medicine (IOM) to achieve a healthcare system that is: *safe, effective, patient centred, timely, efficient and equitable* (Institute of Medicine 2001). These recommendations support the creation of a system where it is easier 'to do things right than to do things wrong' and underscore the importance of teamwork and communication in relation to patient safety. This is especially true within a complex and critical environment like the operating theatre (OT).

Errors in OT can have serious consequences for patients and families but also for healthcare professionals themselves and the entire healthcare organization. Poor communication and collaboration between OT members, being one of the major causes for incidents, renders the team itself to be the most critical resource to improve surgical safety (Sexton et al. 2006). In addition to technical knowledge and skill, good communication and teamwork are critical for teams to be effective in complex and critical environments like the OT (Yule et al. 2006). Good teamwork depends on each individual team member having a better understanding of what others do, to anticipate the needs of other team members, adjust to each others actions, and have a shared understanding of the procedure (Baker et al. 2006). Establishing a high level of situational awareness is one of the conditions for teams to work effectively. Yet most teams in OT have had little team training and cannot rely on adequate work structures to improve effective teamwork and improve patient safety.

The aim of the project TOP*plus* is to improve situational awareness, decision-making, transparency and cooperation among team members; characteristics that are key in the requirements of the World Health Organization (WHO) Guidelines for Safe Surgery (World Health Organization 2008). Improvement of these characteristics helps individual team members to make the transition from autonomous professional to team player and overcome one of the barriers to achieve safe care. Healthcare professionals must be open to others with respect to problems and anticipate accordingly. This also requires looking at care process as a system including other departments like the clinical ward (Amalberti et al. 2005). This in turn leads to reliable processes where a team of healthcare professionals work together for the benefit of the patient and *structurally* decrease the number of incidents and preventable deaths. It is at this specific team level where the proposed intervention TOP*plus* is situated, the level that is also the least well understood level of the structure of healthcare (Batalden and Splaine 2002).

TOPplus *and Underlying Principles*

TOP*plus* is based on the principles of crew resource management (CRM). CRM training encompasses a wide range of knowledge, skills and attitudes including communication, situational awareness, problem solving, decision-making, and teamwork (also referred to as non-technical skills).

In aviation, where links between teamwork and performance are paramount, CRM has successfully been used for teaching error management to flight crews, 'error management' meaning:

> Using all available data to understand the causes of errors and taking appropriate actions, including changing policy, procedures, and special training to reduce their incidence of error and to minimize the consequences of those that do occur. (Helmreich 1998, p. 1)

One of the underlying principles of error management is the recognition of the inevitability of human error and the adoption of a blame-free environment.

Most of the time commercial pilots fly as ad hoc teams and often work with unfamiliar team members, with different skills and knowledge and different tasks and responsibilities. Circumstances that are similar to the multidisciplinary teams that work together in OT. Like flight crews, operating teams need good, easy-to-transfer non-technical skills in order to work effectively.

As healthcare is a high risk and technically complex industry, cooperation between professionals is crucial to assure safety and reliability of care processes. Although interdependency is high and teamwork essential, teamwork is often poorly developed (Leggat 2007). One of the barriers for teamwork is partly due to the individual's formal education and training. Professional education forms a solid base for proficiency in technical knowledge and skills and standardization of processes, but also creates job boundaries and 'status' thus stifling communication (Boonstra 2004). Another barrier for teamwork has to do with the culture of the medical profession, like stress recognition. Healthcare professionals have a tendency to deny the influence of stressors such as fatigue, danger, and personal problems on performances. Denial of these stressors leads to defensive reasoning, blaming the environment rather than reflecting critically on one's own work performance (Argyris 1991, pp. 99–109).

Another important contributing factor to teamwork is the organizational context in which the teams operate. This directly affects the design of teams and the training and resources available to them (Lemieux-Charles and McGuire 2006). The linkages between the different systems and levels must be seamless, timely, efficient and reliable (Nelson et al. 2002). One of the main contributors of effective teamwork in the organizational context is the influence of leadership (Mickan and Rodger 2005). Leadership at all levels of the organization – senior leaders, team leaders as well as the front line staff – plays an important role in the strategy for leading change and creating the desired culture (Pronovost et al. 2006).

The main factors influencing teamwork are these non-technical, behavioural skills rather than a lack of technical knowledge and skills. Teams make fewer mistakes when they know each other's responsibilities, are able to anticipate the needs of others, adjust to each others actions, and have a shared understanding of a certain procedure (Baker et al. 2006).

Introduction of Crew Resource Management in the Operating Theatre

Non-technical skills, individual as well as team skills are directly related to failures and patient safety (Flin and Maran 2004). These skills are difficult to measure and difficult to change. However, there is emerging evidence that interventions, like pre-operative briefings (also called 'time out') have a positive effect on teamwork climate and the reduction of incidents (Makary et al. 2006). In 2003, the Joint Commission on Accreditation of Health Care Organizations (JCAHCO) introduced the Universal Protocol based on three primary components: (1) the pre-operative verification process, (2) marking the operative site, and (3) taking a 'time out' immediately before starting the procedure (Joint Commission on Accreditation of Health Care Organizations 2003).

After introduction of the time out in the 'Eye Hospital, Rotterdam' in 2004, wrong site incidents were reduced to zero. The introduction of a time out in Intensive Care Units (ICUs) at New York's public hospitals drastically reduced the number of serious infections (Hartocollis 2008). In a recent Canadian study it was concluded that inter-professional checklist briefings reduced the number of communication failures and promoted proactive and collaborative team communication (Lingard et al. 2008). Rather than introducing the whole CRM-concept including team training, development of checklists and a time out at once, it was decided to introduce the time out and a debriefing as the first step, called TOP*plus* (Time Out Procedure *plus* Debriefing).

TOP*plus: Development and Introduction of a Time Out Procedure and Debriefing*

TOP*plus* is designed to support team learning and engage the OT team in double-loop learning. Both the time out (briefing) and the debriefing put a strong emphasis on reflection, which is one of the main principles of adult learning. Leading to reflection *in* action and reflection *on* action, moving from single-loop learning to double-loop learning.

Double-loop learning occurs when error is detected and corrected in ways that involve the modification of an organization's underlying norms, policies and objectives (Argyris and Schön 1978, pp. 2–3; Smith 2001).

In case incidents occur because of a lack of technical skills or knowledge, or because of negligence, team members need their non-technical skills to solve the problem. The team member being 'lower' in the traditional hierarchy should know how to address the other team member who, in turn, needs to know how to react on suggestions for improvement. Also, the team member higher in hierarchy should know how to address technical shortcomings from other team members in a positive way. All this implies the combination of highly specialized technical expertise with the ability to work effectively in teams, form productive relationships and critically reflect on and then change organizational practices

(Argyris 1991). Therefore TOP*plus* is team- and dialogue-based and involves the use of a structured communication protocol.

Registration of TOP*plus* provides structured and reliable information on incidents as well as on communication and teamwork, which is an important condition to support error management. The time out is the final step in a series of checks, which start when the patient leaves the clinical ward, and is performed in OT just before incision. In the debriefing, just before closing the wound, incidents occurred during surgery are reported. These data provide a reliable base for a reporting system, which in turn provide the ability to learn from failures and enhance patient safety. If incidents are reported, analysis might show similarities and patterns in sources of risk that may otherwise go unnoticed. This in turn leads to knowledge and actions for improvement: 'Ultimately it is the action we take in response to reporting – not the reporting itself – that leads to change' (World Health Organization 2005b, p. 3).

According to the WHO (World Health Organization 2005b, p. 49), guidelines for safety reporting and learning system must:

- be safe for the individuals who report;
- lead to constructive response and meaningful analysis;
- have a solid base of adequate expertise and financial resources.

The reporting system must be capable of disseminating information on hazards and recommendations for changes.

To support TOP*plus,* a poster was developed to structure and support the time out and debriefing. This was based on The Universal Protocol of the JCAHCO (Joint Commission on Accreditation of Health Care Organizations 2003), the WHO recommendations on Safe Surgery (including their safety checklist) (World Health Organization 2008), and expert opinions of the 'Eye Hospital, Rotterdam'. The aim of the TOP*plus* procedure was to include *all* members of the operating team and double-check important factors related to the surgical procedure and patient characteristics. The poster was developed to structure the process, ensure the participation of all team members and improve the dialogue between team members. The objectives of TOP*plus* were:

- to reduce the number of incidents;
- to improve communication and teamwork;
- to reduce hierarchical structures.

Questionnaire: Communication and Teamwork

In order to measure the change in perceptions and opinions of team members on communication and teamwork, a questionnaire was developed comprising four teamwork characteristics: Teamwork and Communication, Decision-making, Situational Awareness and Leadership. The questionnaires' characteristics were based on the research on identification of non-technical skills and the development of behavioural markers for anaesthetist, surgeons and OT-teams (Fletcher et al. 2003, Undre and Healey 2006, Yule et al. 2006). The questionnaire 'Communication and Teamwork in Operating Theatre' consisted of 59 questions. Table 10.1 shows the design of the questionnaire. All questions had to be rated on a five-point scale, ranging from fully disagree to fully agree. At the end of each questionnaire, comments could be written down.

Team learning starts with dialogue, the capacity of team members to suspend assumptions and enter in a genuine 'thinking together' (Senge 1990). A factor that might inhibit this kind of learning is the perception of communication and teamwork, which like the perception of leadership, varies considerably among the different team members. Where physicians rate teamwork as high, nurses at the same time perceive it as mediocre (Makary et al. 2006). A cross-sectional survey including physicians and nurses from teaching and general hospitals revealed that, unlike physicians, nurses reported that it is difficult to speak up, disagreements are not appropriately resolved, more input into decision-making is needed and nurse input is not well received (Thomas et al. 2003). All this might inhibit team learning and thus sustainable improvement and patient safety. Therefore, measuring the effect of TOP*plus* on improving communication and teamwork and the reduction of the hierarchical structures is as important as measuring the effect on the reduction of incidents. In the research final project ten hospitals are participating, following the protocol for implementation shown in Table 10.2.

Table 10.1 **Overview questionnaire communication and teamwork in operating theatre**

Number of questions	Subject
6	General information (age, sex, hospital, years working in function in particular hospital)
1	Who does the team regard as the leader during the surgical procedure?
52	'Communication and Teamwork' (based on the definitions of the NOTSS and ANTS rating systems) subdivided into:
18 & 11	– *Communication and Teamwork:* Skills for working in a team context to ensure that the team has an acceptable shared picture of the situation and can complete the tasks effectively.
8	– *Situational Awareness:* Developing and maintaining a dynamic awareness of the situation in theatre based on assembling data from the environment (patient, team, time, displays, and equipment); understanding what they mean and thinking ahead what might happen next.
11	– *Decision-making*: Skills for diagnosing the situation and reaching a judgement in order to choose an appropriate course of action.
4	– *Leadership*: Leading the team and providing direction, demonstrating high standards of clinical practice and care, and being considerate about the needs of individual team members.

Table 10.2   Time frame TOP*plus* project

Month 1–2	Visit hospital to provide additional information about TOP*plus* Distribute questionnaire 'Communication and Teamwork in OT' (T0) (Week 1 – Distribution, Week 3 – Reminder, Week 4 – Closure)
Month 2	Introduction TOP*plus* in OT according to poster Perform TOP*plus* during 100 surgical procedures Analyse response questionnaire
Month 3	Analyse data and evaluate registrations of TOP*plus* Adapt poster to local context if necessary Present analysis of questionnaire (T0) and TOP*plus*
Month 4–6	Resume TOP*plus* in OT according to (adapted) poster
Month 7	Redistribute questionnaire 'Communication and Teamwork in OT' (T1) (Week 1 – Distribution, Week 3 – Reminder, Week 4 – Closure)
Month 8	Analyse data and evaluate registrations of TOP*plus* Analyse questionnaire T1 and compare to T0
Month 9	Present data on incidents and questionnaire

Material and Methods

Pilot TOPplus in Operating Theatre

The project was piloted at three locations: the ambulatory care department of an academic hospital, a teaching hospital and a community hospital. TOP*plus* consisted of three interventions: (1) a questionnaire 'Communication and Teamwork in OT', (2) a time out, and (3) a debriefing. The main objective of the pilot was to test the poster, which was designed to support the time out and debriefing procedures. The main objective of the questionnaire was to measure the effect of TOP*plus* on the perception of teamwork and communication of the individual team members. The first results of the questionnaire will be used for validation of the Dutch translation and will not be elaborated in this chapter.

The objectives of the pilot study were the following:

- Improve patient safety and efficiency during the surgical procedure.
- Improve communication involving *all* team members.
- Test the design of the time out and debriefing: layout of the poster, structure and the designation of specific team members to certain questions and answers.
- Test the registration of incidents that occur during surgery.
- Measure how much time the time out and the debriefing take.

Implementation

Poster A feasibility study was initiated to test the design and the usability of the poster. In all three participating hospitals the use of the poster was presented and explained to representatives of the OT team. They in turn explained the project's aim and use of the poster to all team members verbally by means of meetings and/or presentations. In addition, all participants received a letter with more detailed information.

The poster was developed based on literature and expert opinions (Figure 10.2) (Joint Commission on Accreditation of Health Care Organizations 2003,

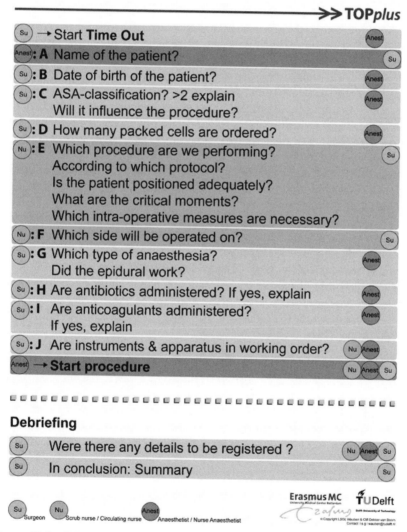

Figure 10.2 TOP*plus* **poster, first version tested during pilot**

World Health Organization 2008). Participants were asked to comment on the layout and structure of the poster. Furthermore, they were asked to comment on the designation of the different team members to ask or answer specific questions. The questions were all related to the formal responsibility of each team member in the operative process. Participants were invited to propose suggestions for improvement.

The shaded bars and corresponding bullets preceding the questions indicated the team member intended to *ask* the question. The purpose of the questions was to engage the dialogue between the team members, and was not to memorize the questions. The bullets at the end of each line indicated the team member(s) intended to *answer* the question.

The surgeon starts the time out. Then the anaesthetist or anaesthetic nurse starts with the first question: 'What is the name of the patient?' The surgeon is supposed to answer. Then the surgeon will ask the next question, and so on according to the poster.

Time out   The time out was initiated when all operating team members were present in OT, just before the first incision. Because the time out is a double-check, the patient did not have an active role, as he/she was already under anaesthesia or pre-medicated in addition to a regional block anaesthesia.

During the time out the anaesthetic nurse (demanding a special qualification, which is unknown outside the Netherlands) filled out a registration form, which included the following aspects:

- Did the designated team member *ask* the question?
- Did the designated team member *answer* the question?
- Were the questions asked as stated on the poster or in a different way?
- Did all team members participate? If not, please indicate which person did not.
- The time it took to perform the time out.

Debriefing   The debriefing had to take place just before closing the wound. This particular moment in the surgical procedure was chosen because, in academic and most teaching hospitals, the supervising surgeon will leave the OT. The surgeon initiated the debriefing by asking: 'Were there any details to be reported?' All team members were invited to report incidents related to the operative process or related to communication and teamwork.

As in the time out, the anaesthetic nurse filled out the registration form. This form included the following aspects:

- the time it took to perform the debriefing;
- the remarks/incidents mentioned by the different team members.

Results

Implementation of TOP*plus*

This section represents the results of the pilot of the time out and debriefing in three participating hospitals during 308 surgical procedures (academic n=28, teaching n=180, community n=100).

The time out was performed and reported in 206 out of the 308 procedures. In reality the time out was performed during more procedures, but was not reported. No specific reason was given for not reporting the time out.

Did the designated team member ask the question? An important aspect was the layout of the poster. The layout was directly related to each person's tasks and responsibilities and was meant to involve the whole team in the discussion. Usually checks are performed individually and team members exchange little information, partly due to the strong hierarchical structure in OT. The time out is a relatively small intervention in the operative process but, because of this specific structure, a rather drastic one. Information from the team members directly involved provides important information on the feasibility of the project.

The designated team member asked most questions (Figure 10.3). Differences in a team member asking questions than the one indicated on the poster, were minor and improved during the course of the implementation process. If the designated team member did not ask the question, other team members took the initiative.

Did the designated team member answer the question? The designated team member answered most questions (Figure 10.4). In those cases where a team

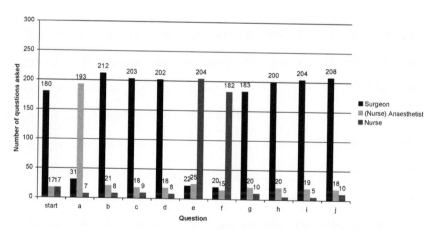

Figure 10.3   Questions asked by team members as indicated on the poster

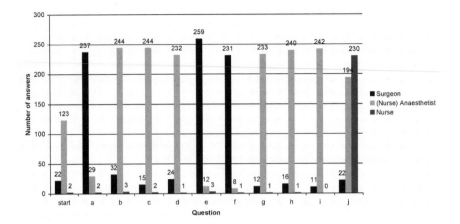

Figure 10.4   Answers given by the team members as indicated on the poster

member other than the designated one answered the question, most of the time the surgeon answered.

Were the questions asked as stated on the poster or in a different way?   One of the pilot's objectives was to find out which layout would best support the time out and debriefing, and support the involvement of the whole team. In one location, two versions of the poster were used: one version with unabbreviated questions (1), and a second version presenting short remarks (2), more resembling a checklist. It was expected that the questions in version 1 would be abbreviated to short remarks. However, the results (n=28) showed no significant difference in usage between the two versions. Both questions were asked and answered as indicated on the poster. In addition to the pilot in one location, representatives of the different OT teams were asked which poster they preferred. All OT teams in the participating hospitals decided to use the poster with the unabbreviated questions, as these full sentences would support the communication and dialogue within the team.

In most cases (n=160) questions were asked according to the poster, in 68 cases it was unknown and in 80 cases a different way of questioning was followed. During almost half of these, differences were reported. The most frequent ones were:

- The team members asking the questions were not reported, only the ones answering the questions (n=27).
- The questions were shortened (n=7).
- The content of the question asked was identical to the one on the poster, but the question was formulated differently (n=4).

Did All Team Members Participate? If Not, Please Indicate who Did Not In 157 cases all team members participated in the time out. In 76 cases no additional information was given on team members' participation. In 101 cases where not all team members participated, the specific team member was reported (surgeon n=11, nurse n=14, anaesthetist n=61, anaesthetist in training n=1, anaesthetic nurse n=14). The high number of anaesthetists not participating (61 out of 101 cases) was mainly the result of working structures. This structure entails that he/she works in two OTs concurrently. A qualified anaesthetic nurse mans both rooms. Therefore the anaesthetist did not participate in the time out because he/she was not present in OT at that specific moment.

How long does it take to perform the time out? The time out took an average of 1.6 minutes (95.58 seconds, see Table 10.3). When the time out took significantly more time, most incidents reported were related to instruments or material missing. There was no specific explanation found for the duration of the time out taking longer in the academic and the teaching hospital.

How long does it take to perform the debriefing? The registration of the debriefing was carried out in the academic and community hospital. There is a significant difference in time/duration needed to perform the debriefing between the two locations (Table 10.4). The debriefing in the academic hospitals took twice as much time (52.2 seconds) as the debriefing in the community hospital (24.31 seconds). As with the time out no particular reason was indicated.

Table 10.3   Duration of the time out (in seconds)

	Average (sec)	STDEV (sec)	n=	other	missing data
1. Academic	101.79	65.49	28	-	-
2. Teaching	98.61	67.19	122	4	54
3. Community	86.35	59.09	78	1	21
Total	**95.58**	**63.92**	**228**	**5**	**75**

Table 10.4   Duration of the debriefing (in seconds)

	Average (sec)	STDEV (sec)	n=	other	missing data
1. Academic	52.22	28.33	28	–	–
2. Teaching	–	–	–	–	–
3. Community	24.31	31.04	70	9	21

What were the remarks/incidents mentioned during the debriefing? Several remarks and incidents were reported; the most reported ones are described below, subdivided into the categories used in the questionnaire.

- Communication and teamwork (n=44)
    - Improving communication between all team members, improving information on patient characteristics, surgical day schedule, necessary equipment, and surgical approach (32 per cent of the remarks 'communication & teamwork').
    - Improve team spirit and teambuilding (20 per cent).
    - Show respect for your all OT-members and be honest (11 per cent).
- Situational awareness (n=30)
    - Improving information on the surgical day schedule, better preparation of surgery (including instrument set-up), improve written communication, introduce pre-operative team meeting (33 per cent).
    - Update on status of surgery (7 per cent).
    - Implement standards and protocols, including communicating this to all team members (7 per cent).
- Decision-making (n=1)
    - Improvements should be implemented faster.
    - Leadership (total 5 remarks).
    - Less hierarchy, more commitment, increase consultation and direct communication (60 per cent).

Discussion

The results of the pilot provide important information for implementing TOP*plus* on a wider scale and ensure that it supports its objectives. Some elements of the poster are still subject to discussion. The main conclusions are presented below. In general, four topics for discussion were reported:

1. The moment of the time out just before incision, rather than before administering total or local anaesthesia.
2. Performing a debriefing with patients under local anaesthetic.
3. Performing a time out and debriefing when three or more similar and relatively simple surgical procedures are scheduled successively.
4. The content of the time out being context specific (as expected).

The recently published 'Surgical Safety Checklist' of the WHO (World Health Organization 2008, p. 153) splits the checking process in three parts:

- Before induction of anaesthesia: including patient data confirmed by patient himself/herself, surgical site, anaesthesia safety check completed?, pulse oximeter on patient and functioning?, allergies?, difficult airway/ aspiration?, and risk of blood loss?

- Before skin incision: similar to TOP*plus*.
- Before patients leaves OT: nurse verbally confirms name of procedure reported, instruments, sponge and needles correct?, correct labelling specimen?, equipment problems?, and review by the whole team on key concerns for recovery and management of this patient.

TOP*plus* focused on Part 2. The hospitals that participated in the pilot are now analysing their pre-operative and post-operative process and adding checks related to these phases to their checks. Therefore, TOP*plus* acted as a catalyst for improving and checking the care process.

Topic 1: Performing a time out after the patient has been given a local or general anaesthetic and is ready for surgery raised questions. Some incidents might result in postponement of surgery for one or two hours or even another day which might harm the patient, physically as well as mentally. However, one of the problems is the presence of the whole team as a requirement for the time out. Especially for the surgeons being present before anaesthesia as this means a drastic change in routine procedures. At the moment, in one of the hospitals a pilot is carried out to report incidents related to the moment of the time out just before incision.

Team members participating in the pilot suggested several solutions:

- Starting the time out before total or local anaesthesia is administered, with the whole team present including the surgeon.
- Starting the time out before total or local anaesthesia is administered, with the whole team present and one of the surgical staff members or one of the residents representing the surgeon.
- Starting the time out just before incision, but reducing the number of questions asked and developing multidisciplinary checklists carried out by two or more professionals during the pre-operative process.

Questions and answers indicated to be asked/answered by the anaesthetist should be adapted to the local situation. In case the anaesthetist is not present, because of different work structures, the anaesthetic nurse can take over.

Topic 2 Free exchange of information during the debriefing when patients are under local anaesthetic, requires good and timely information to the patient and an open and blame-free culture, which takes longer to develop. TOP*plus* by itself is a relatively simple intervention and easy to introduce into daily routines but, in relation to professional and organizational culture, a rather drastic one. Although the first reaction was very positive, it took all participants four to six months to take the appropriate steps for communication with everyone involved and to establish the necessary commitment and support.

Topic 3: In those cases where four or more similar, small and routine surgical procedures were scheduled, and the team remained the same, it was suggested to adapt the time out and debriefing:

- Before the whole session: Perform *one* overall time out, discussing surgical procedures and patients' characteristics with the whole OT-team AND perform a reduced time out with every surgical procedure, just before incision.
- Perform *one* overall debriefing of all patients after all scheduled surgeries.

However, this subject is still open to discussion.

Topic 4: Some questions were considered irrelevant and some questions were not addressed in the time out, but perceived as being important in a specific local context. The questions asked during the time out, and therefore stated on the poster, should be relevant to all team members. The most important adjustments were the following:

- Questions were adjusted to the ambulatory department such as the anaesthetic procedure, blood products ordered or ASA classification (physical status classification of the American Society of Anesthesiologists).
- Specific questions on subjects such as allergies, antibiotics or thrombo-prophylaxis were added according to the needs of the local OT teams.
- Sometimes questions were added to the poster because these were related to specific projects in the hospital such as infection prevention.

The ability to discuss the questions and adapt the content subsequently was much appreciated and is an important condition for establishing commitment and support of all parties involved. This is one of the principles of adult learning where personal involvement is crucial and in line with one of the basic rules of change management, to create powerful guiding coalitions:

> Efforts that lack a sufficiently powerful guiding coalition can make apparent progress for a while. The organizational structure might be changed, or a reengineering effort might be launched. But sooner or later, countervailing forces undermine the initiatives. (Kotter 1996, p. 6)

In the course of the pilot one adjustment to the poster was made. It concerned the registration of the incidents reported in the debriefing. Analysing the incidents showed that a more detailed registration of incidents was necessary for adequate reporting. It was decided to create four categories: incidents related to surgery, anaesthesiology, materials and instruments, and communication and teamwork (Figure 10.5).

As mentioned before several initiatives were started by the hospitals to include checks in the whole care process.

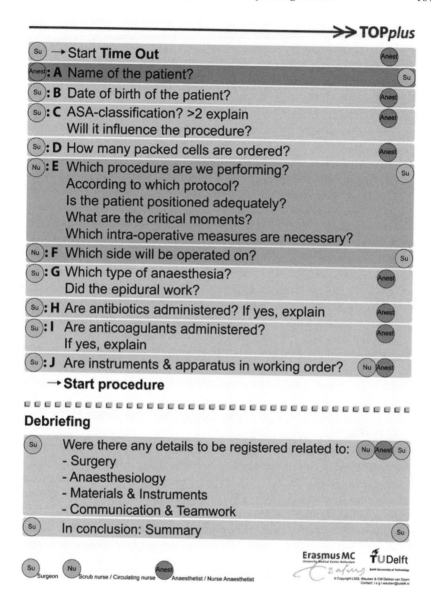

Figure 10.5   Final version of the poster

Conclusion

Most professionals received the development of TOP*plus*, introducing a time out and a debriefing in OT, as a very good initiative. Especially the specific design of the time out (team-based and dialogue-based) and the objective to make it evidence-based created many positive reactions. The objective was to include two non-academic hospitals in the study. At this moment ten Dutch hospitals are participating in the project and a few more have shown interest.

Although results from the final research project are not yet available, some conclusions can be drawn from the pilot study. Conditions for successful implementation are:

- The ability to adjust the poster to the local context in regard to the questions as well as the designated team members is important for successful implementation, because ambulatory care, clinical care and some specific medical specialties have different requirements. The poster should provide a template including basic questions (an 'in addition to' format). Hospitals and departments should then add specific questions and topics relating to their local context and wishes. The questions on the poster should be 'owned' by all OT-team members.
- Good and timely information to the patient about the objectives of the time out and debriefing.
- Creating a blame-free and safe environment. This means that the registration of the incidents should be kept confidential and should be related to the kind of incidents and frequency and not to specific team members.

The precise moment of the time out and consequences for the questions asked is still open to discussion. These questions will be addressed in the final research project. There might be a concern about the time it takes to perform the time out and debriefing. One concern is related to the difference between the academic and community hospital. The second has to do with the total time it takes to perform the time out and debriefing.

A logical explanation for the difference in time between the two hospitals might be the number of people present in OT because of the teaching aspect. Another factor might be new residents joining the OT team rather frequently, as they change hospitals every few months during their medical specialist training. This might influence the time it takes for new work procedures like the time out to become a standard operating procedure. Finally, some hospitals used a different method of time recording during the time out. For example, when a specific instrument was not present, some hospitals recorded the time until the instrument was actually in OT, while others did not include this in their time recordings. Another explanation might be the fact that a correction for patient case-mix was not applied in the analysis. In general 20–30 per cent of the patients hospitalized in academic and maybe a little less in teaching hospitals, consists of tertiary referrals in general, including more complex patients where standard protocols are not applicable. Tertiary referrals are rare in community hospitals.

The total time it takes to perform both the time out and debriefing with every surgical procedure might become a concern. With an average production of 20,000–25,000 surgical procedures per annum, the total time adds up to quite an investment. Comparing the costs of the time invested in the time out and debriefing with the costs of incidents might help to overcome financial barriers. Healthcare associated infections in the United Kingdom are estimated to cost £1 billion (€1.26 billion) a year. In the United States, the estimate is between £2.3–3 billion (€3–3.7 billion) per year (World Health Organization 2005a). The average costs for a surgical site infection amounts to £5393 (€6780) (World Health Organization 2005a). Furthermore, a re-operation to restore iatrogenic ductal injury after a laparoscopic cholecystectomy costs 4.5–6 times the initial cost of an uncomplicated surgery (Savader et al. 1997). All these costs involve hospital budget. Besides, there are also costs involved for society, such as loss of wages of the patient and caretakers, additional treatment in an outpatient department, and additional medication. Also, medical claims due to medical liability lead to cost increase.

In conclusion, TOP*plus* is a feasible instrument which, once adapted to the local context, improves teamwork and communication and in the end improves patient safety. Although it requires some extra time, this will be compensated by fewer incidents in the end.

References

Amalberti, R., Auroy, Y., Berwick, D. and Barach, P. (2005) Five system barriers to achieving ultrasafe health care. *Annals of Internal Medicine* 142(9), 756–64.

Argyris, C. (1991) Teaching smart people how to learn. *Harvard Business Review* May–June.

Argyris, C. and Schön, D. (1978) *Organizational Learning: A Theory of Action Perspective.* Reading, MA: Addison Wesley.

Baker, D.P., Day, R. and Salas, E. (2006) Teamwork as an essential component of high-reliability organizations. *Health Services Research* 41(4), Pt 2, 1576–98.

Batalden, P. and Splaine, M. (2002) What will it take to lead the continual improvement and innovation of health care in the twenty-first century? *Quality Management in Health Care* 11(1), 45–54.

Boonstra, J.J. (2004) *Dynamics of Organizational Change and Learning.* Forlag: Wiley and Sons Ltd.

Cuschieri, A. (2006) Nature of human error. Implications for surgical practice. *Annals of Surgery* 244(5), 642–8.

de Bruijne, M.C., Zegers, M., Hoonhout, L.H.F. and Wagner, C. (2007) *Unintended Harm in Dutch Hospitals. Dossier Study of Hospital Admissions in 2004. [Onbedoelde schade in Nederlandse ziekenhuizen. Dossieronderzoek van ziekenhuisopnames in 2004.]* Utrecht: EMGO Institute Amsterdam and NIVEL.

Fletcher, G., Flin, R., McGeorge, P., Glavin, R., Maran, N. and Patey, R. (2003) Anaesthetists Non-Technical Skills (ANTS): Evaluation of a behavioural marker system. *British Journal of Anaesthesia* 90(5), 580–8.

Flin, R. and Maran, N. (2004) Identifying and training non-technical skills for teams in acute medicine. *Quality of Safety in Health Care* 13 Suppl 1, i80–4.

Grol, R. (2001) Successes and failures in the implementation of evidence-based guidelines for clinical practice. *Medical Care* 39(8), Suppl 2, ii46–54.

Hartocollis, A. (2008) In hospitals, simple reminders reduce deadly infections. *The New York Times* 19 May.

Helmreich, R.L. (1998) Error management as organizational strategy. *Proceedings of the IATA Human Factors Seminar*. Bangkok, Thailand.

Institute of Medicine (2001) *Crossing the Quality Chasm: A New Health System for the 21st Century.* Washington, DC: National Academic Press.

Joint Commission on Accreditation of Health Care Organizations (2003) Universal Protocol For Preventing Wrong Site, Wrong Procedure, Wrong Person Surgery, <http://www.jointcommission.org/NR/rdonlyres/E3C600EB-043B-4E86-B04E-CA4A89AD5433/0/universal_protocol.pdf> [accessed August 2008].

Kotter, J.P. (1996) *Leading Change.* Boston, MA: Harvard Business Press.

Leggat, S.G. (2007) Effective healthcare teams require effective team members: Defining teamwork competencies. *BMC Health Services Research* 7, 17.

Lemieux-Charles, L. and McGuire, W.L. (2006) What do we know about health care team effectiveness? A review of the literature. *Medical Care Research Review* 63(3), 263–300.

Lingard, L., Regehr, G., Orser, B., Reznick, R., Baker, G. R., Doran, D., Espin, S., Bohnen, J. and Whyte, S. (2008) Evaluation of a preoperative checklist and team briefing among surgeons, nurses, and anesthesiologists to reduce failures in communication. *Archives of Surgery* 143(1), 12–7; discussion 18.

Makary, M.A., Sexton, J.B., Freischlag, J.A., Holzmueller, C.G., Millman, E.A., Rowen, L. and Pronovost, P.J. (2006) Operating room teamwork among physicians and nurses: Teamwork in the eye of the beholder. *Journal of the American College of Surgeons* 202(5), 746–52.

Mickan, S.M. and Rodger, S.A. (2005) Effective health care teams: A model of six characteristics developed from shared perceptions. *Journal of Interprofessional Care* 19(4), 358–70.

Nelson, E.C., Batalden, P.B., Huber, T.P., Mohr, J.J., Godfrey, M.M., Headrick, L.A. and Wasson, J.H. (2002) Microsystems in health care: Part 1. Learning from high-performing front-line clinical units. *Joint Commission Journal on Quality Improvement* 28(9), 472–93.

Pronovost, P.J., Berenholtz, S.M., Goeschel, C.A., Needham, D.M., Sexton, J.B., Thompson, D.A., Lubomski, L.H., Marsteller, J.A., Makary, M.A. and Hunt, E. (2006) Creating high reliability in health care organizations. *Health Services Research,* 41(4) Pt 2, 1599–617.

Reason, J. (2005) Safety in the operating theatre – Part 2: Human error and organisational failure. *Quality of Safety in Health Care* 14(1), 56–60.

Savader, S.J., Lillemoe, K.D., Prescott, C.A., Winick, A.B., Venbrux, A.C., Lund, G.B., Mitchell, S.E., Cameron, J.L. and Osterman, F.A. (1997) Laparoscopic cholecystectomy-related bile duct injuries: A health and financial disaster. *Annals of Surgery* 225(3), 268–73.

Schuster, M.A., McGlynn, E.A. and Brook, R.H. (1998) How good is the quality of health care in the United States? *Milbank Q* 76(4), 517–63, 509.

Senge, P.M. (1990) *The Fifth Discipline: The Art and Practice of the Learning Organization.* New York: Doubleday.

Sexton, J.B., Makary, M.A., Tersigni, A.R., Pryor, D., Hendrich, A., Thomas, E.J., Holzmueller, C.G., Knight, A.P., Wu, Y. and Pronovost, P.J. (2006) Teamwork in the operating room: Frontline perspectives among hospitals and operating room personnel. *Anesthesiology* 105(5), 877–84.

Smith, M.K. (2001) *Donald Schön: Learning, Reflection and Change.* Available at: <www.infed.org/thinkers/et-schon.htm> [accessed September 2008].

Thomas, E.J., Sexton, J.B. and Helmreich, R.L. (2003) Discrepant attitudes about teamwork among critical care nurses and physicians. *Critical Care Medicine* 31(3), 956–9.

Undre, S. and Healey, A.N. (2006) *Observational Teamwork Assessment for Surgery (OTAS). User Manual.* London: Imperial College.

Wagner and de Bruijne (2007) Utrecht: EMGO Institute Amsterdam and NIVEL.

World Health Organization (2005a) *Global Patient Safety Challenge: Clean Care is Safer Care.* Geneva: WHO Press, pp. 1–35.

World Health Organization (2005b) *WHO Draft Guidelines for Adverse Event Reporting and Learning Systems.* Geneva: WHO Press, pp. 1–80.

World Health Organization (2008) *WHO Guidelines for Safe Surgery* 1st edition. Geneva: WHO Press, pp. 1–173.

Yule, S., Flin, R., Paterson-Brown, S., Maran, N. and Rowley, D. (2006) Development of a rating system for surgeons' non-technical skills. *Medical Education* 40(11), 1098–104.

PART II
Observational Studies of Anaesthetics

Chapter 11

Integrating Non-Technical Skills into Anaesthetists' Workplace-based Assessment Tools

Ronnie Glavin and Rona Patey

Introduction

In this chapter, the authors will provide a brief account of the development of the Anaesthetists' Non-Technical Skills (ANTS) system and then consider how this system may find a suitable home in the UK anaesthetic curriculum (*Anaesthetists' Non-Technical Skills System Handbook*).

But first, what are non-technical skills (NTS)? Within the context of anaesthesia they have been defined as behaviours in the operating theatre environment, which are not directly related to the use of medical expertise, drugs or equipment (Fletcher et al. 2003). They encompass both interpersonal skills (e.g., communication, team working and leadership) and also cognitive skills (e.g., situation awareness and decision making) (*Anaesthetists' Non-Technical Skills System Handbook*). NTS are important because we need them to function effectively in our professional lives. As with many important aspects of living, we really only notice them when they are absent or poorly performed. Then, our practice is not so effective and may become dangerous. In anaesthesia, and many other professions, studies of adverse incidents consistently suggest that the underlying factors are more likely to be due to difficulties with the application of NTS rather than a lack of basic knowledge or practical skill (Flin et al. 2008). Is it then reasonable to ask: 'If NTS are so important why have they not featured prominently in anaesthetic training?' One might reply that they might have done had we known what they were exactly in the context of anaesthesia. Until now NTS have been elusive and difficult to describe or pin down. This inability to accurately define or describe NTS has resulted in them generally only being considered under a broad umbrella category of 'soft skills'. However, there is nothing soft about these skills. The platform they provide, along with the knowledge and skills from more conventional areas of the curriculum, is the solid base required for the development of anaesthetic practice.

So far, we have referred to NTS as if they were a generic set of skills found across many circumstances and professions. Bob Helmreich, emeritus psychologist at University of Texas, Austin, played a key role in the early NASA work in this field of key human factors and then oversaw the development of the concept from infancy to maturity in other industries. He reminds us that there is no generic set of NTS and has warned that different organizations/professions and cultures have their own variations of NTS (Helmreich 2000). Therefore, whilst NTS identified in other professions can give us a flavour of those used in anaesthesia, we cannot just assume that they cross directly into our practice. With this in mind, in 1999, having confirmed that such work was not already under way, a research team comprising clinical anaesthetists (including both authors) and psychologists set about the business of identifying the non-technical skills important for anaesthetic practice (funded by NHS Education for Scotland).

Development of the Anaesthetists' Non-Technical Skills System

How did we do this? We believed that anaesthetists had always learned and used NTS but that this was largely an unconscious process. Therefore, we could not simply ask anaesthetists 'What non-technical skills are important in your practice?' Nor would the quantitative or positivistic approach, which was the research tradition that the clinical anaesthetists in the team were familiar with, be appropriate. This was not an investigation where quantitative measurement, such as where a new technique is developed to impact on blood pressure or cardiac output, would help. A different approach was required. A set of task analysis techniques was used with questionnaires, observations and interviews. For the last, a form of cognitive task analysis was employed (Crandall et al. 2006, Fletcher et al. 2004). This is a qualitative research method whereby the researcher uses a set of probes, usually in the form of questions, to help the interviewee (in this case consultant anaesthetists) describe one or more episodes of clinical practice. The interviews contained the raw data and were analysed by extracting all the behaviours and skills that were mentioned. These approaches allowed access to behaviours which may not otherwise have impinged upon the consciousness of the participants. These elicited behaviours do not come neatly ordered, and so for clarity and ease of use, a system has to be assembled from the data. For this, a series of iterative steps took place where the research team developed a prototype categorization of the principal behaviours and took rudimentary versions of the system into the workplace and studied their apparent effectiveness. After several iterations the current Anaesthetists' Non-Technical Skills (ANTS) system was arrived at (see Table 11.1).

The next step was to evaluate some key properties of this system. Was it valid? Could it be used in a reliable manner – would different assessors give similar scores to the same performance? At an even more fundamental level, could clinical anaesthetists actually use the system? To address these questions, 50 consultant anaesthetists across Scotland took part in a study. They attended a one-day session comprising a morning of teaching and familiarization with the concepts behind the system and the system itself followed by an afternoon of applying the system to eight video-recorded anaesthetic scenarios that had been conceived, performed and produced by the research team. The findings have been published elsewhere

Table 11.1   The ANTS system: categories and elements

Category	Element
Task management	Planning and preparing Prioritizing Providing and maintaining standards Identifying and utilizing resources
Team working	Coordinating activities with team members Exchanging information Using authority and assertiveness Assessing capabilities Supporting others
Situation awareness	Gathering information Recognizing and understanding Anticipating
Decision-making	Identifying options Balancing risks and selecting options Re-evaluating

(Fletcher et al. 2003), but the main conclusions were that the clinical anaesthetists could use the system and could provide broad consensus on the scores awarded, and that the system captured the NTS observed. However, these anaesthetists were scoring performances while observing them on videotape, without any other distractions. It was important to assess if the system could be used in the workplace. Here, if trainers were to apply the system to assess the performance of a trainee in order to provide feedback, they would also be required to continue to monitor the patient and the operating theatre environment.

Of the original volunteers, 17 participated in the usability study. The consultant anaesthetists and the trainees being supervised were asked to complete questionnaires at the end of the theatre session. The results of this usability study, which are detailed elsewhere, were positive (Patey et al. 2005). It seemed that the system could be used in the workplace and furthermore participating trainers and trainees responded in a very positive manner to use of the system as a way of providing formative assessment and teaching of NTS. Was the anaesthetic community in the UK now ready to adopt the ANTS system into routine training?

Early Experiences of Promoting the ANTS System

The body responsible for standards of anaesthetic practice and training of anaesthetists in the UK is the Royal College of Anaesthetists. Presentations on the ANTS system to the relevant committees and bodies of stakeholders produced a very positive response. Following this, the next hurdle was how to best assimilate the ANTS system into the teaching and assessment of anaesthetists. The usability study had shown that individual consultant anaesthetists could use the system, but could the ANTS system be incorporated into the teaching practice of a whole hospital department of anaesthesia?

The proposed strategy for introduction to a department was to use a cascade system for training the trainers. One of the authors of this chapter would visit several UK anaesthetic departments that had volunteered to trial the use of the ANTS system and deliver a one-day teaching session for local enthusiasts. The cascade approach was based on the notion that those who had attended the one-day course would use the system, become more familiar with its application and then reach a stage where they would be comfortable to instruct their consultant colleagues. Similar to the initial system evaluation study, the training day would consist of a morning going over the background to NTS, followed by familiarization with the ANTS system. In the afternoon, the performance of anaesthetists in video-recorded scripted scenarios would be assessed allowing practice using the system. The afternoon differed from the research work in that the participants were encouraged to discuss their scores to allow calibration to take place. When the participants reached consensus and awarded very similar scores then that part of the session ended. Would this cascade approach work?

Although NTS could be identified and discussed by consultants during ANTS training sessions, on the whole the cascade approach was not successful. It seems from discussion with consultants that the reasons for this were multifactorial (Dodd 2005). Firstly, most consultants only had limited familiarity with NTS and experience with the ANTS taxonomy (only the single day of training and some recommended reading) and wanted further opportunities and support to become more familiar with the tool before using it in the workplace. Accurately observing behaviours is a skill, like any other, which requires deliberate practice, and although consultants regularly participated in clinical training they had not received training in behavioural observation. Where the consultants had no formal training or experience in providing structured feedback (which was often the case), they were particularly uncomfortable. In all probability, too many new changes were introduced at one time but it is worth exploring the intended training approach and barriers to its success in greater detail.

A conventional approach to instructing anaesthetic trainees in the use of the NTS highlighted in the ANTS system would be to incorporate the underlying theoretical concepts into classroom-style teaching and then build on that base during clinical training by demonstrating application of those principles. Knowledge and practice would then be formally assessed in some kind of examination. We were adopting an entirely different approach, where the system was being used to score the performance of a trainee anaesthetist in the workplace. The scores awarded for the relevant categories and elements were intended to form the basis for a discussion between consultant and trainee as a way of drawing attention to the trainees' existing strengths and limitations in the use of NTS and then plan for further development. We had made the assumption that consultant anaesthetists were used to assessing trainees on accompanied theatre lists and then providing structured feedback. However, although consultants had considerable experience assessing the performance of trainees this was done in a very informal manner. Many consultants in the UK had little experience in the use of formal workplace-based assessment tools. This was not surprising because no such tools were in widespread use in the UK.

Workplace-Based Assessment and the Curriculum in Anaesthesia

One result of this limited use of workplace-based assessment tools is that little attention has previously been paid to the requirements to support consultants in providing structured feedback in the workplace. Consultant training, to highlight the essential role of feedback in both optimal learning and in the use of effective feedback techniques, has been limited. In addition, it can be difficult during a busy working day for the consultant and trainee to identify time for feedback. If time can be identified, perhaps at the end of the day, it may not be close to the event under consideration, and at this time both parties may be concerned with other duties such as post-operative or pre-operative visiting. The conditions during a training session in operating theatres are also not ideal. The presence of the whole theatre team can be inhibiting, particularly where there is discussion to be had on an area where there are difficulties. The authors have noted that this seems to cause particular concern where NTS are concerned and consultants perceive that they are commenting on personality-related matters. These various factors all conspire to make it easy to delay a feedback discussion.

When time can be identified for feedback, use of the ANTS system should actually reduce the anxiety of commenting on a trainee's personality traits. The system allows discussion and emphasis on specific NTS behaviours either observed or thought to be deficient or absent, rather than comments which are difficult to interpret or may be interpreted as personality assessments. Discussion can then follow on how these specific behaviours impact on the ANTS system elements and categories. The consultant can then encourage the trainee to consider why these behaviours were observed or not. However, as we have previously noted, providing feedback is not the only skill in which consultant anaesthetists lack training. Accurately observing behaviour is a skill in itself and requires deliberate practice for learning.

This situation, where there is limited use of formal workplace-based assessment, is changing in the UK in response to the processes brought about under the umbrella of Modernising Medical Careers (The Foundation Programme). The body with regulatory powers for postgraduate medical training (the Postgraduate Medical and Training Board, referred to as PMETB) with the right to approve curricula, including assessment tools, is promoting workplace-based assessment tools as one method for providing evidence that trainees are achieving the appropriate competencies for their respective curricula (The Postgraduate Medical Education and Training Board). The proposed workplace-based tools are being modified from tools introduced in the UK in 2005 for use during the first two years of postgraduate training (the UK

Foundation Training programme). These tools are the Mini Clinical Evaluation Exercise (MiniCEX), the Directly Observed Procedural Skills (DOPS), the Case Based Discussion (CBD) and a form of 360° feedback. The MiniCEX can deal with many aspects of interaction with a patient including history taking, conducting an examination or explaining benefits and risks of procedures. The DOPS focuses on procedural skills including the decision-making, preparation and set up of the procedure. The CBD is intended to look at decision-making processes by referring to information recorded by trainees in the patient's case notes, while the 360° allows peers and other colleagues from a range of professions to comment on professional attitudes and teamworking skills. Specially modified versions of these tools are now described for anaesthetic speciality training (The Royal College of Anaesthetists, *Workplace-based Assessment*).

At the time of writing, there is a sense of concern in the anaesthetic community with regard to these tools. Consultant anaesthetists have embraced the principles behind workplace-based assessment. However, as we found when considering use of the ANTS system, consultants have expressed concern about the level of their training, support and preparation for using these tools. Moreover, for many who have not yet considered NTS, these reactions have been focused on areas of anaesthetic practice which have been traditionally assessed (technical skills). It is therefore hardly surprising that asking consultants to conduct workplace-based assessments of NTS, an area in which they had no previous experience, was a step too far. It is also likely that the cascade approach was overambitious in that too much was asked of too few people without ongoing support (Grant and Stanton 1999). Nevertheless, despite the cascade approach having had limited success, the Royal College of Anaesthetists has continued to support the concept of using the ANTS system and it featured as one of the assessment tools submitted to PMETB for approval.

Using the ANTS System to Frame Teaching

However, the difficulty with the cascade approach to incorporating NTS into anaesthetic training was not just a problem of becoming familiar with observing behaviours, using the ANTS system and considering how best to give feedback. There were barriers because of the very nature of clinical training in the UK. In this training system the trainee spends regular time providing anaesthetic care with a trainer, gradually taking a more central role in the clinical work in a wider range of clinical settings. This would seem to be ideal in that there are regular opportunities for the trainer to observe the trainee's practice and provide feedback. The method of use of the ANTS system which was favoured by the 17 anaesthetists during the usability study was to allocate the perioperative management of a particular patient to the trainee accompanying them on the theatre list. They would then assess the performance of the trainee and, using the observed behaviours, provide feedback after the case. The consultant, of course, retained overall responsibility and could step in and make changes if necessary but, in the absence of concerns about patient or trainee safety, would let the trainee handle the management of the patient. This approach had some implications. The trainer does not only have the trainee to observe but also the clinical work. As a senior trainee has more experience than a junior trainee, the consultant is more likely to have confidence that the trainee will identify the key issues involved with the management of a wider range of patients for either the whole anaesthetic management or specific parts of a case. There are therefore more opportunities to delegate responsibility to a senior trainee than a junior trainee. Consultant participants in the study reported that they were better able to use the system with senior rather than junior trainees. There is some apparent logic in this finding. If we want to look at ANTS categories such as decision-making then it is necessary to let trainees make decisions, therefore you have to delegate that responsibility. This message was also conveyed when evaluating the cascade training.

One might therefore imagine that the system could be used satisfactorily with senior trainees at least. However, frequently senior trainees are given responsibility not only for individual patients but for a complete surgical list, either intentionally to provide them with required clinical experience, or to cover for leave or sickness. Although a consultant anaesthetist will have supervisory responsibility for that trainee, they may be occupied elsewhere and unable to give continuous personal supervision. These factors limit the operating lists where a consultant and a senior trainee work together, and participants in the cascade training initiative listed this as another factor contributing to their difficulties in using the ANTS system. In addition, often, no sooner had a trained consultant explained the system than the trainee was re-allocated to another theatre list.

Given the various difficulties which had been encountered with the cascade approach, it was important to consider whether there were further approaches which could be used in addition. As the clinical anaesthetists in the research team continued to use the system in their own practice, some other uses began to become apparent. It was possible to use the system as a framework on which to base both the NTS elements and also the more conventional technical tasks during anaesthesia. The reluctance of consultants to use the ANTS system with junior trainees was partly based on a concern that anaesthetists in the early stages of training have large areas of knowledge and practical skills to assimilate and struggle to cope with an additional load of considering NTS. However, if the teacher or instructor was using the ANTS system as a framework or mental model then he or she need not communicate that framework to the learner. The consultant as instructor could use the system to provide scaffolding for the trainee without this being visible to the trainee. Some examples will help to clarify this process.

Let us begin with the category of 'Situation Awareness'. One of the elements in the ANTS system category Situation Awareness is *gathering information*. A key technical skill to be mastered by novice anaesthetists is taking an anaesthetic history from a patient. This skill resembles the history taking skills that medical undergraduates have to master but there is sufficient difference to require specific additional instruction. When not familiar with the ANTS system, the trainee will view this skill as history taking, not as gathering information. Of course there is more to gathering information for situation awareness than history taking from the patient. Information about the intended surgical procedure is required to formulate a suitable anaesthetic plan. Trainees are traditionally taught to ask for the information about the proposed surgical procedure that they require, such as how long will it take; what position will the patient be in; does the surgeon need access to the abdominal, chest or pelvic cavities; what is the anticipated blood loss? This information may be gathered from a variety of sources such as the surgeons and the operating department nursing staff. The trainee is now *exchanging information* and *coordinating activities with team members*, which are elements from the category Team Working.

As a further example, during the course of anaesthesia there will be episodes where the anaesthetic trainee needs to focus on surgical events, such as when the surgeon makes the skin incision. At this time the anaesthetist should be observing the response of the patient to confirm that the depth of anaesthesia is appropriate for that patient. The relevant elements are *gathering information* and *anticipation* from Situation Awareness, *prioritizing* from Task Management and *exchanging information* from Team Working. Prioritization is included because the anaesthetist should not be involved in other activities that are less essential (such as drawing up antibiotic drugs). The anaesthetist should anticipate the skin incision by observing the progress of the prepping of the surgical field and the placing of sterile drapes around the surgical field. They should be alert for an exchange of information (a surgeon with appropriate NTS will ask if it is all right to perform the incision and the anaesthetist should be in a position to reply).

Taking this method further, the relevant NTS behaviours can be discussed during procedural skills training and the key role of NTS for safety can be highlighted. To illustrate this technique, consider the insertion of a central venous line. The trainee is taught to attach cardiac monitoring so that they can be aware of arrhythmia generation should the guide wire be passed too far. Of course this allows *information gathering* to provide more accurate Situation Awareness of how the technical procedure is proceeding. There can be discussion of where the monitor is best placed for *information gathering*. As this is sometimes found to be out of clear sight for the person inserting the cannula, the trainee may suggest that they would ask an assistant (*exchanging information*) to watch the monitor during the insertion (*coordinating activities*). It is not uncommon for trainee anaesthetists to assume that their assistants in theatre are familiar with all their activities. In this situation the trainee may assume that the assistant will understand both what to look for and when to look at the monitor. In fact this is often not so, and facilitating discussion with ANTS elements and categories clarifies the importance of the exchange of information and coordination of activities so that the trainee and his/her assistant have shared situation awareness and the safety of the procedure for the patient will be enhanced.

At this time, in the earliest stages of postgraduate training, it is likely that most UK medical graduates will not be aware of the concept of NTS. The novice trainee may not see the behaviours being highlighted in the examples given above as NTS. They may just be seen as behaviours to be copied and applied as part of the initiation into the profession of anaesthesia. However, where the instructor carries the framework and uses it to structure the components of practice, this can help direct the behaviours of the novice into good habits of practice. Then, when the trainee is introduced to the theoretical aspects of NTS, there are examples of clinical practice readily available to be used for illustrative purposes. Furthermore, when trainees have familiarity with the ANTS system, they can be asked to incorporate NTS when they articulate discussion of cases or events.

To summarize, we can say that a trainer who is familiar with the ANTS system can use that system as a framework to help trainees acquire non-technical skills from the earliest stages of training. It will also have become obvious that there can be considerable overlap between anaesthetists' technical and non-technical skills. A trainee anaesthetist can only anticipate what will happen during an operation if they have acquired some experience of that procedure. In a similar vein a trainee can only anticipate what impact a particular drug will have on a patient if that trainee has the necessary understanding of physiology and pharmacology. It may now become a little clearer why in the early days of applying the ANTS system the emphasis was on use with more experienced trainees.

Future Directions

So, where do we go from here? Let us review the position briefly.

1. The ANTS system can be used in the clinical workplace.
2. The cascade model introduced by the Royal College of Anaesthetists to introduce the ANTS system as a tool to be used at departmental level has not been successful.
3. Workplace-based assessment tools are now being introduced into postgraduate medical training in the UK.
4. The proposed assessment tools have been adapted from existing tools and are being modified for purpose.
5. There appears to be an overlap between technical and non-technical skills in anaesthesia.

One possible strategy is to incorporate appropriate aspects of the ANTS system into the miniCEX, DOPS and CBD workplace-based assessment tools. As anaesthetists learn to use these tools in the workplace they can begin to include NTS in the manner outlined previously. In this way, we may assist consultant anaesthetists in becoming more familiar with the ANTS system. An experimental MiniCEX form (Figure 11.1 and 11.2) was designed in a collaborative venture between UK and New Zealand departments. Results from the UK limb are in the process of being collected and analysis is awaited.

Mini CEX Trainee Assessment, Victoria Infirmary

Demographics

Trainee name: [   ] Assessor name: [   ]

Date: [   ] Stage of training: [   ]

Case Details

Surgical subspecialty: [   ] Surgical complexity: minimal moderate high

ASA: [   ] Age: [   ] Focus of Encounter: [   ]

Grading

Grade the following, *taking into account the level of training* (NB a descriptor for each competency is outlined overleaf)

	Unsatisfactory			Satisfactory			Superior			
CATEGORY	1	2	3	4	5	6	7	8	9	UC
Patient assessment/preparation										
Equipment and theatre preparation										
Management plan										
Technical skills										
Communication skills – Patient										
Communication skills – Staff										
Clinical judgement										
Organization/efficiency										
Professionalism										
Overall clinical care										

Assessor's Comments

What did the trainee do well? [   ]

Areas for improvement: [   ]

Agreed Action: [   ]

Feedback

	1	2	3	4	5	6	7	8	9	10
Trainee satisfaction with Mini CEX										
Assessor satisfaction with mini CEX										

Assessor training (circle as many as apply)

None   written training   web-based training   face-to-face training

Time taken (in minutes)   observation of trainee: [   ]   feedback: [   ]

Interval between observation and feedback: [   ]

Figure 11.1   Mini CEX trainee assessment, Victoria Infirmary

Mini CEX Competency Descriptors

Patient assessment/ preparation	Elicits relevant information from history and examination of patient Gathers information from patient's notes and investigations including medication history and allergies Orders further investigations or treatment appropriately
Equipment and theatre preparation	Carries out machine check Ensures that equipment necessary for case is working and is prepared, including fluid warming devices, invasive monitoring, airway equipment, equipment for regional or local anaesthesia Prepares emergency drugs Confirms that relevant personnel are present
Management plan	Formulates an appropriate plan for the perioperative care of the patient, including back-up plans for possible complications
Technical skills	Proficiency in application of monitoring, vascular access, regional technique, airway skills, patient positioning
Communication skills – patient	Explores patient's perspective, jargon free, open and honest; agrees management plan with patient
Communication skills – staff	Communicates anaesthesia plan to appropriate staff Maintains open communication with surgical team Fosters effective team communication (open, two-way, clear, concise, closes communication loop)
Clinical judgement	Monitors patient, procedure, progress and personnel Maintains anaesthesia satisfactorily Responds appropriately to changes in patient status/unanticipated events Makes appropriate diagnoses and formulates suitable plans Orders/performs appropriate diagnostic studies or interventions, considers risks and benefits Anticipates and prepares for future events Plans for and appropriately manages transition to post-operative care
Organization/efficiency	Prioritizes, is timely, succinct Well-organized workspace, efficient use of time without compromising patient care Good standard of record keeping
Professionalism	Shows respect, compassion and empathy for patients and establishes trust Attends to patient's needs and comfort Respects confidentiality Behaves in an ethical manner, aware of legal frameworks for consent Shows integrity Aware of own limitations including risk of fatigue, impairment Commitment to quality and safety (e.g. practices to reduce medical error, complies with hospital protocols) Responsible use of resources
Overall clinical care	During period of observation demonstrates satisfactory clinical judgement, synthesis of information, caring and clinical effectiveness Demonstrates efficiency, appropriate use of resources Balances risks and benefits Good communication and teamwork Aware of own limitations

Figure 11.2   Mini CEX competency descriptors

It is important to note that use of the approach outlined above does not suggest that the MiniCEX, DOPS or CBD should replace the ANTS system. However the training of consultant anaesthetists to become trainers in the use of the ANTS system could then build upon the experience gained with the other workplace-based assessment tools. There is likely to be a need for the use of the ANTS system for trainee assessment in its entirety when further exploring the non-technical skills of underperforming anaesthetists. In addition, if specific classroom training in NTS is provided, and perhaps this should be happening at an undergraduate stage, the order and structure of the ANTS system will help trainees learn about the observable non-technical skills considered important for anaesthetic practice.

Summary

In this chapter we have attempted to outline the journey so far to incorporate non-technical skills into the training of UK anaesthetists and to make some suggestions for the next stages of development. The ANTS project allowed us to identify NTS, describe them using a common language and develop a taxonomy of the non-technical skills which are considered crucial for good practice by the anaesthetic community. This was an important first step. Currently there remain a number of hurdles to be overcome before non-technical skills are fully integrated into training. It is apparent that there is a need for further support and training in workplace-based assessment for consultants for all clinical activities, not just for non-technical skills training. The changes in the UK training system which require the use of a variety of workplace-based assessment tools are helping to drive this process forward.

References[1]

Anaesthetists' Non-Technical Skills (ANTS) System Handbook (2003). Industrial Psychology Research Centre, University of Aberdeen. Available at: <http://www.abdn.ac.uk/iprc /ANTS> [last accessed March 2009].

Crandall, B., Klein, G. and Hoffman, R.R. (2006) *Working Minds: A Practitioner's Guide to Cognitive Task Analysis.* Boston: The MIT Press.

Dodd, F. (2005) *Assessment of Anaesthetic Non-Technical Skills.* Presentation delivered at the Society for Education in Anaesthesia (UK) Annual Scientific Meeting: Newcastle-upon-Tyne.

Fletcher, G., Flin, R., McGeorge, P., Glavin, R., Maran, N. and Patey, R. (2003) Anaesthetists Non-Technical Skills (ANTS): Evaluation of a behavioural marker system. *British Journal of Anaesthesia* 90(3), 580–8.

Fletcher, G., Flin, R., McGeorge, P., Glavin, R., Maran, N. and Patey, R. (2004) Rating non-technical skills: Developing a behavioural marker system for use in anaesthesia. *Cognition, Technology and Work* 6, 165–71.

---

1   At the time of writing there are major changes taking place in postgraduate medical training in the UK and documents from the bodies concerned with training continue to evolve. Please note that the training documents cited may have been subsequently replaced.

Flin, R., O'Connor, P. and Crichton, M. (2008) *Safety at the Sharp End: A Guide to Non-Technical Skills*. Aldershot: Ashgate.

Grant, J. and Stanton, F. (1999) *The Effectiveness of Continuing Professional Development: A Report for the Chief Medical Officer's Review of Continuing Professional Development in Practice.* Edinburgh: Association for the Study of Medical Education.

Helmreich, R.L. (2000) On error management: Lessons from aviation. *British Medical Journal* [online] 320(7237): 781–5.

Patey, R., Flin, R., Fletcher, G., Maran, N. and Glavin, R. (2005) Anaesthetists' non-technical skills (ANTS). In K Henriks (ed.) *Advances in Patient Safety: From Research to Implementation*. Washington: Agency for Quality and Safety in Healthcare.

Modernising Medical Careers, NHS. *The Foundation Programme Curriculum* (June 2007). Available at: <http://www.foundationprogramme.nhs.uk/pages/home/key-documents> [last accessed March 2009].

The Postgraduate Medical Education and Training Programme (July 2008), *Standards for Curricula and Assessment Systems*. Available at: <http://www.pmetb.org.uk/index.php?id=scas> [last accessed November 2008].

The Royal College of Anaesthetists. *Workplace-Based Assessment – Blueprint, Forms, Guidance and Portfolio* (Updated 17 March 2009). Available at: <http://www.rcoa.ac.uk/index.asp?PageID=982> [last accessed March 2009].

Chapter 12

Using ANTS for Workplace Assessment

Jodi Graham, Emma Giles and Graham Hocking

Introduction

Around the world, administrative bodies of medical specialities are faced with the challenge of assessing their trainees. While different forms of assessment have been used for many years, assessment in the workplace is thought to be the most meaningful. The challenge is to create and test tools that will be robust enough to perform high stakes assessments.

In 2006, the Australian and New Zealand College of Anaesthetists (ANZCA) offered grants for projects investigating tools to assess trainee behaviour in the workplace. ANZCA hopes to add summative workplace-based assessment to the current primary and final examinations and to replace the formative and subjective in-training assessment (ITA). In-training assessment is used currently to assess workplace performance but has low reliability and is prone to rater bias (Spike et al. 2000) particularly since there is no assessor training within ANZCA. Grants were offered to investigate three tools – Anaesthetists' Non-Technical Skills (ANTS), Directly Observed Procedural Skills (DOPS) and Mini Clinical Evaluation Exercise (mini-CEX). We successfully tendered for a grant to quantitatively assess the reliability and qualitatively assess the feasibility of ANTS.

There is growing appreciation amongst medical educators that medical competencies need to be broader than simply medical expertise (CanMEDS 2000). There is a reciprocal growing appreciation amongst certifying bodies in medicine that examinations, isolated from the complexities of the clinical environment, do not comprehensively examine a doctor's true performance (Hays et al. 2002). Medicine is practised in multidisciplinary teams and has an increasing reliance on technology. The introduction of safer, thus shorter, working hours has led to discontinuity of care and interdependence with other colleagues. Medical practice can now rarely be modelled as an expert having a simple one-on-one relationship with a patient.

There are a range of attributes which should be common to all doctors, and these are being addressed through projects such as CanMEDS (CanMEDS 2000) and the Australian Curriculum Framework for Junior Doctors (Gleason et al. 2007). Each speciality, however, will have additional specific attributes. Many of these attributes can be taught and ideally, all should be testable. The developers of ANTS have fully explored the domains of non-technical practice in anaesthesia, creating a tool with high content and face validity (Fletcher et al. 2004).

The reliability of ANTS has previously been investigated using videos of simulated conduct of anaesthesia, with the assessed raters being anaesthetists involved in either training or assessment of anaesthesia trainees. If ANTS were to be adopted as an assessment tool, we felt these parameters would change. Performance in simulated settings could take away the dynamism of the environment, and could be unfeasible to implement with limited access to medium or high fidelity simulators. Widespread trainee assessment would require involvement of significant numbers of assessors who are less experienced in education. These changes have previously been postulated to reduce reliability (Downing 2004). This would be a stumbling block for such a high stakes assessment where a reliability coefficient should be over 0.9 in a defensible programme (Downing 2004).

We were also interested in the feasibility of introducing such a tool but had specific concerns regarding the complex issues its introduction would bring, which included; difficulty in training raters, acceptance by anaesthetists of ANTS as a valid tool, and time and resource allocation redirected from patient care.

Methodology

Our hypothesis was that 'Anaesthetists can be trained to use ANTS at an assessor level in one day'. We designed a pilot study because the one site restriction of our ANZCA grant limited the scope of the project. We were aiming to achieve inter-rater reliability. An assessor level of agreement was determined to be an r_{wg} (within group inter-rater agreement) of 0.7, although for high stakes assessment, $r > 0.8$–0.9 is desirable (Downing 2004). Previous research with minimally trained ANTS raters has demonstrated an r_{wg} of 0.5–0.7 (Fletcher et al. 2004).

Study Design

The study was divided into stages. A series of videos were made of anesthetists' real-time performance and these were used for rater training. A rater training day was then developed and implemented. Reliability data were calculated from ratings of performance collected from five separate videos. Pre- and post-workshop questionnaires were handed out with the intention of gathering qualitative information. Demographic data were collected; questions asked by the Scottish group (Fletcher et al. 2004) were repeated, other questions added and acceptability by the participants of ANTS as a summative assessment tool was determined.

Video

This aspect of our research has generated an enormous amount of interest as it seems that many people would like to video workplace performance. There are many administrative, ethical and some legal requirements to overcome. Described below is the process we followed, with very little trouble. Of course, different countries and even other Australian states have differing laws to consider.

Consent for Video

During the design phase of this project, the feasibility of using real-time video in the operating theatre was investigated. Looking back, this was probably one of the most significant steps in the design of this project. Ensuring the video process was possible before embarking on the study ensured that we were able to complete the project on time.

Investigating the use of video was achieved by contacting the chief executive officer (CEO) of our hospital for advice. Ensuring that our audio-visual department was willing and able to produce the videos was essential. Advice from our CEO indicated that we must gain written consent from both the patient and the principal anaesthetist taking part in the video. Patient protection was foremost in all our minds. Protecting the hospital from potential litigation was also going to be of major concern. Therefore, the consent process and any conditions were focused specifically around the patient.

The consent process was simpler for the anaesthetist and theatre staff. Written consent was obtained from the main anaesthetist in the video and verbal consent from other theatre staff. Any staff member who did not wish to be seen on video either left the theatre or was edited out if they appeared.

The documentation was based on the standard hospital consent form, but had to state a number of items concerning use of the video. These included where the videos would be stored (e.g., locked cabinet), how long they would be stored for, and who would see them. The specificity of where the videos would be stored was of paramount importance. Consent could be withdrawn at any time.

To ensure the video could not be used as evidence by the patient if there was a mishap of some kind, the research was registered as a quality assurance project. By doing this, the hospital was satisfied that any evidence captured on video would not be discoverable.

Recruitment

Video production was divided into phases. Volunteers were found amongst our anaesthesia registrars and consultants at Sir Charles Gairdner Hospital. We were able to find enough volunteers to film the 20 videos required for the project. Our colleagues who allowed us to video them at work have our gratitude. We now realize that what seemed simple at the time has in fact been very difficult for others to achieve. We suspect the strong focus on education at our institution led to our success.

The audio-visual department made a number of posters which were displayed in the clinic where patients undergo pre-operative assessment. The posters were also seen in the day surgery admission centres and elsewhere patients may be entering the hospital for surgery. The posters explained briefly that some patients might be asked if their anaesthetist could be filmed during the start of their anaesthetic. Brief details of the project were included. This ensured that when patients were approached, they were already aware of the project. Patients were more than willing to take part in the videos and no patient refused a request. Some even commented they were disappointed not to be asked so it seems there is a budding film star in all of us!

Our hospital predominantly performs elective surgery, making it somewhat easier to recruit patients pre-operatively. Even those who asked questions were pleased to participate in a project that was ultimately aimed at improving patient safety. Some requested a copy but were politely declined, understanding the reason for this when it was explained. Following the end of video production, patients were still enquiring about participating in the video after seeing the signs. Unfortunately, we had to inform them that the project had been completed.

Video Production

Video production commenced in January 2007 and took seven months. The videos were produced by the audio-visual department at Sir Charles Gairdner Hospital. They did an outstanding job, especially considering they were sometimes required to attend at relatively short notice. The quality of the video produced was very high, ensuring that the raters had the opportunity to observe even subtle behaviours.

When assessing videoed performance, the sound and picture quality are crucial since the people on screen are being assessed on their behaviours. What the assessor sees and hears will determine their assessment. Care must be taken by the cameraman and editor to ensure behaviours are not missed.

To achieve the quality required, two high quality tripod mounted video cameras were used and these were handled by professionals, not your average home video maker. One zoomed camera followed the subject anaesthetist/s and the other recorded the wider theatre view. This allowed us to choose the footage that best exhibited what needed to be seen. For example, if the anaesthetist's behaviour was being influenced by the other theatre staff then we were able to see this. Alternatively, if what they were doing was influencing other theatre staff, we could also observe this.

Each subject anaesthetist was asked to wear a lapel microphone. The rest of the conversation and noise in theatre was captured by a separate camera mounted microphone. The lapel microphone enabled the viewer to clearly hear almost all that was going on. Prior to the start of this project we had taken a test video with a small camera. Although adequate, it was difficult to hear all that was required. Sound is one of the most important aspects of video production for this purpose.

The video taken was of anaesthetists' real-time performance. This was chosen instead of simulated crises for a number of reasons. Simulation is not a standard assessment tool and while crisis management is relevant, this is something we may revisit in the future. Assessment in the workplace is something that can occur any day in each hospital. It is familiar and accessible. For this reason we chose to train our raters viewing real anaesthesia. All videos were unscripted as it was important that we were able to observe real behaviours since subtleties in behaviour are often lost by non-professional actors acting to a script.

Twenty videos were decided upon for the purposes of both this project and any future projects to stem from the original. The number was not completely arbitrary. Initially, the number required for the rater training day was calculated and thereafter, the number of videos required to catch a range of behaviours to use as examples was agreed. From prior use of ANTS we knew approximately how often the less common behaviours would occur. Twenty videos were thought to be enough to allow us not only some choice, but some good examples of particular behaviours.

Editing of the footage was performed by the expert raters and staff members of the audio-visual department using Final Cut Pro (Apple Inc.).

The two experts rated each video. These were used as the reference points for calibration on the training day. At the time of editing, a selection of excerpts was also chosen to illustrate particular behaviours.

The videos were used for many aspects of our rater training day. These included performance dimension training, behavioural observation training and calibration compared to expert raters. These aspects of the rater training are described in detail later in this chapter.

ANTS Rater Training

Development of the rater training day was the second phase of our project. There has been much previous research in the area of rater training. A simple search of psychology literature will reveal a large body of work on this topic. We based our training on that used in other industries (Salas et al. 2001, Woehr and Huffcutt 1994).

Some of the issues surrounding rater training include:

- Time taken to train raters to the standard that is required for reliable and accurate assessment.
- Rater calibration, frequency accuracy and inter-rater agreement required between assessors.
- Homogeneity of assessor training to ensure standards are maintained.

Rater training for behavioural marker systems has been used in aviation and other industries for a number of years. An adequate level must be achieved in their assessment to continue working or re-training must occur.

Rater training aims to improve rater accuracy and agreement between raters. Strategies to improve rater training include:

- *Rater Error Training (RET)*: The goal is to reduce rating error and produce more normally distributed ratings.

- *Performance Dimension Training (PDT)*: Increase rating accuracy by facilitating dimension-relevant evaluations.
- *Behavioural Observation Training (BOT)*: Increase rating accuracy by focusing on the observation of behaviour.
- *Frame of Reference training (FOR)*: Increase rating accuracy by focusing on the different levels of performance (Salas et al. 2001).

Reportedly, it is seemingly straightforward to train a single group of raters and achieve a relatively high level of inter-rater agreement and accuracy when compared to a standard set rated by an expert (Salas et al. 2001). The potential sources of error means that it is not as easy to translate this to many groups who are trained in separate centres or by different trainers. The rate of between-group rater agreement and accuracy is known to drop significantly without addressing such errors.

Salas et al. (2001) outlined guidelines for training raters in the use of behavioural markers. These guidelines have been developed to try and minimize the sources of error described above. There is limited recent evidence on effective rater training in the medical domain and so these guidelines were followed to develop our rater training for ANTS. These guidelines were previously followed by Flin and Glavin's research group (Fletcher et al. 2003) to evaluate inter-rater agreement for ANTS.

Baker et al (2001) employed an eight-hour rater training programme for a behavioural marker system. They achieved an adequate level of inter-rater agreement and accuracy in this time frame. Workpackage Report 7 from the University of Aberdeen investigating ANTS reports a four-hour training programme (Fletcher et al. 2002). With this minimal amount of training, inter-rater agreement of rwg = 0.55–0.67 was achieved at an elemental level, and 0.56–0.65 for a categorical level. This was also without feedback and calibration.

During the initial evaluation of ANTS by the Scottish team, feedback from experts and calibration were deliberately excluded from rater training to isolate the impact of these on inter-rater agreement. In this way, the training provided to their participants was intentionally limited to try and isolate the reliability of the tool itself. With our research we hoped to move this forward a phase by including feedback from experts to test calibration, and thus improve inter-rater agreement.

Rater Training Day

When planning the project we aimed to train 15 participants as raters. This was the number we reasonably thought we could expect since we were only able to recruit from our own department. We chose a single day of training as a feasible length. Were the college to have a widespread roll-out of ANTS as an assessment tool, a short course would be necessary if many assessors were to be trained.

Surprisingly, 26 participants applied and attended the training which was held at a venue with excellent audio-visual capacity, desk space and good catering for participants and trainers.

Pre-reading was sent out prior to the workshop including the *ANTS Handbook* (<www.abdn.ac.uk/ANTS>) and 'Recommendations for the use of behavioural markers' (Klampfer et al. 2001).

An outline of the rater training is as follows:

- welcome and introduction;
- ANTS background information;
- Behavioural Observation Training;
- Rater Error Training;
- Performance Dimension and Frame Of Reference training;
- assessment practice and calibration.

The attendees found the behavioural observation training to be an enjoyable experience. This session involved observing continuity errors in films, amongst other activities. The performance dimension and frame of reference training utilized the excerpts that were selected from the videos. This was the first opportunity our raters had to practise their assessment skills.

Five videos were shown in the afternoon for the purpose of practice assessment and calibration. ANTS scores from these five videos were collected for statistical analysis. Score sheets were collected from each rater prior to any discussion about the video. Expert ratings and a discussion followed for the purpose of calibration. Many of the learning points that we gained from this project arose during these sessions and will be discussed later.

Results

Participants rated performance in the five test videos, scoring in each case for 15 identified skill elements. Following lengthy discussion with our statistician, intra-class correlation (ICC) (Shrout and Fleiss 1979) was chosen to demonstrate agreement between the 26 raters. ICC allows different sources of variability to be included and is essentially another way of calculating inter-rater agreement. By choosing ICC we were able to include multiple sources of variability. This reflects the many sources of variability that are introduced when investigating inter-rater agreement.

$$ICC = var(target) / var(target) + var(judge) + var(residual).$$

Intraclass correlations were calculated for each element of ANTS (see Figure 12.1). A random effects linear model approach was used to estimate variance components and to ultimately estimate the ICC. None even reached the minimal acceptable value of 0.7, let alone the higher value of 0.9 that would be considered necessary for a high stakes assessment. We therefore showed a lack of reliability. As you will see later in this chapter, we learnt a number of lessons while trying to achieve inter-rater reliability with such a large group.

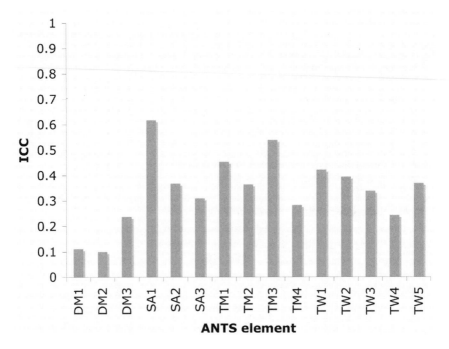

Figure 12.1   Intraclass correlations calculated for each component of ANTS

Comparison of scores with those of the 'expert raters' also showed unsatisfactory results.

Qualitative Data

Pre-workshop Questionnaire

All participants were involved in the supervision of ANZCA trainees with a range of experience in terms of supervision from 1–30 years. Of the 26 participants, eight had one year or less of supervising experience.

Only seven participants already had a system for assessment in the workplace. Of these, one was a regional education officer, and the others were generally experienced (5–30 years as a consultant). New supervisors were less likely to have a method for assessment. However, there were still some experienced anaesthetists amongst those who felt they had no real system for assessment.

The most common aims the participants identified for the workshop were to 'provide better or constructive feedback', and 'to have a systematic method for assessment' (22 out of 26). No one felt that the elements of the current in-training assessment process were useful for assessment.

Post-workshop Questionnaire

All participants thought ANTS was a useful system for structuring assessment and the majority found the system easy to use. Four participants found it difficult to place appropriate rating scores next to the observed behaviour.

Pre-reading was universally helpful and one participant even requested extra pre-reading. The level for most of the training was scored at 'just right'. The amount of information in each section was 'just right' for the majority of participants. Specific comments about the training were few, but noted to adapt future training sessions.

Most participants felt they needed more practice before using ANTS for assessment. Despite this, most felt they had received enough training to use the ANTS system.

All participants felt that ANTS was useful for consultants to give training to junior anaesthetists. One comment was that it sets a 'gold standard' for behaviours in theatre. All felt it is important for trainees to have or develop these skills.

Each participant felt that ANTS was useful as a formative assessment tool. The comments associated with this question included the fact that it was useful to give structured feedback. Most also felt that it would highlight the importance of non-technical skills.

The question as to whether ANTS was suitable as a summative assessment tool divided the participants. Thirteen raters thought it was suitable as a summative assessment tool and 13 thought more work should be done. During which year of training summative assessment of non-technical skills should be performed also divided opinion. This could be determined by a future project but would require large numbers of both trainees and raters. The comments associated with this question give an insight into what the average ANZCA fellow may think about using ANTS in its current form.

Comments from ANZCA fellows regarding the use of ANTS as a summative assessment tool:

- Only a small number of expert raters should perform this assessment.
- Such an assessment may have severe implications for supervision of trainees.
- This should only be used for trainees who are already struggling.
- Anaesthesia trainees should be exposed to non-technical skills training early to encourage good behaviours.

Discussion

It seems unusual that the Scottish team investigating ANTS achieved an inter-rater reliability of $r=0.5–0.7$ with minimal training yet, in comparison, our correlation is so poor. What was different? We were hoping to see the introduction of ANTS as a summative assessment tool and unfortunately, this does not look to be a great start.

We believe there are a number of reasons why we could not achieve sufficient agreement between raters in one day. Some of these were obvious from the discussion during calibration on the training day, and some have become clearer afterwards.

Following the viewing of each video, the expert ratings were discussed to see if we could achieve further agreement amongst the group before the next video. We observed a number of interesting opinions, discussions and thoughts about using ANTS from our raters. At the time we thought we were seeing potential problems with our rater training, but what we actually saw were some warnings for the use of workplace-based assessment in general.

Misclassification

When discussing the viewed scenario it seemed that everybody was seeing the same behaviours yet there was a definite lack of agreement. This was because the behaviours were being placed into different elements.

Anybody who has used the ANTS system will know that one behaviour can potentially be placed beside more than one element. When behaviours are placed beside a different set of elements by raters, it can result in different ratings for each element. This will ultimately result in a lack of agreement.

Disagreement on Safety Standards

Not everyone agrees on safety standards within anaesthesia. An example of this is 'test ventilation'. Some anaesthetists believe this is mandatory practice, while others think it is dangerous. This is a problem that is directly relevant to the future of workplace assessment. Since ANTS is essentially based on patient safety, it is vital that assessors agree on what is 'safe' if they are to enforce this view on trainees.

We believe these two problems were mainly responsible for the lack of inter-rater agreement. This was obvious from some of the 'lively' discussions during calibration. However, this still does not account for the large difference between the Scottish raters and the Australian ones.

Herein lies the next difference. When we designed our study, we kept in mind the fact that ANTS could be used, in the future, on a large scale and by a variety of anaesthetists.

The participants in our rater training day were all specialist anaesthetists of varying experience, but without specific training in education or simulation. In fact, most of them play no formal role in education or training. All the anaesthetists in the Scottish study had some involvement in education and training activities (Fletcher et al. 2002). The large difference in inter-rater agreement could be an effect of education. The same argument that holds for teaching anaesthesia trainees formally about non-technical skills, if we are to assess them, may apply to consultants doing the assessing.

The Scottish raters were also assessing acted scenarios as opposed to the real cases that our raters observed. This may be yet another source of bias that was introduced. We learnt many lessons from our rater training day, and realized how many sources of bias can be introduced.

Lessons Learnt

1. ANTS as an appropriate instrument for workplace-based assessment for anaesthetists-in-training:
   a.   *Validity.* Content validity was established in previous work on ANTS. Our trainee raters agreed in the post-workshop questionnaire. Criterion validity is almost impossible to establish due to a lack of gold standard. We compressed the data to improve our reliability. Whilst this appears to have face validity, we have not formally assessed the validity of this approach.
   b.   *Reliability.* We failed to demonstrate acceptable inter-rater reliability with the level of training we offered. Acceptable reliability could be gained by compressing the data. If the data are compressed to an average score from each rater then the inter-rater agreement substantially increases. A longer course may offer higher reliability but may not be feasible. Reliability is difficult to demonstrate because variability is multifactorial. Addressing it would require larger sample sizes or greater control over video content. Changing the latter would detract from the validity of the real world experience.
   c.   *Acceptability.* There was high acceptability of this tool amongst both video subjects and workshop participants. However, the voluntary nature of the participation introduces bias. Data from these motivated individuals may not translate to a wider population. Resistance to implementation could be predicted to occur with many of the stakeholders. This would include trainees needing to accept the importance of this dimension of their practice and qualified anaesthetists, who work with trainees, having to incorporate the principles of ANTS explicitly in their practice. Those involved with the central examination process would need to accept devolution of their power and local centres would have to accept an increase in non-clinical workload. Trainees may also worry about the introduction of local bias into their assessment, a process which until now, has been central and viewed as impartial.
   d.   *Feasibility.* ANTS does not appear to be a feasible tool to use for summative assessment in its current state. Significant training and practice are likely to be needed, leading to low interest in potential assessors. A widespread implementation would require large human and financial resources. Potentially, it could be used as a screening tool by assessors with limited training and using a compressed scoring system. Those rated as underperforming could be assessed further

by a small number of highly trained and committed assessors. The validity of this modification would also need to be examined.

2. General lessons learnt about implementation of a workplace-based assessment tool.

   a.   The use of video footage was invaluable to teach potential assessors, though still failed to show all the information the audience wanted. High audiovisual quality was critical. Video has been shown to have similar validity and reliability to real-time observation (Hays et al. 2002) but is unlikely to be useful in our setting for trainee assessment due to the increased cost.

   b.   The workshop demonstrated that techniques borrowed from other industries were appropriate in this setting. The dynamics of the group impacted more on results than we would have expected, with vigorous discussion becoming unhealthy at times. We appeared unable to dislodge preconceptions about some behaviours, despite others in the group making it clear these beliefs were held by only a very small minority. Observations of those with dissenting opinions in the group tallied closely with their standing as an outlier in the rating process. The workshop can therefore also be an opportunity to decide who is reliable enough to become an assessor.

Conclusion

The overriding strength of ANTS is its content validity, with effective coverage of the domains of non-technical practice of anaesthesia. This coverage is also its downfall, giving it a complexity that limits its feasibility as a summative assessment tool. The poor inter-rater reliability that we demonstrated is likely to be a feature of any workplace-based assessment tool for anaesthesia as the subtleties of medical practice make maintaining high validity and reliability together difficult. Simplifying ANTS can improve reliability and may do this without impairing validity although successfully applying the tool will remain complex. The well-mapped-out domains of anaesthesia practice should make this an ideal speciality to pioneer workplace-based assessment in medicine. Given our responsibility to government and patients to provide safe, appropriately trained anaesthetists, it seems unfeasible to not introduce an appropriate comprehensive assessment programme.

References

Baker, D., Mulqueen, C. and Dismukes, R. (2001) Training raters to assess resource management skills. In E. Salas, C. Bowers and E. Edens (eds), *Improving Teamwork in Organizations* (pp. 131–45). Mahwah, NJ: Lawrence Erlbaum Associates.

CanMEDS (2000) Extract from the CanMEDS 2000 Project Societal Needs Working Group Report. *Medical Teacher* 22(6), 549–54.

Downing, S.M. (2004) Reliability: On the reproducibility of assessment data. *Medical Education* 38(9), 1006–12.

Fletcher, G., Flin, R., McGeorge, P., Glavin, R., Maran, N. and Patey, R. (2002) *WP7 Report: Evaluation of the Prototype Anaesthetist's Non-Technical Skills (ANTS) Behavioural Marker System: University of Aberdeen Workpackage Report for SCPMDE.* Available from <http://www.abdn.ac.uk/iprc/ants> [last accessed March 2009].

Fletcher, G., Flin, R., McGeorge, P., Glavin, R., Maran., N and Patey., R. (2003) Anaesthetists' Non-Technical Skills (ANTS): Evaluation of a behavioural marker system. *British Journal of Anaesthesia* 90(5), 580–8.

Fletcher, G., Flin, R., McGeorge, P., Glavin, R., Maran, N. and Patey, R. (2004) Rating non-technical skills: Developing a behavioural marker system for use in anaesthesia. *Cognition, Technology and Work* 6, 165–71.

Gleason, A.J., Daly, J.O. and Blackham, R.E. (2007) Prevocational medical training and the Australian Curriculum Framework for Junior Doctors: A junior doctor perspective. *Medical Journal of Australia* 186(3), 114–16.

Hays, R.B., Davies, H.A., Beard, J.D., Caldon, L.J.M., Farmer, E.A., Finucane, P.M., McCrorie, P., Newble, D.I., Schuwirth, L.W. and Sibbald, G.R. (2002) Selecting performance assessment methods for experienced physicians. *Medical Education* 36(10), 910–17.

Klampfer, B., Flin, R., Helmreich, R.L., Hausler, R., Sexton, B., Fletcher, G., Field, P., Staender, S., Lauche, K., Dieckmann, P. and Amacher, A. (2001) *Enhancing Performance in High Risk Environments: Recommendations for Using Behavioural Markers.* Zurich: Group Interaction in High Risk Environments. Swissair Training Centre.

Salas, E., Bowers, C.A. and Edens, E. (eds) (2001) *Improving Teamwork in Organizations: Applications of Resource Management Training.* Mahwah, NJ: Lawrence Erlbaum Associates.

Shrout, P.E. and Fleiss, J.L. (1979) Intraclass correlations: Uses in assessing rater reliability. *Psychological Bulletin* 86(2), 420–8.

Spike, N., Alexander, H., Elliott, S., Hazlett, C., Kilminster S., Prideaux, D., and Roberts, T. (2000) In-training assessment – its potential in enhancing clinical teaching. *Medical Education* 34(10), 858–61.

Woehr, D.J. and Huffcutt, A.I. (1994) Rater training for performance appraisal: A quantitative review. *Journal of Occupational and Organizational Psychology* 67(3), 189–205.

Chapter 13
Measuring Coordination Behaviour in Anaesthesia Teams During Induction of General Anaesthetics

Michaela Kolbe, Barbara Künzle, Enikö Zala-Mezö, Johannes Wacker and Gudela Grote

Introduction

Working in groups is widespread in medicine, especially in the operating room. Anaesthesia is a classic small-group performance situation where a variety of organizational, group process and personality factors are crucial to outcomes such as patient safety. Human factors such as breakdown in the quality of teamwork have been identified as a main source of failures in medical treatment (Arbous et al. 2001, Cooper et al. 2002, Gaba 2000, Helmreich and Davies 1996, Lingard et al. 2004, Reason 2005, Sexton et al. 2000). There is growing evidence that the ability of medical teams to deal with the required complex work processes strongly depends on adaptive team coordination (e.g., Manser et al. 2008, Risser et al. 1999, Rosen et al. 2008, Salas et al. 2007b, Schaafstal et al. 2001, Zala-Mezö et al. 2009). Coordination has been defined as the 'structured patterning of within-group activities by which groups strive to achieve their goal' (Arrow et al. 2000, p. 104). However, for anaesthesia teams, there is very little empirical evidence in which specific coordination behaviours can help teams maintain effective clinical performance – especially in transitions from routine situations to the management of non-routine events. In our ongoing work, we attempt to fill this gap by analysing coordination behaviour and clinical performance in routine and non-routine events. In this chapter, we will analyse the relevance of adaptive coordination in anaesthetic work and present our approach to measuring team coordination behaviour in anaesthesia.

Teamwork in Anaesthesia

The induction of anaesthesia is particularly demanding compared to the other tasks involved in the anaesthetic process (see Phipps et al. 2008). Clinical team performance is influenced by a variety of factors such as team member experience or the patient's condition. Specifically, on the *individual level*, relevant factors include technical competence, heterogeneous knowledge (Rosen et al. 2008), high work commitment (Nyssen et al. 2003) and a variety of attitudes towards the interpersonal aspect of one's work and the effects of stress on performance (Flin et al. 2003). On the *team level*, anaesthetic teams are mostly crew-like (Arrow et al. 2000, Tschan et al. 2006) – structured with traditional hierarchies, varying size, sometimes no previous experience as a team and almost no formal training in teamwork or interaction with one another. Finally, the *context* of anaesthetic teamwork usually includes highly structured organizations and the necessity to be attentive to a range of tasks (Leedal and Smith 2007). Tasks are characterized by routine procedures as well as by rapidly shifting priorities, requiring the handling of high risks where failures can potentially endanger human life. Thus, as suggested by functional models of teamwork (Hackman and Morris 1975, Marks et al. 2001, Wittenbaum et al. 2004), team and task variants influence clinical team performance via the *interaction* of the anaesthetic team members. Hence, this interaction requires coordination in order to realize effective clinical team performance (Dickinson and McIntyre 1997, Tschan et al. 2006). Besides individual medical skills, experience and patient factors, *coordination within the team* is a crucial factor influencing the quality and timeliness of a reaction to unexpected complications. This coordination requirement can actually be exacerbated by the crew structure (e.g., MacMillan et al. 2004). In other words, without appropriate coordination and effective communication beyond hierarchical constraints, the team interaction could cause process losses which in turn would negatively impact team performance (Marks et al. 2002, Steiner 1972). The following section outlines mechanisms of anaesthesia team coordination.

Adaptive Coordination in Anaesthesia Teams

Coordination Requirements in Anaesthesia Teams

Performing joint actions requires coordination in the sense of orchestrating the 'sequence and the timing of interdependent actions' (Marks et al. 2001, p. 363). However, it is not only the coordination of *actions* but also the coordination of *information* (e.g., sharing information regarding a patient's allergy and discussing its implication for medication) that is important for clinical performance (Arrow et al. 2000). For example, failure to appropriately communicate relevant information (e.g., patient allergies) to all team members is a frequently reported incident in anaesthesia (Catchpole et al. 2008) and problems in information transfer are generally well known in the domain of healthcare (Cook et al. 2000, Murff and Bates 2001). This might be due to the fact that in medicine, task-relevant information is often unshared and has to be obtained either from the patient, other team members, written notes or from several monitors in the operating room.

These complex information requirements (Hirokawa 1990) pose high demands on team coordination.

After having defined *what* has to be coordinated during team interaction, questions arise on *when* – during interaction – specific coordination is appropriate. As stated above, anaesthesia is characterized by routine as well as by non-routine procedures in the sense of rapidly shifting priorities. In non-routine situations, teams have to manage unexpected and unfamiliar problems potentially endangering the system or outcome (Waller et al. 2004). This is a significant point as a non-routine event (NRE) in anaesthesia is by the definition of Weinger and Slagle (2002, p. S59) '*any* event that is perceived by care providers or skilled observers to be unusual, out-of-the-ordinary, or atypical'. NREs include critical incidents as well as a broad range of events that might not lead to immediate adverse outcomes but nevertheless could be early heralds of post-operative patient outcomes (Oken et al. 2007). A recent survey in anaesthesia has shown that NREs occur in 30.4 per cent of reported cases (Oken et al. 2007). By their very nature, NREs are likely to be ill-defined problems resulting from ambiguous cues and therefore requiring diagnostic effort to define the problem. Interestingly, studies from a comparable domain, aviation, showed that non-routine situations require more communication than routine situations (e.g., Orasanu 1993). The question arises as to how these results can be transferred to anaesthesia and how anaesthetic teams can coordinate actions and information *adaptively* to routine and non-routine situations.

Adaptive Coordination

Team adaptation means a change in team performance in response to a salient cue leading to a functional outcome for the entire team (Burke et al. 2006). For example, teams perform better when their members adapt their role behaviour in response to unanticipated change (LePine 2003) or when they change leadership behaviour depending upon the level of routine of a situation, the degree of standardization or experience of team members (Künzle et al. in press). As Manser and co-authors (2008) pointed out, adaptive coordination occurs on different organizational levels. Adaptability has been found to be fundamental to establishing safety (Salas et al. 2007b) and has been examined as one of the core components of effective teamwork and a prerequisite for coordination (Salas et al. 2005). In our work, we focused on adaptive coordination on the team level and argue that adaptability can be considered a coordination process in and of itself rather than simply a prerequisite to coordination. Similar to contingency models of leadership (e.g., Fiedler 1964), the concept of *adaptive coordination* implies that different coordination mechanisms are appropriate in different situations. The core idea of adaptive coordination lies in the dynamic use of coordination mechanisms in accordance with the workload of a given situation (Entin and Serfaty 1999, Grote et al. 2004, Rico et al. 2008, Salas et al. 2007a, Serfaty and Kleinman 1990). Here, workload describes a relationship between available resources such as information processing capacity and task demands (Byrne et al. 1998, Young et al. 2008) and refs to how a given situation is perceived by the person facing the task (Grote et al. 2003). However, it is not only the coordination behaviour in either routine or non-routine situations which is linked to team performance. Rather, it is the adaptive transition from routine to non-routine and vice versa which seems to have significant effects on team performance (Waller et al. 2004). The question then arises of how coordination should be changed in the adaptive transitions and by which behavioural means it can be executed.

Means of Adaptive Coordination

Within the literature on team coordination, scholars have differentiated between *explicit* and *implicit* coordination mechanisms (Entin and Serfaty 1999, Espinosa et al. 2004, Kolbe and Boos 2009, Grote et al. 2003, Wittenbaum et al. 1998, Zala-Mezö et al. 2009).

- *Explicit coordination* is behaviour that is intentionally used for the purpose of team coordination and mostly executed by means of verbal or written communication (Espinosa et al. 2004, MacMillan et al. 2004, Wittenbaum et al. 1998) or by transferring information and resources upon request (Serfaty and Kleinman 1990) and can be used prior to or during team interaction (Wittenbaum et al. 1998). In medicine as well as in other high reliability contexts, a typical form of explicit *pre-coordination* is standardization of behaviour through rules (Grote et al. 2004). *During* the interaction, the team process can be explicitly coordinated by mechanisms such as commands or affirmations (Marsch et al. 2004). It was found that healthcare teams which successfully treated a cardiac arrest showed more explicit coordination than poorly performing teams (Marsch et al. 2004). Explicit coordination can also be used to support group decision processes, for instance by repeating task-relevant information (Kolbe 2007). Explicit coordination is clear and generally understandable but involves communicative effort and time. It can be executed by every team member on every hierarchical level or in the sense of shared leadership.

- *Implicit coordination* is postulated to be primarily based on shared cognition and on the anticipations of the actions and needs of the team members (MacMillan et al. 2004, Rico et al. 2008, Serfaty and Kleinman 1990, Toups and Kerne 2007, Wittenbaum et al. 1996) and is also related to team situation awareness (Manser et al. 2008, Salas et al. 2005). In a recent study of anaesthesia teams, it was found that transactive memory (knowing who knows what) predicted team members' perceptions of team effectiveness, and also affective outcomes such as team identification and job satisfaction (Michinov et al. 2008). Compared to explicit coordination, implicit coordination is less time intensive, but is only effective if the team members have not only shared but accurate mental models of the task and the team interaction. If one of these two requirements is not met, reliance on implicit coordination can be very risky. This is in line with the proposals by Wittenbaum et al. (1998) who postulated that implicit coordination can be ineffective in complex and interdependent tasks. They suggested that the more coordination required (e.g., divergent goals, unequal information distribution, ambiguity of opinions and preferences), the more group members need to coordinate explicitly. In fact, explicit coordination has been considered to be a prerequisite of implicit coordination (Orasanu 1993). Given the fact that both implicit and explicit team coordination modes have advantages and disadvantages, the suggestion is that they be used according to the situational demands (Grote et al. 2004). However, in medical teams there seems to be an inherent preference for implicitness as the silver bullet of coordination styles and reluctance against being explicit. As Heath and colleagues (2002) observed in operating theatres, team members would rather unobtrusively encourage others to perform certain actions with the underlying assumption that explicitly asking them for assistance or consideration was inappropriate or would interrupt activities in which they were already engaged. This tacit assumption that 'the more implicit the communication, the more effective it is' could be problematic in non-routine situations where explicit coordination is required (Wittenbaum et al. 1998). To ensure that such needs for explicitness are identified, it seems that heedful interrelating can be a useful mechanism of adaptive team coordination.

The idea of *heedful interrelating* was introduced by Weick and Roberts (1993) and has received considerable attention. It includes certain attitudes and behaviours towards the team and the situation in order to act in close alignment with situational and team requirements. Being a heedful team member implies being mindful of the team goal and one's own contribution to it (Dougherty and Takacs 2004). This means that while being heedful, the team members constantly reconsider their own contributions in relation to the team goals (Grommes and Grote 2001, Weick and Roberts 1993). It also means that rather than acting only habitually, team members act purposefully with regard to the joint situation (Dougherty and Takacs 2004) and are well aware of how their actions fit into the overall team goal (Wears and Sutcliff 2003). This form of mindfulness is especially relevant for complex and tightly coupled systems (Vogus and Welbourne 2003). Recent research results have shown that heedful interrelating mediates the relationships of trust in team members and monitoring by team members with future team performance (Bijlsma-Frankema et al. 2008). Heedful interrelating consists of three different actions: (1) the individual *contribution* by providing own actions, (2) the *representation* of the system of joint actions and (3) the final interrelation or *subordination* of own actions within the envisaged system (Dougherty and Takacs 2004, Grommes and Grote 2001, Weick and Roberts 1993). Thus, heedful interrelating is related to the anticipation of the needs of other team members but can be regarded as a coordination mechanism that goes beyond mere implicit coordination because it can allow team members to identify needs for explicit coordination (Grommes and Grote 2001). For instance, one team member might realize that his or her own or someone else's actions are not in line with the team goal and therefore the work process has to be reorganized. Heedful interrelating also extends team orientation (see Salas et al. 2005), because the latter is confined to an attitudinal preference for working with others and enhancing individual performance while working with others. Furthermore, heedful interrelating can prevent team members from narrowly following protocols or from over-learned responses (Wears and Sutcliff 2003) and might allow team members the flexibility to speak up when necessary which in turn enhances learning and adaptability (Edmondson 2003), as well as the overall effectiveness of the team.

Still, some authors argue that heedful interrelating refers to a way in which behaviour is enacted rather than to the behaviour itself (Druskat and Pescosolido 2002). In line with this, only a few studies have analysed concrete behaviours or communication by which heedful interrelating could be enacted (Cooren 2004, Grommes and Grote 2001, Grote et al. 2003, Zala-Mezö et al. 2009). A recent study on coordination in anaesthesia teams showed that heedful interrelating occurred more in situations of high workload than in low workload phases (Zala-Mezö et al. 2009). Thus, we need to know more about the interplay of explicit and implicit coordination and how heedful interrelating facilitates the adaptive transitions between these coordination modes.

Measuring Adaptive Team Coordination Behaviour in Anaesthesia

The objective of our current research on anaesthetic team coordination is to gain a broad perspective of anaesthetic team behaviour coordination during routine and non-routine and relate it to clinical performance. This requires detailed analyses of team processes which have proven to be costly in both time and effort. However, some authors suggest that not doing these analyses would be even more costly because one would then be forced to forego key information regarding comparative team dynamics and adaptation behaviours (McGrath and Altermatt 2002). As Weingart (1997) concluded, gaining knowledge regarding what anaesthetic teams actually do, how they complete their work and the resulting levels of success increased our understanding of which processes (in this case, coordination) influence group performance, specifically clinical effectiveness. However, measuring explicit and implicit team coordination as well as heedful interrelating is far from being a straightforward endeavour that allows us to draw on a variety of existing methods. Even though implicit team coordination has been analysed experimentally (Wittenbaum et al. 1996) and by using self-report measures (Rico et al. 2008), studies on behaviour observations of implicit coordination are rare (Entin and Serfaty 1999, Grote et al. 2003, Kolbe 2007, Serfaty et al. 1993, Zala-Mezö et al. 2009), a fact that might be due to the tacit nature of implicitness.

Thus, the necessity to investigate effective and adaptive team coordination and the lack of suitable observation methods led us to develop a taxonomy of explicit and implicit team coordination and heedful interrelating behaviour.

Taxonomy of Explicit and Implicit Team Coordination and Heedful Interrelating Behaviour

The taxonomy we developed for our research on adaptive coordination in anaesthesia teams consists of three main categories: *explicit and implicit coordination, heedful interrelating* and *other behaviour* (Figure 13.1). The main category of *explicit and implicit coordination* includes two sub-categories: *coordination of information exchange* and *coordination of actions* (Arrow et al. 2000). Within these sub-categories we differentiate *explicit* from *implicit* coordination mechanism, as shown in Figure 13.1. The applied taxonomy was developed to measure coordination mechanisms with regard to explicitness, implicitness and heedfulness. Its strength lies in the precise yet practical description of behaviour patterns specifically found in anaesthesia teams.

The subcategories were developed in an iterative process based on previous work (Grote and Zala-Mezö 2004, Grote et al. 2003, Grote et al. 2004), on team coordination literature (Arrow et al. 2000, Bowers et al. 1998, Espinosa et al. 2004, Kolbe 2007, Marks and Panzer 2004, Marsch et al. 2004, Rico et al. 2008, Salas et al. 2005, Serfaty et al. 1993, Serfaty and Kleinman 1990, Toups and Kerne 2007, Tschan et al. 2006, Wittenbaum et al. 1996, Wittenbaum et al. 1998), and on literature regarding heedful interrelating and related concepts (e.g., Bijlsma-Frankema et al. 2008, Dougherty and Takacs 2004, Druskat and Pescosolido 2002, Grommes and Grote 2001, Rhee 2006, Toups and Kerne 2007, Vogus and Welbourne 2003, Weick and Roberts 1993). Table 13.1 gives definitions and examples of these coordination mode categories.

Data were coded using INTERACT (Mangold 2007), a coding software which allows for marking and coding events within a digitalized video without the need for transcribing the communication. In order to analyse the dynamic coordination process and determine whether a certain coordination act is followed by another coordination act and how long each act lasts, *focal sampling* (observing the whole group for a specified amount of time such as the induction to anaesthesia) and *continuous coding* are required (Bakeman 2000, Bakeman and Gottman 1986, Martin and Bateson 1993). However, in doing so, the procedure of (1) defining coding units (amount of behaviour that is assigned to one category) and (2) coding these units into categories were confounded because the coding units are defined with reference to the categories (McGrath and Altermatt 2002), a practice which usually impairs the reliability of an observation method (Kolbe 2007). But, since there were no appropriate unitizing rules for verbal *and* non-verbal interaction, we had to define the coding units as utterances or actions by a team member that fit into a single category.

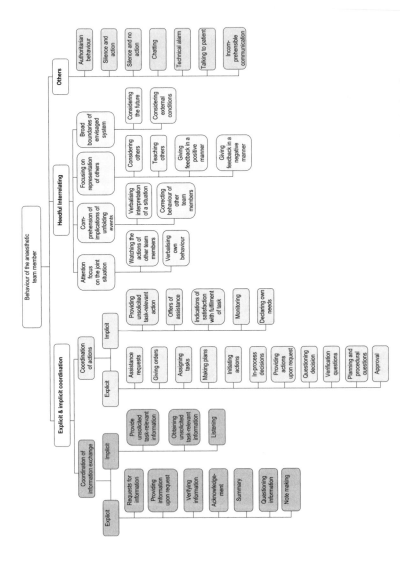

Figure 13.1   A taxonomy of explicit and implicit team coordination and heedful interrelating behaviour

Note: Coding units are here defined as utterances or actions by team members that fit into one category (Bales 1950, Beck and Fisch 2000, Marby and Attridge 1990). For each act, the actor, the target, and the duration are coded.

Table 13.1   Definitions and examples for categories

Category	Definition	Example
Explicit coordination of information exchange		
Requests for information	Checklist questions asked of team members or questions addressed to the patient.	'Where's the defibrillator?' 'Do you have any allergies?'
Providing information upon request	Includes answering direct questions. Information is given only in response to direct questions.	'The defibrillator is right behind you.'
Verifying information	Includes repeating information or giving verbal confirmations regarding fulfilled actions.	'Electrodes are checked.'
Acknowledgements	Includes verbal statements indicating one has heard or understood given information.	'Okay.' 'Um hm.'
Summary	Includes statements regarding state of affairs or processes.	'We had an asystole in reaction to laryngoscopy. We treated it with atropine and 30 seconds of heart massage.'
Questioning information	Includes statements expressing doubts about the accuracy or source of information.	'Are you sure he has no allergies?'
Note making	Coded when a team member fills out the patient's chart.	
Implicit coordination of information exchange		
Providing unsolicited task-relevant information	Providing information without being asked to do so.	'Blood pressure is okay.'
Obtaining unsolicited task-relevant information	Includes actively garnering information without being asked to do so.	Reading patient's chart.
Listening	Includes obviously and attentively listening to another team member or patient with undivided attention.	
Explicit coordination of actions		
Assistance requests	Include explicitly asking for help.	'Can you help me with this?'

Table 13.1   *Continued*

Category	Definition	Example
Giving orders	Include directives, commands, or instructions.	'Can you hold this?' 'Give him the fentanyl.'
Assigning tasks	Coded when subtasks are assigned to team members.	'I'll intubate, you watch the monitor.'
Making plans	Include verbalizations of non-immediate considerations regarding what should be done and when.	'When we've finished intubation we'll call for an OR nurse.'
Initiating actions	Include statements or behaviours which initiate actions (not orders or decisions).	'We could give him more fentanyl.'
In-process decisions	Include statements of decision such as defining timing of intubation initiation.	'We can intubate now.'
Providing actions upon request	Includes behaviour that is performed because asked to do so.	After the physician has asked the nurse to administer the fentanyl, the nurse accepts the order and administers the drug.
Questioning decisions	Occurs when somebody expresses doubts concerning a decision, order or proposal.	'Are you sure you want to intubate right now?'
Verification questions	Include somebody asking a question to make sure they are about to do the right thing.	'I'll start now, is that alright?' 'You've already administered the atropine, right?'
Planning and procedural questions	Include questions concerning procedure and further courses of action.	'How much fentanyl do you want me to give?'
Approval	Includes short verbalizations of acceptance in reaction to a proposal.	'Good idea.'

Implicit coordination of actions

Providing unsolicited task-relevant actions	Include task-relevant actions completed without being asked to do so.	After the physician announces he/she is going to intubate, the nurse holds out the laryngoscope.

Table 13.1   *Continued*

Category	Definition	Example
Offers of assistance	Coded when somebody verbally offers help.	'Can I help you with this?'
Indications of satisfaction with fulfilment of task	Include statements of general agreements.	'Fine.' 'Okay.' 'Good.'
Monitoring (patient or machine)	Codes when a team member checks the monitor or behaviour of the patient.	Reading indicators on a monitor.
Declaring own needs	Includes verbal statements expressing personal need for something (without asking another person for it).	'I don't have gloves.' 'I'm so thirsty.'

Heedful interrelating

Category	Definition	Example
Watching actions of other team members	Coded when a team member observes the actions of his/her colleagues.	Team member watches what another team member is doing.
Verbalizing own behaviour	Occurs when personal task action is verbally communicated.	'I'm calling the attending.' 'I'm turning the alarm down.'
Verbalizing interpretation of a situation	Includes declarations or assessments of a situation.	'That was close!' 'Now he seems to feel better.'
Correcting behaviour of other team members	Includes actions that correct the behaviour of a colleague.	'No, you should plug it in here.'
Considering others	Includes attention given to another's condition influencing task fulfilment.	'Are you okay?' 'Thanks.'
Teaching others	Includes detailed explanations or demonstrations beyond the mere correcting of a behaviour of another team member.	'The way you did that wasn't wrong but it's easier if you do it this way.'
Giving feedback in a positive manner	Includes friendly reassurances to a team member.	'That was a very good reaction.'
Giving feedback in a negative manner	Includes providing feedback in a less-than-sincere manner.	'This was not too bad.'
Considering the future	Includes considering the consequences of personal or other's actions.	'We have to be careful with this tube because we have to put him in a prone position afterwards.'

Table 13.1 *Concluded*

Category	Definition	Example
Considering external conditions	Includes considerations of conditions outside the team and their consequences.	'They're already waiting for us.'
Others		
Authoritarian behaviour	Includes behaviours which are aimed at underlining power and status.	Grabbing an instrument out of the hand of a team member without explanation.
Silence and action	Includes situations where team members work silently and independently.	
Silence and no action	Coded if a person is obviously doing nothing at all – not even observing.	A team member stands around without paying attention to the process.
Chatting	Includes non-task-relevant talk.	Team member talks about the weather.
Technical alarm	Includes technical (acoustic) warning signals from one of the machines.	An alarm goes off.
Talking to patient	Includes communicating with the patient beyond garnering or imparting clinical information.	'You will start to feel very sleepy.'
Incomprehensible communication	Serves as a category for anything that is acoustically incomprehensible.	

In an ongoing research project, we investigate the relationship between adaptive coordination processes, non-technical skills ratings (Fletcher et al. 2003) and clinical performance of anaesthesia teams in both simulated and live settings during routine situations, as well as when confronted with non-routine events. Within this project we tested the taxonomy of explicit and implicit team coordination and heedful interrelating behaviour presented in Figure 13.1 for inter-rater reliability. This required that two coders independently coded two out of 15 simulated inductions of general anaesthesia. Analyses of Cohen's Kappa values showed fair to substantial reliability (for *Explicit coordination of information exchange* κ = .67; for *Explicit coordination of actions* κ = .63; for *Implicit coordination of information exchange* κ = .32; for *Implicit coordination of actions* κ = .76; heedful interrelating (κ = .60) (Landis and Koch 1977).Indeed, these results indicate that the taxonomy we developed for various modes of anaesthesia team behaviour allowed reliable measurement of explicit and implicit coordination and heedful interrelating behaviour. In particular, implicit action coordination which is by definition difficult to observe was able to be measured reliably. Only the fair Kappa value for implicit information coordination points out the need for further refining of the respective categories. The specific strengths of the taxonomy are (a) the precise assessment of explicit as well as implicit team coordination behaviour in the anaesthetic work environment in routine as well as non-routine situations and (b) the measurement of heedful behaviour which might serve as a mechanism facilitating the transition between explicit and implicit coordination. With regard to manageability, the hierarchical organization of the taxonomy simplifies the coding procedure. Furthermore, the categories are detailed enough to allow for determination of successful coordination behaviour, which in turn helps to design team training interventions.

Outlook

Within our current research project, we compare the above coordination taxonomy with the observation system developed by Manser and colleagues (2008) and test their sensitivity in detecting teams' behavioural differences between phases with varying workload in simulated as well as in live clinical settings in anaesthesia. In comparing these two observation methods for coordination behaviour, it is our intention to investigate the main differences between the two systems and how they can complement each other (see also Chapter 14 in this volume by Manser et al.). For instance, the observation system of Manser and colleagues (2008) records not only coordination behaviour but also clinical activities performed by the anaesthesia team and records actions carried out simultaneously. On the other hand, the taxonomy presented in Figure 13.1 focuses particularly on coordination of information exchange and of joint actions and provides a more detailed account of explicit and implicit coordination mechanisms and heedful interrelating. The comparison of the two observation systems will provide the data necessary for us to develop an integrated behaviour and communication observation system and improve methods for analysing team coordination behaviour in the operating room.

By exploring the relationships between routine and non-routine event coordination behaviour, non-technical skills and clinical performance with the sketched methodology, the research project is expected to contribute to both our knowledge of adaptive team coordination behaviour and the development of appropriate and reliable methods for studying human factors influencing levels of effectiveness in anaesthesia. This will allow for improvements in training anaesthesia teams and for enhancing organizational support for adaptive coordination.

Acknowledgement

We gratefully acknowledge the financial support for this project by Swiss National Science Foundation. Also, we thank Raphael Agosti and Silja Barbara Sollberger for their assistance in behaviour coding. The first author thanks Margarita Neff-Heinrich for her helpful comments on an earlier version of this chapter.

References

Arbous, M.S., Grobee, D.E., van Kleef, J.W., de Lange, J.J., Spoormans, H.H.A.J.M., Touw, P., Werner, F.M. and Meursing, A.E.E. (2001) Mortality associated with anaesthesia: A qualitative analysis to identify risk factors. *Anaesthesia* 56, 1141–53.

Arrow, H., McGrath, J.E. and Berdahl, J.L. (2000) *Small Groups as Complex Systems: Formation, Coordination, Development, and Adaption.* Thousand Oaks: Sage.

Bakeman, R. (2000) Behavioral observation and coding. In H.T. Reis and C.M Judd (eds) *Handbook of Research Methods in Social and Personality Psychology.* New York, NY: Cambridge University Press.

Bakeman, R. and Gottman, J.M. (1986) *Observing Interaction: An Introduction to Sequential Analysis.* Cambridge: Cambridge University Press.

Bales, R.E. (1950) *Interaction Process Analysis: A Method for the Study of Small Groups.* Cambridge, MA: Addison-Wesley.

Beck, D. and Fisch, R. (2000) Argumentation and emotional processes in group decision-making: Illustration of a multi-level interaction process analysis approach. *Group Processes and Intergroup Relations* 3, 183–201.

Bijlsma-Frankema, K., de Jong, B. and van de Bunt, G. (2008) Heed, a missing link between trust, monitoring and performance in knowledge intensive teams. *The International Journal of Human Resource Management* 19, 19–40.

Bowers, C.A., Jentsch, F., Salas, E. and Braun, C.C. (1998) Analyzing communication sequences for team training needs assessment. *Human Factors* 40, 672–9.

Burke, C.S., Stagl, K.C. and Salas, E. (2006) Understanding team adaptation: A conceptual analysis and model. *Journal of Applied Psychology* 91, 1189–207.

Byrne, A.J., Sellen, A.J. and Jones, J.G. (1998) Errors in anaesthetic record charts as a measure of anaesthetic performance during simulated critical incidents. *British Journal of Anaesthesia* 80, 58–62.

Catchpole, K., Bell, M.D.D. and Johnson, S. (2008) Safety on anaesthesia: A study of 12606 reported incidents from the UK national reporting and learning system. *Anaesthesia* 63, 340–6.

Cook, R.I., Render, M. and Woods, D.D. (2000) Gaps in the continuity of care and progress on patient safety. *British Medical Journal* 320, 791–4.

Cooper, J.B., Newbower, R.S., Long, C.D. and McPeek, B. (2002) Preventable anesthesia mishaps: A study of human factors. *Quality and Safety in Health Care* 11, 277–83.

Cooren, F. (2004) The communicative achievement of collective minding. *Management Communication Quarterly* 17, 517–51.

Dickinson, T.L. and McIntyre, R.M. (1997) A conceptual framework for teamwork measurement. In M.T. Brannick, E. Salas and C. Prince (eds) *Team Performance Assessment and Measurement*. Mahwah, NJ: Lawrence Erlbaum.

Dougherty, D. and Takacs, C.H. (2004) Team play: Heedful interrelating as the boundary for innovation. *Long Range Planning* 37, 569–90.

Druskat, V.U. and Pescosolido, A.T. (2002) The content of effective teamwork mental models in self-managing teams: Ownership, learning and heedful interrelating. *Human Relations* 55, 283–314.

Edmondson, A.C. (2003) Speaking up in the operating room: How team leaders promote learning in interdisciplinary action teams. *Journal of Management Studies* 40, 1419–52.

Entin, E.E. and Serfaty, D. (1999) Adaptive team coordination. *Human Factors* 41, 312–25.

Espinosa, A., Lerch, F.J. and Kraut, R.E. (2004) Explicit vs. implicit coordination mechanisms and task dependencies: One size does not fit all. In E. Salas and S.M. Fiore (eds) *Team Cognition: Understanding the Factors That Drive Process and Performance*. Washington, DC: American Psychological Association.

Fiedler, F.E. (1964) A contingency model of leadership effectiveness. In L. Berkowitz (ed.) *Advances in Experimental Social Psychology*. New York: Academic Press.

Fletcher, G., Flin, R., McGeorge, P., Glavin, R., Maran, N. and Patey, R. (2003) Anaesthetists' Non-Technical Skills (ANTS): Evaluation of a behavioural marker system. *British Journal of Anaesthesia* 90, 580–8.

Flin, R., Fletcher, G., McGeorge, P., Sutherland, A. and Patey, R. (2003) Anaesthetists' attitudes to teamwork and safety. *Anaesthesia* 58, 233–42.

Gaba, D.M. (2000) Anaesthesiology as a model for patient safety in health care. *British Medical Journal* 320, 785–8.

Grommes, P. and Grote, G. (2001) Coordination in action. Comparing two work situations with high vs. low degrees of formalization. In R. Kühnlein, A. Newlands and H. Rieser (eds) *Proceedings of the Workshop on Coordination and Action at Esslli 01*. Helsinki: University of Helsinki.

Grote, G. and Zala-Mezö, E. (2004) *The Effects of Different Forms of Coordination in Coping with Work Load: Cockpit Versus Operating Theatre*. Zürich: Eidgenössische Technische Hochschule Zürich, Institut für Arbeitspsychologie.

Grote, G., Zala-Mezö, E. and Grommes, P. (2003) Effects of standardization on coordination and communication in high workload situations. *Linguistische Berichte, Sonderheft* 12, 127–55.

Grote, G., Zala-Mezö, E. and Grommes, P. (2004) The effects of different forms of co-ordination on coping with workload. In R. Dietrich and T.M. Childress (eds) *Group Interaction in High Risk Environments*. Aldershot: Ashgate.

Hackman, J.R. and Morris, C.G. (1975) Group tasks, group interaction process, and group performance effectiveness: A review and proposed integration. In L. Berkowitz (ed.) *Advances in Experimental Social Psychology*. New York: Academic Press.

Heath, C., Sanchez Svensson, M., Hindmarsh, J., Luff, P. and vom Lehm, D. (2002) Configuring awareness. *Computer Supported Cooperative Work* 11, 317–47.

Helmreich, R.L. and Davies, J.M. (1996) Human factors in the operating room: Interpersonal determinants of safety, efficiency and morale. *Bailliere's Clinical Anaesthesiology* 10, 277–95.

Hirokawa, R.Y. (1990) The role of communication in group decision-making efficacy. A task-contingency perspective. *Small Group Research* 21, 190–204.

Kolbe, M. (2007) *Coordination of Decision-making in Groups. The Importance of Explicit Coordination Mechanisms.* [*Koordination von Entscheidungsprozessen in Gruppen. Die Bedeutung expliziter Koordinationsmechanismen.*] Saarbrücken: VDM.

Kolbe, M. and Boos, M. (2009) Facilitating group decision-making: Facilitators' subjective theories on group coordination. *Qualitative Research on Intercultural Communication* 10, doi: 0114-fqs0901287. Available at: <http://nbn-resolving. de/urn:nbn:de:0114-fqs0901287> [last accessed March 2009].

Künzle, B., Zala-Mezö, E., Kolbe, M., Wacker, J., and Grote, G. (in press). Substitutes for leadership in anaesthesia teams and their impact on leadership effectiveness. *European Journal of Work and Organizational Psychology*.

Landis, J.R. and Koch, G.G. (1977) The measurement of observer agreement for categorial data. *Biometrics* 33, 159–74.

Leedal, J.M. and Smith, A.F. (2007) Methodological approaches to anaesthetists' workload in the operating theatre. *British Journal of Anaesthesia* 94, 702–709.

LePine, J.A. (2003) Team adaptation and postchange performance: Effects of team composition in terms of members' cognitive abilities and personality. *Journal of Applied Psychology* 88, 27–39.

Lingard, L., Espin, S., Whyte, S., Regehr, G., Baker, G.R., Reznick, R., Bohnen, J., Orser, B., Doran, D. and Grober, E. (2004) Communication failures in the operating room: An observational classification of recurrent types and effects. *Quality and Safety in Health Care* 13, 330–4.

MacMillan, J., Entin, E.E. and Serfaty, D. (2004) Communication overhead: The hidden cost of team cognition. In E. Salas and S.M. Fiore (eds) *Team Cognition. Understanding the Factors That Drive Process and Performance.* Washington, DC: American Psychological Society.

Mangold, P. (2007) Interact. Unpublished manual, Mangold Software and Consulting.

Manser, T., Howard, S.K. and Gaba, D.M. (2008) Adaptive coordination in cardiac anaesthesia: A study of situational changes in coordination patterns using a new observation system. *Ergonomics* 51, 1153–78.

Marby, E.A. and Attridge, M.D. (1990) Small group interaction and outcome correlates for structured and unstructured tasks. *Small Group Research* 21, 315–32.

Marks, M.A., Mathieu, J.E. and Zaccaro, S.J. (2001) A temporally based framework and taxonomy of team processes. *Academy of Management Review* 26, 356–76.

Marks, M.A., Sabella, M.J., Burke, C.S. and Zaccaro, S.J. (2002) The impact of cross-training on team effectiveness. *Journal of Applied Psychology* 87, 3–13.

Marks, M.A. and Panzer, F.J. (2004) The influence of team monitoring on team processes and performance. *Human Performance* 17, 25–41.

Marsch, S.C.U., Müller, C., Marquardt, K., Conrad, G., Tschan, F. and Hunziker, P.R. (2004) Human factors affect the quality of cardiopulmonary resuscitation in simulated cardiac arrests. *Resuscitation* 60, 51–6.

Martin, P. and Bateson, P. (1993) *Measuring Behaviour. An Introductory Guide.* Cambridge: Cambridge University Press.

McGrath, J. E. and Altermatt, T.W. (2002) Observation and analysis of group interaction over time: Some methodological and strategic choices. In M.A. Hogg and S. Tindale (eds) *Blackwell Handbook of Social Psychology: Group Processes.* Boston: Blackwell.

Michinov, E., Olivier-Chiron, E., Rusch, E. and Chiron, B. (2008) Influence of transactive memory on perceived performance, job satisfaction and identification in anaesthesia teams. *British Journal of Anaesthesia* 100, 327–32.

Murff, H.J. and Bates, D.W. (2001) Information transfer. In K.G. Shojania, B.W. Duncan, K.M. McDonald and R.M. Wachter (eds) *Making Health Care Safer: A Critical Analysis of Patient Safety Practices.* AHRQ Publication.

Nyssen, A.S., Hansez, I., Baele, P., Lamy, M. and De Keyser, V. (2003) Occupational stress and burnout in anaesthesia. *British Journal of Anaesthesia* 90, 333–7.

Oken, A., Rasmusson, M.D., Slagle, J.M., Jain, S., Kuykendall, T., Ordonez, N. and Weinger, M.B. (2007) A facilitated survey instrument captures significantly more anesthesia events than does traditional voluntary event reporting. *Anesthesiology* 107, 909–22.

Orasanu, J.M. (1993) Decision-making in the cockpit. In E.L. Wiener, B.G. Kanki and R.L. Helmreich (eds) *Cockpit Resource Management.* San Diego, CA: Academic Press.

Phipps, D., Meakin, G.H., Beatty, P.C.W., Nsoedo, C. and Parker, D. (2008) Human factors in anaesthetic practice: Insights from a task analysis. *British Journal of Anaesthesia* 100, 333–43.

Reason, J. (2005) Safety in the operating theatre – Part 2: Human errors and organisational failure. *Quality and Safety in Health Care* 14, 56–61.

Rhee, S.Y. (2006) Shared emotions and group effectiveness: The role of broadening-and-building interactions. *Academy of Management Best Conference Papers*, B1–B6.

Rico, R., Sánchez-Manzanares, M., Gil, F. and Gibson, C. (2008) Team implicit coordination processes: A team knowledge-based approach. *Academy of Management Review* 33, 163–84.

Risser, D.T., Rice, M.M., Salisbury, M.L., Simon, R., Jay, G.D. and Berns, S.D. (1999) The potential for improved teamwork to reduce medical errors in the emergency department. *Annals of Emergency Medicine* 34, 373–83.

Rosen, M.A., Salas, E., Wilson, K.A., King, H.B., Salisbury, M.L., Augenstein, J.S. Robinson, D.W. and Birnbach, D.J. (2008) Measuring team performance in simulation-based training: Adopting best practices for healthcare. *Simulation in Healthcare* 3, 33–41.

Salas, E., Sims, D.E. and Burke, C.S. (2005) Is there a 'Big Five' in teamwork? *Small Group Research* 36, 555–99.

Salas, E., Nichols, D.R. and Driskell, J.E. (2007a) Testing three team training strategies in intact teams. A meta-analysis. *Small Group Research* 38, 471–88.

Salas, E., Rosen, M.A. and King, H. (2007b) Managing teams managing crisis: Principles of teamwork to improve patient safety in the emergency room and beyond. *Theoretical Issues in Ergonomics Science* 8, 381–94.

Schaafstal, A.M., Johnston, J.H. and Oser, R.L. (2001) Training teams for emergency management. *Computers in Human Behaviour* 17, 615–26.

Serfaty, D., Entin, E.E. and Volpe, C. (1993) Adaptation to stress in team decision-making and coordination. *Proceedings of the Human Factors and Ergonomics Society 37th Annual Meeting*. Santa Monica, CA: Human Factors and Ergonomics Society.

Serfaty, D. and Kleinman, D.L. (1990) Adaptation processes in team decision-making and coordination. *Proceedings of the International Conference on Systems, Man and Cybernetics*. Los Angeles: IEEE.

Sexton, J.B., Thomas, E.J. and Helmreich, R.L. (2000) Error, stress, and teamwork in medicine and aviation: Cross sectional surveys. *British Medical Journal* 320, 745–9.

Steiner, I.D. (1972) *Group Processes and Productivity*. New York: Academic Press.

Toups, Z.O. and Kerne, A. (2007) Implicit coordination in firefighting practice: Design implications for teaching fire emergency responders. *Proceedings of the SIGCHI Conference on Human Factors in Computing Systems*. New York: ACM Press.

Tschan, F., Semmer, N.K., Gautschi, D., Hunziker, P., Spychiger, M. and Marsch, S.U. (2006) Leading to recovery: Group performance and coordinative activities in medical emergency driven groups. *Human Performance* 19, 277–304.

Vogus, T.J. and Welbourne, T.M. (2003) Structuring for high reliability: HR practices and mindful processes in reliability-seeking organizations. *Journal of Organizational Behaviour* 24, 877–903.

Waller, M.J., Gupta, N. and Giambatista, R.C. (2004) Effects of adaptive behaviours and shared mental models on control crew performance. *Management Science* 50, 1534–44.

Wears, R.L. and Sutcliff, K.M. (2003) Promoting heedful interrelating and collective competence in the emergency department. *Focus on Patient Safety. A newsletter from the National Patient Safety Foundation* 6, 4–5.

Weick, K.E. and Roberts, K.H. (1993) Collective mind in organizations: Heedful interrelating on flight decks. *Administrative Science Quarterly* 38, 357–81.

Weingart, L.R. (1997) How did they do that? The ways and means of studying group process. *Research in Organizational Behaviour* 19, 189–239.

Weinger, M.B. and Slagle, J. (2002) Human factors research in anaesthesia patient safety: Techniques to elucidate factors affecting clinical task performance and decision making. *Journal of the American Medical Association* 9, S58–S63.

Wittenbaum, G.M., Stasser, G. and Merry, C.J. (1996) Tacit coordination in anticipation of small group task completion. *Journal of Experimental Social Psychology* 32, 129–52.

Wittenbaum, G.M., Vaughan, S.I. and Stasser, G. (1998) Coordination in task-performing groups. In R.S. Tindale, L. Heath, J. Edwards, E.J. Posavac, F.B. Bryant, Y. Suarez-Balcazar, E. Henderson-King and J. Myers (eds) *Theory and Research on Small Groups*. New York: Plenum Press.

Wittenbaum, G.M., Hollingshead, A.B., Paulus, P.B., Hirokawa, R.Y., Ancona, D.G., Peterson, R.S., Jehn, K.A. and Yoon, K. (2004) The functional perspective as a lens for understanding groups. *Small Group Research* 35, 17–43.

Young, G., Zavelina, L. and Hooper, V. (2008) Assessment of workload using NASA task load index in perianesthesia nursing. *Journal of PeriAnesthesia Nursing* 23, 102–10.

Zala-Mezö, E., Wacker, J., Künzle, B., Brüsch, M. and Grote, G. (2009) The influence of standardisation and task load on team coordination patterns during anaesthesia inductions. *Quality and Safety in Health Care* 18, 127–130.

Chapter 14

Identifying Characteristics of Effective Teamwork in Complex Medical Work Environments: Adaptive Crew Coordination in Anaesthesia

Tanja Manser, Steven K. Howard and David M. Gaba

Introduction

The aim of psychological research on the relationship between human performance and patient safety is to support healthcare professionals and their organizations to provide patient care more safely, in a wider variety of clinical situations, with greater efficiency and with increased satisfaction to both patients and practitioners. Such recommendations require an improved understanding of the performance of clinicians in terms of the strengths and vulnerabilities pertaining to their work environment. Although 'performance' is an intuitively meaningful concept, research on human performance in complex work environments usually has to integrate the complementary pieces of information provided by different research approaches, none of which by itself captures the entire picture (Gaba et al. 1998, Rall and Gaba 2004, Salvendy 2006). Sources of information include retrospective analyses of incident reports (i.e., reconstructive approach to human performance), prospective observation of routine patient care (i.e., naturalistic approach to human performance), prospective observation of the response to simulated events (i.e., quasi-experimental approach to human performance) and objective data from artificial laboratory tasks (i.e., experimental approach to human performance).

Both work/organizational psychology and applied cognitive psychology have successfully developed methodological approaches to address human performance issues in complex work environments. The methodological spectrum ranges from ethnographic field studies to experimental studies in laboratory settings and from qualitative interviews to survey instruments (Bungard and Herrmann 1993, Salvendy 2006). However, methods need to be adapted to the specifics of the complex medical work environment. For example, systems to evaluate the performance of two-person cockpit crews will not capture the dynamics of a multidisciplinary medical team with fluid team membership. In recent years, significant progress has been made in this area. Prominent examples are instruments for non-technical skills rating (Fletcher et al. 2004, Healey et al 2004,

Yule et al 2006) and systematic behavioural task analysis (Manser and Wehner 2002, Weinger et al. 1994).

Team Performance and Patient Safety

The process of providing healthcare is inherently interdisciplinary involving physicians, nurses and allied health professionals from different specialties. In the patient safety literature, it has been widely recognized that team performance is crucial to providing safe patient care and that many of the factors contributing to adverse events in healthcare originate from flawed teamwork rather than from a lack of clinical skills. Thus, teamwork has become a key factor addressed by many system-based interventions to improve patient safety and medical education standards (Carthey et al. 2001, Chassin and Becher 2002, Davies 2001, Donchin et al. 1995, Lingard et al. 2004, Manser 2009, Sutcliffe et al. 2004, Wilson et al. 1995). The quality and efficiency of patient care as well as the confidence of patients in healthcare providers were shown to be affected by poor coordination among providers at various organizational levels (Edmondson 1996, Gerteis et al. 1993, Gittell et al. 2000, Young et al. 1998).

It has been argued that there is much rhetoric about how to set up medical teams while the process of teamwork in patient care has not been studied systematically (Cott 1997). Given the importance of teamwork to safe and efficient patient care, both clinical competence and the ability to work in teams need to be assessed when studying the professional behaviour of healthcare providers (Fletcher et al. 2002, Gaba et al. 1998, Wilson et al. 2005). However, many studies of teamwork in healthcare still centre around the main research themes identified by Nagi (1975): (a) status, power, authority, and influence, (b) roles and professional identities, and (c) decision-making and communication (Manser 2009). In recent years significant progress has been made in research on healthcare teams (Manser 2008, Manser 2009) and this progress is clearly documented by the contributions in this book. Aspects of teamwork that were found to correspond to the quality and safety of patient care are, for example, perceived team climate, leadership behaviour furthering open communication, and adaptive coordination and leadership (Manser, 2009).

Adaptive Coordination as a Key Characteristic of Successful Team Performance in Complex Work Environments

In general, teamwork provides the opportunity for pursuing multiple goals and performing multiple interdependent tasks simultaneously. Thus, teams have to share information and resources, plan and synchronize task execution; they have to coordinate and anticipate errors likely to occur (Brannick et al. 1995, Brannick and Prince 1997, Dickinson and McIntyre 1997, Hackman and Morris 1975, Kontogiannis and Kossiavelou 1999). A multitude of definitions regarding the term 'coordination' has been proposed, such as 'the process by which team resources, activities, and responses are organized to ensure that tasks are integrated, synchronized, and completed within established temporal constraints' (Cannon-Bowers et al. 1995, p. 345) or simply 'some kind of adjustment that one or more of the team members make so that the goal is reached' (Brannick and Prince 1997, p. 4).

Studies in many complex work environments show that successful teams adapt their coordination process to the coordination requirements that vary depending on task characteristics (e.g., task complexity, task interdependence), team characteristics such as familiarity of its members (Foushee et al. 1986, Kanki and Foushee 1989), and the situation (e.g., time pressure, routine vs. non-routine procedure) (Kontogiannis and Kossiavelou 1999). For example, effective teams have been described to increase their communication in emergency situations – specifically information exchange and verbalization of plans (Brehmer 1996, Orasanu 1990, Orasanu and Fischer 1992). However, team adaptation is not limited to coordination behaviour. Integrating evidence from empirical studies conducted in various safety critical domains (Burke et al. 2006) have developed a comprehensive model of team adaptation that includes adaptations concerning a) the input into the teamwork process such as a mobilization of additional resources or a structural reconfiguration of the team as well as b) process adaptations, i.e., changes in coordination mechanism, decision making, and communication patterns in response to unexpected events (Brehmer 1996, Entin and Serfaty 1999, Serfaty et al. 1994, Serfaty et al. 1993).

Investigating Adaptive Coordination in Anaesthesia Crews

This chapter addresses the issue of adaptation and adaptability of coordination processes in anaesthesia in the face of changing situational requirements. We pursued the question of adaptive coordination (i.e., the situational management of coordination requirements) initially via an interview study and then in two observational studies. The main results of the interview study will be summarized briefly because they were used in the development of the taxonomy of coordination behaviour used for the two observational studies.

Collaborative Management of Unexpected Events in Anaesthesia

Little empirical evidence exists about how anaesthetists perceive changes in coordination requirements related to different phases of a procedure or different surgical procedures and which coordination strategies they use to maintain good clinical and team performance. Semi-structured interviews focusing on coordination requirements in cardiac anaesthesia were conducted in a tertiary care hospital in the USA with all six anaesthesia attendings who perform cardiac anaesthesia, five third-year anaesthesia residents who had just completed their cardiac rotation, and the only two cardiac surgeons for the hospital (Manser 2006, Manser et al. 2006). Participants were asked to describe the coordination needs within the anaesthesia crew as well as to other members of the perioperative team (a) during different phases of cardiac anaesthesia, (b) for two different surgical procedures, and (c) how these coordination needs change, for example, in case of unexpected clinical events. A qualitative content analysis of the verbatim transcripts was performed (ATLAS.ti Software, Version 5) deductively applying categories derived from the conceptual framework for a team's response to unexpected events proposed by Wehner and colleagues (2000).

Their model of adaptive collaborative practice (see Figure 14.1) emphasizes that within work processes, *initial coordinatedness* has usually evolved over a long period of time based on division of labour.

Unexpected events or disturbances within work processes demand cooperation. *Corrective cooperation* (e.g., workarounds) can help to restore the original coordinatedness by means of collective process-related and situational action. However, if too much corrective cooperation is needed, a remediation of the initial coordinatedness may be necessary. This remediation process involves either expansive cooperation or co-construction. *Expansive cooperation* takes place if the problem requires an expansion of the range of interaction or the number of interaction partners (e.g., solving problems that occur at organizational boundaries). *Co-construction* is an attempt to generate organizational solutions

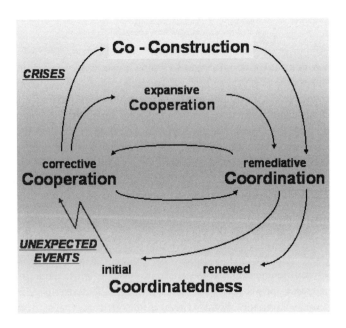

Figure 14.1   Conceptual framework of adaptive collaborative practice (by Wehner et al. 2000)

that transcend single cases (e.g., change projects). In addition to this ideal type of progression, Wehner et al. (2000) outline *self-regulatory processes*, i.e., a short-paced cycle consisting of corrective cooperation and remediative coordination. In this process, the coordinatedness is renewed by means of active coordination behaviour of the local actors, which normally leads to a sufficient adaptation to the situational requirements.

In summary, the results of our interview study show that work processes in cardiac anaesthesia are characterized by interlinked tasks in a multidisciplinary and multiprofessional team that acts within narrow temporal constraints within a complex and highly dynamic work environment. Depending on the surgical procedure and the segment of the case, the task interdependence between anaesthesia crew and surgical crew changes and so do the coordination requirements. Accordingly, there is a high degree of situational variability, not all of which can be planned for in advance but most of which has to be corrected for, swiftly and effectively. This variability and situational flexibility is, to a certain extent, already implemented within the initial coordinatedness. Anaesthetists rely on a combination of initial coordinatedness, anticipation *and* response or reaction to events (i.e., adaptation to situational requirements is achieved mainly through self-regulation as a sub-process of corrective cooperation). All interviewees highlighted the importance of observing the surgical field as it supports the anticipatory handling of unexpected events and of potential breaks in the initial coordinatedness. For example, one anaesthesia attending pointed out that:

> For most procedures [.] you have this kind of ideal course, a template in your brain [.] And then if things start deviating from that template [.] I mean I'm kind of running this program of what should be going on. I'm always comparing it to things that are happening left and right. (A2-1:35)

The adaptation to 'unexpected' events, which not only bear a potential for the breakdown of coordination, but also of harm to the patient, is primarily performed through self-regulatory processes along situational and case-specific peculiarities. The central importance of self-regulation processes is seen in the adaptation of role distribution to situational requirements or in the anticipation of possible breaks in coordinatedness. As the following quote shows, anticipation and adaptation require a detailed knowledge of surgical interventions and therefore a profound understanding of the task procedure linking all team members.

> I think it's really important to recognize that cardiac surgery, cardiac anesthesia is a team sport. It's a team effort and the analogy I frequently make is to ballet. There is a choreography. Everyone has studied it. Everyone knows it. Everyone knows that each has a different part; there's the underlying music. There's the set. Okay, let's go. And then stuff happens. And you know, somebody stumbles or a piece of the set doesn't go where it's supposed to go or whatever. And

so some of what you do is response or reaction. A lot of it is, more of it is anticipation. (A6-2:66)

Development of an Observation System for Adaptive Coordination

The development of this observation system for coordination behaviour in anaesthesia was guided by four aims. Firstly, the observation system should be comprehensive to allow for continuous behaviour coding. Secondly, to allow for a systematic comparison of coordination behaviour and technical as well as non-technical performance ratings in future studies, one key requirement for the observation system was to include only descriptive categories of coordination activities. Thirdly, we decided to include clinical activities performed by the anaesthesia crew in the observation system, because balancing the efforts to coordinate and the efforts to perform the task is a critical aspect of team performance. Finally, the dynamic composition of the anaesthesia crew (i.e., the absence of any of the anaesthesia crew members from the operating room) was recorded because it influences work and coordination patterns.

In developing the observation system we used three information sources: literature review, data from the interviews summarized above and field notes from ethnographic observations.

In a first step, a literature review was conducted focusing on systems to describe and measure coordination behaviour in complex work settings. In our review we included studies from different domains using a spectrum of methodological approaches such as observational studies, verbal protocol analysis, and questionnaires. Ten lists of descriptive categories relevant to coordination behaviour were identified from the literature and analysed to establish which categories they contained and how they were structured (Bowers et al. 1998, Bowers et al. 1993, Grote 2003, Kanki and Foushee 1989, Leedom and Simon 1995, Mackenzie et al. 1993, Marks et al. 2001, Risser et al. 1999, Urban et al. 1995, Xiao et al. 1998, Xiao and LOTAS 2001) (for an overview see Manser et al. 2008). The main difficulties in analysing these systems were that (a) the same concepts were listed on different levels of abstraction in different systems and (b) descriptive categories and evaluation criteria were often summarized within the same system. We integrated the descriptive categories identified from the literature review into a list and then sorted them into groups with common themes at equivalent levels of abstraction.

In a second step, interviews were conducted focusing on strategies for the situational management of coordination requirements in anaesthesia (Manser et al. 2006). The coordination strategies and behaviours derived from this interview study – complemented with field notes prepared during ethnographic observation in the operating room – were used to refine the list of coordination behaviours derived from the literature review and define a prototype of the observation system. In a final step, this prototype was tested and refined using video recordings of anaesthesia inductions for cardiac surgery.

The resulting observation system consisted of 36 mutually exclusive codes that were grouped into observation categories at two levels of abstraction (see Figure 14.2). The category labels for coordination activities were information management, task management, coordination via the work environment, and meta-coordination (i.e., coordination activities team members use to coordinate about their coordination process). To get an accurate picture of the overall communication, we also recorded communication related to teaching (within the anaesthesia crew) and 'other communication' such as coordination activities not related to the actual case but to the overall work process, social communication not related to the task, and non-codable utterances. To allow for an analysis of the distribution of clinical tasks within the anaesthesia crew, the observation system contains three codes for clinical activities: clinical activities performed by anaesthesia crew member A (e.g., the anaesthesia resident), by anaesthesia crew member B (e.g., the anaesthesia attending), or by the (usually) two members of the anaesthesia crew working simultaneously.

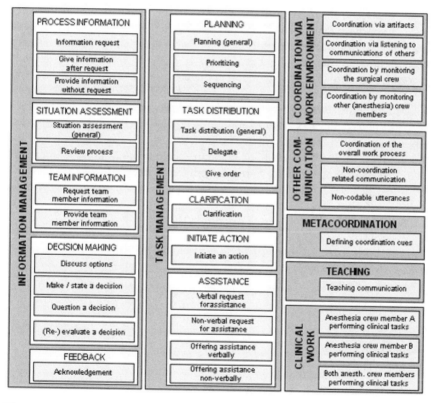

Figure 14.2   Overview of the observation system for coordination behaviour in anaesthesia crews

Data Recording   In both observational studies on adaptive coordination in anaesthesia crews, we used a PDA-based data recording system that allows for the recording of concurrent events such as activities of multiple people as well as multiple activities carried out by one person simultaneously (Held and Manser 2005) (see Figure 14.3). Previously, this data recording system had been used successfully in observational studies of individual anaesthesia care providers (Manser et al. 2007a, Manser and Wehner 2002). The main reason for using this technology was that it can be used for participant observation in the operating room, either in hospital or in a simulation centre, and for behaviour coding using video material. However, the FIT-system software was not originally designed to record as many combinations of behaviour codes including the person performing this behaviour and its target, as needed in this study. As a result, a lot of time-consuming data reformatting and careful checking for any error that may have occurred during this procedure was required.

Coding Reliability   Due to having only one trained observer, a full assessment of the reliability of the coding system has not yet been assessed. We did, however, assess intra-observer agreement over time using randomly selected 10 per cent-segments of videotapes from a full-scale simulator study that were coded a second time six months after the initial coding by the same observer (Manser et al. in press, Manser et al. 2007b). In computing Cohen's Kappa, we: (a) used weights to correct for any influence of the frequency of occurrence, (b) calculated separate values for routine anaesthetic care and crisis management, and (c) allowed for a lag of 2 seconds for onset and offset times as suggested (Bakeman and Gottman 1997) for second by second coding of complex behavioural processes (Held and Manser 2005, Manser et al. 2007a). Good to excellent intra-observer agreement over time was shown for the various observation categories with an overall

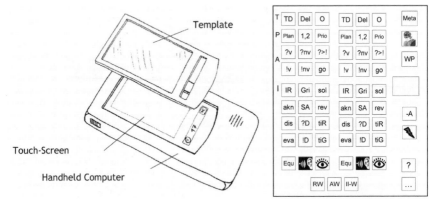

Figure 14.3   System for data recording: FIT-system (left) and template with observation codes including 'buttons' for members of the operating room team (right)

agreement of .85 for routine anaesthetic care and .88 during the management of a simulated anaesthetic crisis (see Table 14.1).

Table 14.1   Intra-observer agreement over time for the observation system reported at the level of observation categories

Observation categories	During routine anaesthetic care	During the management of a simulated anaesthetic crisis
Information management	.80	.86
Task management	.65	.77
Coordination via work environment	.69	.92
Other communication	.86	.57
Metacoordination	.59	Not observed
Teaching	Not observed	Not observed
Clinical work	.92	.92
Overall	**.85**	**.88**

Note: Intra-Observer Agreement given in Cohen's Kappa. Values of .40 to .60 = fair; .60. to .75 = good; over .75 = excellent (Fleiss 1981)

Adaptive Crew Coordination in Anaesthesia: Two Observational Studies

In the following, we summarize the results of two observational studies investigating patterns of adaptive coordination in anaesthesia crews: one field study in the highly complex clinical setting of cardiac anaesthesia and one video-based study of adaptive coordination in the event of a simulated medical emergency. The aims were (a) to test whether the new observation system is sensitive enough to capture adaptation processes in anaesthesia crews, (b) to uncover patterns of adaptive coordination in relation to task characteristics influencing coordination processes (e.g., task interdependence within the perioperative team), and (c) to identify coordination behaviours associated with high clinical performance. In both studies, we focused on the anaesthesia crew. Thus, interactions within the anaesthesia crew, as well as between the anaesthesia crew and other team members (e.g., surgeons, circulating nurse), were recorded. Coordination activities by other members of the operating room team, however, were only recorded when directed towards the anaesthesia crew.

Study 1: Adaptive Coordination in Cardiac Anaesthesia   Study procedure   Over a period of four months in a tertiary care hospital, a trained observer coded the coordination process during 24 cases of cardiac surgery including 16 cases with and 8 without cardiopulmonary bypass (i.e., 123 hours 21 minutes of second-by-second coding of coordination and clinical work processes). In this field study, the anaesthesia crew was equipped with wireless microphones that transmitted to headphones worn by the observer who was positioned adjacent to the anaesthesia workspace. This allowed for accurate coding without disturbing the clinical work process. Data were analysed using the proportion of time spent on each observation category calculated for the overall case duration as well as for each phase of the operation. Multivariate analysis of variance was used to investigate whether different patterns occur during different phases of and between different types of surgical procedures.

Main results   In the following we provide an overview of the results of our field study in cardiac anaesthesia which are reported elsewhere (Manser et al. 2008). In summary, our results indicate that anaesthesia crews dynamically adapt to task requirements. We observed different coordination patterns in response to varying task requirements (a) during different phases of a cardiac anaesthesia case and (b) depending on the type of procedure. We observed a statistically significant increase in both clinical and coordination activity during case segments when the surgical and the anaesthetic task are tightly coupled. Specifically, we found increased coordination activity during the surgical phase including coronary artery bypass grafting. This increase was stronger during coronary artery bypass grafting procedures on the beating heart during which the highest level of interdependence exists between the anaesthesia and the surgical crews due to the criticality of this phase of the procedure (Manser et al. 2006).

Interestingly, the highest level of 'coordination via the work environment' (i.e., an implicit coordination mechanism) was recorded during these periods whereas during other case segments, most time was spent on information management. This result is in line with a key finding of team adaptation research; that teams choose different coordination mechanisms depending on the situational requirements (e.g., explicit vs. implicit coordination mechanisms) (Serfaty et al. 1998, Serfaty et al. 1993, Xiao and LOTAS 2001). Implicit coordination refers to a shared understanding of the task requirements that has usually been established through explicit coordination before engaging in the actual task or during periods of low workload (Orasanu 1990, Orasanu 1993, Wehner et al. 2000, Wittenbaum et al. 1998) and does not necessarily involve verbal communication (MacMillan et al. 2004, Serfaty et al. 1998, Serfaty et al. 1993, Xiao and LOTAS 2001). Implicit coordination is often assumed to be especially effective in high workload situations where resources for explicit coordination may be limited (Entin and Serfaty 1999, Grote et al. 2004). However, empirical evidence on implicit coordination and clinical performance in healthcare teams is scarce and studies show mixed results. Future research needs to systematically include factors potentially mediating these effects. For example, the importance of experience and expertise in effectively using implicit coordination is highlighted by our result that anaesthesia attendings spent more time on coordination and particularly on coordination via the work environment than anaesthesia residents.

Study 2: Adaptive Coordination in the Management of a Simulated Anaesthetic Crisis The goal of this simulator-based study was to systematically analyse the relationship between coordination patterns and clinical performance in the management of a medical crisis situation (Manser et al. 2009).

Study procedure Using the same observation system that was successfully piloted in the field study described above, we coded the coordination processes of anaesthesia crews in 24 scenarios videotaped in a full-scale patient simulator. Study participants were all first-year anaesthesia residents participating in anaesthesia crisis management courses at the Patient Simulation Center of Innovation, VAPAHCS, between 1998 and 2003. The simulator scenario involved a general anaesthetic with a routine phase before the simulated patient experienced an episode of Malignant Hyperthermia (MH). Clinical performance of the anaesthesia crews was rated against the treatment protocol for MH by two independent observers using a time-based scoring system for critical treatment steps (Harrison et al. 2006).

Main results The results of this study are described in detail elsewhere (Manser et al. 2009, Manser et al. 2007b) and are summarized here, with the most important findings highlighted. Firstly, we observed statistically significant changes in clinical work and coordination patterns before and after the declaration of the simulated anaesthetic crisis (i.e., adaptation to the occurrence of a medical crisis). Secondly, the coordination process of anaesthesia crews with higher clinical performance ratings was characterized by significantly less task management, more situation assessment (especially within the anaesthesia crew) and higher levels of information transfer during the first five minutes after declaration of the crisis. Finally, the proportion of monitoring of other anaesthesia crew members – an implicit coordination behaviour aiding in the maintenance of a shared mental model – showed a positive correlation with clinical performance.

Summary and Outlook

The results of the observational studies summarized in this chapter highlight the importance of adaptive patterns of coordination in anaesthesia and complement existing empirical results on coordination in anaesthesia (Grote et al. 2004, Hindmarsch and Pilnick 2002). One aspect of adaptive coordination that has been largely ignored in previous studies (often conducted in work environments with less variation in team composition over time) is the fact that adaptation takes place at different levels of the organization and comprises both process adaptation and structural adaptation (Manser et al. 2008). The observation system described in this chapter has successfully been applied to investigate adaptive coordination behaviour in anaesthesia crews in clinical and simulated work environments. Furthermore, we were able to establish a relationship between certain coordination patterns and clinical performance ratings for a specific anaesthetic crisis in a simulator scenario.

In a current project (see also Chapter 13 by Kolbe et al. in this book), we continue the task-analytic approach to adaptive coordination in anaesthesia crews. This research aims at improving instruments and procedures for team performance assessment by comparing and potentially integrating two observation systems for coordination behaviour. The focus of this project is to empirically evaluate the predictive power of two different observation systems for coordination processes with regard to non-technical skills and clinical performance assessments. Because many assessments of healthcare professionals' work, especially in critical situations, are only possible in a simulator environment, we continue a research strategy using both clinical and simulated research settings to best develop the strengths and counter the limitations associated with either setting. The results of this study will provide an important contribution to improving systems used to assess coordination as a central aspect of team performance. If team performance cannot be assessed accurately, efforts to define specific training needs and to improve team performance may be futile (Manser 2008). In order to define specific competencies that team training should address, to monitor progress, and to finally assess competence, research needs to establish a link between specific behaviours and patient outcome.

Acknowledgements

This research was funded by the Swiss National Science Foundation (PBZH1-100994). We thank the clinical staff at the VAPAHCS, especially the cardiac team and the staff at the Patient Simulation Center of Innovation, for their support in conducting this research. The ongoing study referred to in this chapter is funded by the Swiss National Science Foundation (SNF 100013-116673/1).

References

Bakeman, R. and Gottman, J.M. (1997) *Observing Interaction: An Introduction to Sequential Analysis*. Cambridge: Cambridge University Press.

Bowers, C.A., Morgan Jr, B.B., Salas, E. and Prince, C. (1993) Assessment of coordination demand for aircrew coordination training. *Military Psychology* 5(2), 95–112.

Bowers, C.A., Jentsch, F. Salas, E. and Braun, C. (1998) Analyzing communication sequences for team training needs assessment. *Human Factors* 40(4), 672–9.

Brannick, M.T. and Prince, C. (1997) An overview of team performance measurement. In M.T. Brannick, E. Salas and C. Prince (eds), *Team Performance Assessment and Measurement* (pp. 3–16). Mahwah: Lawrence Erlbaum Associates.

Brannick, M.T., Prince, A., Prince, C. and Salas, E. (1995) The measurement of team process. *Human Factors* 37(3), 641–51.

Brehmer, B. (1996) Dynamic and distributed decision making. *Journal of the Fire Service College* 1(2), 17–36.

Bungard, W. and Herrmann, T. (eds) (1993) Arbeits- und Organisationspsychologie im Spannungsfeld zwischen Grundlagenorientierung und Anwendung [Work and Organizational Psychology in an Area of Tension between Basic and Applied Research]. Bern: Huber.

Burke, C.S., Stagl, K.C., Salas, E., Pierce, L. and Kendall, L. (2006) Understanding team adaptation: A conceptual analysis and model. *Journal of Applied Psychology* 91(6), 1189–207.

Cannon-Bowers, J.A., Tannenbaum, S., Salas, E. and Volpe, C.E. (1995) Defining competencies and establishing team training requirements. In R.A. Guzzo and E. Salas (eds), *Team Effectiveness and Decision Making in Organizations* (pp. 333–80). San Francisco: Jossey-Bass Publishers.

Carthey, J., de Leval, M.R. and Reason, J.T. (2001) The human factor in cardiac surgery: Errors and near misses in a high technology medical domain. *Annals of Thoracic Surgery* 72(1), 300–305.

Chassin, M.R. and Becher, E.C. (2002) The wrong patient. *Annals of Internal Medicine* 136(11), 826–33.

Cott, C. (1997) We decide, you carry it out: A social network analysis of multidisciplinary long-term care teams. *Social Science and Medicine* 45(9), 1411–21.

Davies, J.M. (2001) Medical applications of crew resource management. In E. Salas, C.A. Bowers and E. Edens (eds), *Improving Teamwork in Organizations. Applications of Resource Management Training* (pp. 265–81). Mahwah: Lawrence Erlbaum Associates.

Dickinson, T.L. and McIntyre, R.M. (1997) A conceptual framework for teamwork measurement. In M.T. Brannick, E. Salas and C. Prince (eds), *Team Performance Assessment and Measurement*. Mahwah: Lawrence Earlbaum Associates.

Donchin, Y., Gohper, D., Olin, M., Badihi, Y., Biesky, M., Sprung, C., et al. (1995) A look into the nature and causes of human errors in the intensive care unit. *Critical Care Medicine* 23, 294–300.

Edmondson, A.C. (1996) Learning from mistakes is easier said than done: Group and organizational influences on the detection and correction of human error. *Journal of Applied and Behavioural Science* 32, 5–28.

Entin, E.E. and Serfaty, D. (1999) Adaptive team coordination. *Human Factors* 41(2), 312–25.

Fleiss, J.L. (1981). Statistical Methods for Rates and Proportions. New York: Wiley.

Fletcher, G.C., McGeorge, P., Flin, R.H., Glavin, R.J. and Maran, N.J. (2002) The role of non-technical skills in anaesthesia: A review of current literature. *British Journal of Anaesthesia* 88(3), 418–29.

Fletcher, G., Flin, R., McGeorge, P., Glavin, R.J., Maran, N. and Patey, R. (2004) Rating non-technical skills: Developing a behavioural marker system for use in anaesthesia. *Cognition, Technology & Work* 6, 165–71.

Foushee, H., Lauber, J., Baetge, M. and Acomb, D. (1986) Crew Factors in Flight Operations: III. The Operational Significance of Exposure to Short-haul Air Transport Operations. NASA Technical Memorandum 88322. Washington, DC: National Aeronautics and Space Administration.

Gaba, D.M., Howard, S.K., Flanagan, B., Smith, B.E., Fish, K.J. and Botney, R. (1998) Assessment of clinical performance during simulated crises using both technical and behavioral ratings. *Anesthesiology* 89, 8–18.

Gerteis, M., Edgman-Levitan, S., Daley, J. and Delbanco, T. (1993) *Through the Patient's Eyes: Understanding and Promoting Patient-Centered Care.* San Francisco, CA: Jossey-Bass.

Gittell, J.H., Fairfield, K.M., Bierbaum, B., Head, W., Jackson, R., Kelly, M., et al. (2000) Impact of relational coordination on quality of care, postoperative pain and functioning, and length of stay: A nine-hospital study of surgical patients. *Medical Care* 38(8), 807–19.

Grote, G., Zala-Mezö, E. and Grommes, P. (2003) Effects of standardization on coordination and communication in high workload situations. *Linguistische Berichte* 12, 127–54.

Grote, G., Zala-Mezö, E. and Grommes, P. (2004) The effects of different forms of co-ordination on coping with workload. In R. Dietrich and T.M. Childress (eds), *Group Interaction in High Risk Environments* (pp. 39–55). Aldershot: Ashgate Publishing.

Hackman, J.R. and Morris, C.G. (1975) Group tasks, group interaction process and group performance effectiveness: A review and proposed integration. In L. Berkowitz (ed.), *Advances in Experimental Social Psychology* (Vol. 8) (pp. 45–99). New York: Academic Press.

Harrison, T.K., Manser, T., Howard, S.K. and Gaba, D.M. (2006) Use of cognitive aids in a simulated anesthetic crisis. *Anesthesia and Analgesia* 103(3), 551–6.

Healey, A.N., Undre, S. and Vincent, C.A. (2004) Developing observational measures of performance in surgical teams. *Quality and Safety in Health Care* 13 (suppl 1), i33–40.

Held, J. and Manser, T. (2005) A PDA-based system for online recording and analysis of concurrent events in complex behavioral processes. *Behavior Research Methods, Instruments, & Computers* 37(1), 155–64.

Hindmarsch, J. and Pilnick, A. (2002) The tacit order of teamwork: Collaboration and embodied conduct in anaesthesia. *The Sociological Quarterly* 43(2), 139–64.

Kanki, B.G. and Foushee, H.C. (1989) Communication as group process mediator of aircrew performance. *Aviation, Space, and Environmental Medicine* 60(5), 402–10.

Kontogiannis, T. and Kossiavelou, Z. (1999) Stress and team performance: Principles and challenges for intelligent decision aids. *Safety Science* 33, 103–28.

Leedom, D. and Simon, R. (1995) Improving team coordination: A case for behavior-based training. *Military Psychology* 7(2), 109–22.

Lingard, L., Espin, S., Whyte, S., Regehr, G., Baker, G.R., Reznick, R., et al. (2004) Communication failures in the operating room: An observational classification of recurrent types and effects. *Quality & Safety in Health Care* 13(5), 330–4.

Mackenzie, C.F., Horst, R.L., Mahaffey, M.A. and LOTAS (1993) Group decision-making during trauma patient resuscitation and anesthesia. *Proceedings of the Human Factors and Ergonomics Society 37th Annual Meeting* (pp. 372–6). Santa Monica, CA: Human Factors and Ergonomics Society.

MacMillan, J., Entin, E. and Serfaty, D. (2004) Communication overhead: The hidden cost of team cognition. In E. Salas and S.M. Fiore (eds), *Team Cognition: Understanding the Factors that Drive Process and Performance* (pp. 61–82). Washington: American Psychological Association.

Manser, T. (2006) Selbstregulation als zentrales Element des kooperativen Umgangs mit unerwarteten Ereignissen in komplexen Arbeitssystemen [Self-regulation as a central mechanism to collaboratively manage unexpected events in complex work systems]. In A. Vollmer (ed.), *Kooperatives Handeln zwischen Kontinuität und Brüchen in neuen Tätigkeitssytemen* (pp. 46–80), Lengrich: Pabst.

Manser, T. (2008) Team performance assessment in healthcare: Facing the challenge. *Simulation in Healthcare* 3(1), 1–3.

Manser, T. (2009) Teamwork and patient safety in dynamic domains of healthcare: A review of literature. *Acta Anaesthesiologica Scandinavica* 53(2), 143–151.

Manser, T. and Wehner, T. (2002) Analysing action sequences: Variations in action density in the administration of anaesthesia. *Cognition, Technology and Work* 4, 71–81.

Manser, T., Howard, S.K. and Gaba, D.M. (2006) Self regulation as a central mechanism to collaboratively manage unexpected events in complex work environments. Paper presented at the 13th European Conference on Cognitive Ergonomics (ECCE) Trust and Control in Complex Socio-technical Systems, Zurich.

Manser, T., Dieckmann, P., Wehner, T. and Rall, M. (2007a) Comparison of anaesthetists' activity patterns in the operating room and during simulation. *Ergonomics* 50(2), 246–60.

Manser, T., Harrison, T.K., Howard, S.K. and Gaba, D.M. (2007b) Coordination patterns and clinical performance levels in the management of a simulated anesthetic crisis. In *Proceedings of the 51st Human Factors and Ergonomics Society*, 1–5 October, 2007 (pp. 658–62). Baltimore: Human Factors and Ergonomics Society.

Manser, T., Howard, S.K. and Gaba, D.M. (2008) Adaptive coordination in cardiac anaesthesia: A study of situational changes in coordination patterns using a new observation system. *Ergonomics* 51(8), 1153–78.

Manser, T., Harrison, T.K., Gaba, D.M. and Howard, S.K. (2009) Coordination patterns related to high clinical performance in a simulated anesthetic crisis. *Anesthesia and Analgesia* 108, 1606–1615.

Marks, M., Mathieu, E. and Zaccaro, S.J. (2001) A temporally based framework and taxonomy of team processes. *Academy of Management Review* 26(3), 356–76.

Nagi, S.Z. (1975) Teamwork in health care in the U.S.: A sociological perspective. *The Milbank Memorial Fund Quarterly. Health and Society* 53(1), 75–91.

Orasanu, J. (1990) *Shared Mental Models and Crew Decision Making* (No. 46). Princeton, NJ: Princeton University Cognitive Science Laboratory.

Orasanu, J.M. (1993) Decision making in the cockpit. In E. Wiener, B. Kanki and R. Helmreich (eds), *Cockpit Resource Management* (pp. 137–72). San Diego: Academic Press.

Orasanu, J. and Fischer, U. (1992) Distributed cognition in the cockpit: Linguistic control of shared problem solving. In *Proceedings of the Fourteenth Annual Conference of the Cognitive Science Society*, July 29 to August 1, 1992, Indiana University, Bloomington (pp. 189–794). Hillsdale, NJ: Lawrence Erlbaum Associates

Rall, M. and Gaba, D.M. (2004) Human performance and patient safety. In R.D. Miller (ed.), *Anesthesia*, 6th edition (pp. 3021–72). New York: Elsevier.

Risser, D.T., Rice, M.M., Salisbury, M.L., Simon, R., Jay, G.D. and Berns, S.D. (1999) The potential for improved teamwork to reduce medical errors in the emergency department. The MedTeams Research Consortium. *Annals of Emergency Medicine* 34(3), 373–83.

Salvendy, G. (ed.) (2006) *Handbook of Human Factors and Ergonomics*, 3rd edition. New York: Wiley-Interscience.

Serfaty, D., Entin, E. and Volpe, C. (1993) Adaptation to stress in team decision making and coordination. Proceedings of the Human Factors and Ergonomics Society 38th Annual Meeting (pp. 1228–32). Santa Monica, CA: Human Factors and Ergonomics Society.

Serfaty, D., Entin, E. and Deckert, J.C. (1994) Implicit coordination in command teams. In A.H. Lewis and I.S. Lewis (eds), *Science of Command and Control: Part III: Coping with Change* (pp. 87–94). Fairfax, VA: AFCEA Press.

Serfaty, D., Entin, E. and Johnston, J.H. (1998) Team coordination training. In J.A. Cannon-Bowers and E. Salas (eds), *Making Decision under Stress* (pp. 221–45). Washington: APA Press.

Sutcliffe, K.M., Lewton, E. and Rosenthal, M.E. (2004) Communication failures: An insidious contributor to medical mishaps. *Academic Medicine* 79, 186–94.

Urban, J.M., Bowers, C.A., Monday, S.D. and Morgan Jr, B.B. (1995) Workload, team structure, and communication in team performance. *Military Psychology* 7(2), 123–39.

Wehner, T., Clases, C. and Bachmann, R. (2000) Co-operation at work: A process-oriented perspective on joint activity in inter-organizational relations. *Ergonomics* 43(7), 983–97.

Weinger, M.B., Herndon, O.W., Zornow, M.H., Paulus, M.P., Gaba, D.M. and Dallen, L.T. (1994) An objective methodology for task analysis and workload assessment in anesthesia providers. *Anesthesiology* 80(1), 77–92.

Wilson, K.A., Burke, C.S., Priest, H.A. and Salas, E. (2005) Promoting health care safety through training high reliability teams. *Quality and Safety in Health Care* 14(4), 303–309.

Wilson, R.M., Runciman, W.B., Gibberd, R.W., Harrison, B.T., Newby, L. and Hamilton, J.D. (1995) The Quality in Australian Health Care Study. *Medical Journal of Australia* 163(9), 458–71.

Wittenbaum, G.M., Vaughan, S.I. and Stasser, G. (1998) Coordination in task-performing groups. In R.S. Tindale, J. Edwards and E.J. Posavac (eds), *Social Psychological Applications to Social Issues: Applications of Theory and Research on Groups* (pp. 177–204). New York: Plenum Press.

Xiao, Y. and LOTAS (2001) Understanding coordination in a dynamic medical environment: Methods and results. In M. McNeese, E. Salas and M.R. Endsley (eds), *New Trends in Collaborative Activities: Understanding System Dynamics in Complex Environments* (pp. 242–58). Santa Monica: Human Factors and Ergonomics Society.

Xiao, Y., Mackenzie, C.F., Patey, R. and LOTAS (1998) Team coordination and breakdown in a real-life stressful environment. Proceedings of the Human Factors and Ergonomics Society 42nd annual meeting (pp. 186–90). Santa Monica: Human Factors and Ergonomics Society.

Young, G.J., Charns, M.P., Desai, K., Khuri, S.F., Forbes, M.G., Henderson, W., et al. (1998) Patterns of coordination and clinical outcomes: A study of surgical services. *Health Services Research* 33(5 Pt 1), 1211–36.

Yule, S., Flin, R., Paterson-Brown, S., Maran, N. and Rowley, D. (2006) Development of a rating system for surgeons' non-technical skills. *Medical Education* 40(11), 1098–104.

Chapter 15

Teams, Talk and Transitions in Anaesthetic Practice

Andrew Smith, Catherine Pope, Dawn Goodwin and Maggie Mort

Introduction

Effective communication skills are required for the practice of anaesthesia as they are for any branch of clinical medicine. Despite their importance in practice (Kopp and Shafer 2000, Smith and Shelly 1999) and training (Harms et al. 2004), published work tends to deal with formal, explicit teaching of specific skills such as patient handover (Solet et al. 2005). Communication with patients takes place preoperatively when the anaesthesiologist first meets the patient, on induction of anaesthesia, during surgery (if the patient is conscious), on emergence from anaesthesia and again with the patient postoperatively. Communication also takes place between members of the anaesthetic team – by which we mean anaesthesiologists, their assistants and the recovery room staff. What anaesthesiologists say at these points has seldom been formally studied, and does not feature in traditional textbook teaching on anaesthesia, but seems instead to be learned as part of the informal 'unofficial syllabus' of anaesthetic knowledge (Smith 2007). Further, the issue of how communication is shared between anaesthesiologists and other members of the anaesthetic team does not appear to have been explored. In this chapter we will present data from the Lancaster anaesthetic expertise study, looking at communication between members of the anaesthesia team at a number of transition points: induction of anaesthesia, emergence from anaesthesia and handover of the patient in the recovery room.

Methods

The approval of the local research ethics committees was granted for this study, and written informed consent obtained from patients being cared for by the anaesthesiologists under observation. The study was conducted principally in a medium-sized district hospital in the north-west of England, with shorter periods of observation at a university hospital in the south-west of England. We adopted an ethnographic approach, grounded in detailed observation (Atkinson et al. 2001), followed by a series of in-depth interviews. Ethnography is often used for the in-depth study of complex phenomena within the social context they occur and, as in this study, typically combines a range of methods including observation, interviews and documentary analysis (Pope 2005, Savage 2000). The Lancaster study aimed to explore the ways different types of knowledge are acquired and used in anaesthetic practice. It focused mainly on the operating theatre environment, and included observation of and interviews with anaesthesiologists, operating department practitioners (ODPs)[1] and nurses working in the operating theatre and recovery room (Pope et al. 2003, Smith et al. 2003a). Operating sessions were purposively sampled to cover a range of different types of surgery and anaesthetic practice and levels of anaesthetic expertise.

Most commonly, an individual anaesthesiologist was observed during the course of a routine operating theatre session. We also focused on physical areas, such as the recovery room, and on operating lists where trainer–trainee interactions were taking place. All anaesthesiologists and operating theatre staff were aware of the study. The anaesthesiologists taking part all had the opportunity to decline to be involved either in the study as a whole or in individual observation. The researcher would obtain consent before each observation session. Typically, observation started in the anaesthetic room before the patient arrived and, in some but not all cases, continued until after the patient had been transferred to the recovery room. Conversation between all those in the anaesthetic room – patients, members of the anaesthesia team, surgeons and others who entered the room during this time – was recorded in the form of near-verbatim notes. Observation further continued to include emergence from anaesthesia and then the handover to the recovery room nurse. The researchers recorded, with note book and pencil, the events, talk and behaviour of the anaesthesiologists and other anaesthesia personnel. They aimed to capture the complexity of anaesthesia practice. Immediately after the observation session, these were expanded and annotated, then transcribed for analysis. The interviews we conducted were carried out on a purposively selected cross-section of anaesthesia personnel – physicians, nurses and ODPs.

The analysis was directed towards classifying the communication which occurred at induction, emergence and handover and began with individual close readings and annotations of the observational transcripts by all members of the project team, looking for recurring patterns of talk, behaviour and interaction. These were subsumed into broader categories and themes (Silverman 2001). Discordant data – instances where observed or reported communication differed from the norm or was deemed to be inappropriate in some way – were noted and discussed in detail. Such cases usually stand out in the analysis as they appear contradict the emerging explanation of the phenomena under study and they therefore help to refine the analysis by focussing attention on aspects of the

---

1   The operating department practitioner is a grade of theatre staff unique to the UK. Their two/three-year training course prepares them for three aspects of theatre work: assisting the surgeon, assisting the anaesthesiologist and working in the theatre recovery room.

data which might otherwise have gone unnoticed. Differences in communication between expert and inexperienced practitioners were deliberately sought and examined. These can be especially valuable when a phenomenon such as tacit knowledge in anaesthesia is being studied, as this knowledge may be more easily visible when it is poorly developed or still being formed, as in the observation of trainees at work. The aim of ethnographic research is to produce an account of what is being observed that makes sense to the participants being studied – to get 'under the skin' of what is going on (Pope 2005) and to develop concepts or analytical categories that can be applied to other settings, rather than to produce statistical generalizations. Typically such studies have smaller samples (Silverman 2001, Pope et al. 2000) and a judgement is made that sufficient data have been collected when further analysis of new data yields no new categories or emerging themes ('data saturation': Miles and Huberman 1994). To check the accuracy of our interpretations and findings, some of the research participants were invited to examine the analysis and to tell us if the picture we presented of anaesthetic practice reflected their own experiences and understandings.

Results

Approximately three observation periods were carried out per month over one year, yielding a total of 39 sessions comprising 133 hours of data. At the time we made our observations, there were 12 consultant anaesthesiologists in the department and ten trainees. We observed all but one of the consultants at least once. Of the 31 observations in the operating theatres at the primary site, 13 were of consultants working alone, 12 were a consultant/trainee pair and 6 were of trainees working alone. Nineteen interviews were conducted (Smith et al. 2003a) with anaesthesiologists, anaesthetic and recovery nurses. These interview data were used to supplement and cross-reference the findings from the workplace observation, which was the main focus of our inquiry.

The study as a whole illuminated, for the first time, the interplay of different types of knowledge in professional anaesthetic practice, and how such knowledge is acquired and used. Apart from the general aspects of anaesthetic expertise, we have also been able to draw out more specific aspects of expertise in relation to the use of electronic monitoring (Smith et al. 2003b), regional anaesthesia (Smith et al. 2006a) and the definition and reporting of critical incidents (Smith et al. 2006b), as well as enlightening the sociological discourses of human–machine interaction and distribution of work in interprofessional settings (Goodwin et al. 2005, Mort et al. 2005).

For the purpose of this chapter, we focus on observations of the induction of general anaesthesia on 54 occasions, and of 31 patients emerging from anaesthesia. (The imbalance here arose from the fact that the observers were primarily following the anaesthesiologist, and many patients had been handed over to recovery room personnel before emergence (waking up) from the anaesthetic (Smith et al. 2005)).

We also observed 45 handovers, of which 35 took place in the recovery room, 6 in the operating theatre and 2 in the theatre corridor leading to the recovery room. These involved 17 anaesthetists (9 consultants, 7 trainees and one non-consultant career grade) and 15 recovery nurses (Smith et al. 2008). Illustrative quotes have been selected from this larger pool of data.

Transitions

We noted a number of transitions. There were transitions related to physical movement – from ward, to anaesthetic room, into theatre, into recovery and then back to the ward. There was also movement of the patient from his/her bed onto trolleys, then onto the operating table and back. There were corresponding movements in terms of responsibility for patient care as the patient passes from the nurse, to (in the UK at least) a doctor during the period of anaesthesia, then back to the care of the nurse. There were changes of consciousness, from awake to anaesthetized and back to awake, with some time also spent in liminal interstates, especially in the recovery room. The changes in consciousness are accompanied by the loss of control as patients surrender the management of their vital functions to others, then regain that control on awakening. There are social transitions too, as patients lose their personality and social identity and become more of a physiological object whilst anaesthetized. Along with this goes a degree of intimacy which in 'normal' life would be quite out of place and ways of interacting which treat patients as less competent and/or passive.

Induction of Anaesthesia

We noted three main styles of communication during induction: evocative, descriptive and functional. These three categories arose from the data early in the analysis, suggesting that we reached data saturation readily, and examples of each are given below.

Evocative   These communications seem intended to invoke reassuringly pleasant or familiar images. The effects of sedative or analgesic drugs given before induction are compared to those associated with drinking alcohol. Other calming metaphors are also referred to. For instance, even though time 'stands still' for the patient during anaesthesia, anaesthesiologists often refer to its continuing progress.
Examples:

> Are you sitting comfortably? Then we'll begin.[2]

> (Observation session 27, consultant anaesthesiologist)

---

2   This quote was used to introduce the story in each edition of a British radio programme for pre-school children called 'Listen with Mother', which was popular in the third quarter of the twentieth century.

Descriptive   Here, the anaesthesiologist explains to the patient what he/she might expect to feel:

> 'I'm just going to give you something that will make you feel a little bit drowsy then we'll give you some oxygen to breathe and send you off to sleep.'

> (Observation session 23, consultant anaesthesiologist)

> The anaesthesiologist stands on the left hand side of the patient and continues to inject propofol into the drip tubing. The drug shows white in the tubing. A single snore is heard from the patient. 'You'll start to feel very sleepy.'

> (Observation session 2, consultant anaesthesiologist)

Functional   Here, the talk is largely geared to assessing the depth of anaesthesia or maintaining physiological stability (for instance, by inviting patients to take deep breaths of oxygen from a mask):

> The anaesthesiologist tells the patient to keep the mask on. He attaches the propofol syringe to the cannula. 'Keep your eyes open as long as you can.' (He injects about 10 ml propofol.) 'Are you still with us?' The patient is talking – muffled. He injects another 5 ml. 'Open your eyes Margaret...'

> (Observation session 20, consultant anaesthesiologist)

The three elements were often blended together, as in the following extract, where a pleasant image is curtly interrupted by a more prosaic question about drug allergies:

> Anaesthesiologist: 'I'm sure this will give you a feeling of vodka ... magic milk, coconut rum ... you're not allergic to anything?'

> Patient: 'No.'

> Anaesthesiologist: 'As you go off to sleep ... oxygen over your face ...'
> Anaesthetic assistant: '... magic milk ... cold in your arm ... take you off to dream land ... think about something very pleasant...'

> (Observation session 31, senior house officer)

The above excerpt is also notable for the contribution of the anaesthesiologist's assistant, which was another common finding in our observations. Talk unites the anaesthetic team both in the sense that they may all participate in it, but also because it signals to the rest of the team how the process of induction is progressing. When this is absent, the smooth, predictable sequence of events can be disrupted:

> There have been a couple of other cases where I've felt uneasy really. In one particular instance, the anaesthesiologist gave the anaesthetic without warning the patient and the patient panicked. I felt uneasy then, I felt very uneasy because the patient sat bolt upright and started grabbing hold of her throat and I felt bad because I hadn't warned the patient. I thought the anaesthesiologist was going to do it … the patient was scared stiff … if that was me I would have quite a phobia about coming into theatres now.

> (Interview 11, ODP)

Another case was described where a similar loss of continuity might have occurred, but the assistant realized sooner and was able to act to try to 'repair' the situation:

> While we are waiting for the next patient, (Brian), an ODP, talks to the researcher in the corridor. He talks about what happened with the previous patient. He points out how the anaesthesiologist set the propofol infusion going but didn't tell either him or the patient that she was going off to sleep, he just noticed the infusion going, so he quickly moved to the side of the patient to hold her steady, as she was lying on her side, and reassure her.

> (Notes recorded in theatre during observation session 32)

Anaesthesiologists and the other members of their team thus tend to make use of highly individual communication 'routines' on induction of anaesthesia. Despite their ubiquity, nowhere in our study did we observe these being discussed or taught formally.

Emergence from Anaesthesia

At the end of the surgical operation, the anaesthesiologist must allow the patient to regain consciousness and control of his/her vital functions once more. At the end of anaesthesia, we observed anaesthesia personnel talking loudly to patients, as if talking to the hard of hearing, and usually addressing them by name. Communication tended to fall into the functional category above, as it focused on establishing that the patient was awake – that is, responding to voice or command – and had regained vital physiological functions such as muscle strength, protective airway reflexes and breathing. We also observed some descriptive communication, where an attempt was made to re-orientate or reassure the patient. In some cases, recovery room nurses were the ones who spoke to the patient on emergence. In this extract of a typical routine emergence, the anaesthesiologist and recovery nurse both happen to be present just as the patient is waking up:[3]

A1 disconnects the breathing circuit and connects the portable oxygen.

S1 'Have we got a wedge, she's going to dislocate that hip if we don't put one in…'

RN1 [recovery nurse] enters.

A1 'Freda.'

The scrub nurse hands over to RN1.

A1 'Shall we go then?'

RN1 takes the brakes off the bed.

RN1 'Freda, open your mouth.'

Patient opens her eyes.

A1 holds the patient's hands, repositions the pulse oximeter.

A1 'Looks a bit blue.'

RN1 'Pinking up a bit now.'

RN1 'Open your mouth, nice and wide.'

RN1 removes the laryngeal mask (LM). A1 disconnects the oxygen from the LM and points it at the patient's nose, RN1 connects it to a face mask and puts it on the patient.

A1 'PCA.'

RN1 'I shall connect it if you have prescribed it.'

RN1 changes the pulse oximeter position again.

Pulse oximeter reads 64 per cent … 85 per cent.

---

3   A key to the abbreviations used in the extended transcript extracts can be found at the end of this chapter.

A1 'Nice deep breaths now.' (nudging the patient's shoulder)

RN1 'Relax, operation's finished. All right?'

Patient nods.

(Observation session 29, senior house officer)

Here, both members of the team take part in an unscripted yet collaborative effort. In the next extract, however, the operation finished earlier than expected, leaving the patient temporarily weak from the residual effect of the muscle relaxant drug given at the beginning of the procedure:

A2 'Brian!' (loudly)

10.25

The anaesthetic machine is beeping, ODP1 is tidying up.

A2 '… reversed…'

A2 draws up the drug to reverse the action of the muscle relaxant. A2 replaces the pulse oximeter, it reads 100 per cent. The patient is wheeled to Recovery.

10.26

RN2 is at the head of the patient. The patient is still breathing loudly and laboured, it sounds like a kind of wheeze and a kind of snore, the patient's shoulders move as if it is taking a lot of effort to breathe. The patient's eyes open and close. RN3 attaches some of the monitoring.

A2 '… bit jerky…' (about the patient)

A3 draws up some more reversal agent. RN2 attaches some monitoring.

A2 'I think he might not be completely reversed, RN2, the operation ended rather sooner than we thought …'

A3 gives the reversal agent. Patient twitching.

A2 'Brian, you're in Recovery, do you feel a little bit weak? You will be back to normal in a couple of minutes, just concentrate on your breathing, nice slow deep breaths.'

A2, A3 and RN2 wait, looking at the patient.

A2 'Brian, you're feeling a bit weak, you'll be back to normal in a short while'.

The patient seems to acknowledge this and says yes. After a few moments the patient quietens down, as if he's gone back off to sleep, not struggling to breathe so much. Condensation is seen on the oxygen mask. A2 talks to A3.

A2 'Get an explanation …' The patient opens his eyes and twitches a little bit, not as much as before.

A2 'All right Brian, your operation's finished.'

A3 leaves Recovery. A2 goes to connect the PCA but cannot find the keys initially. Finds the keys and checks the programme. The patient starts to take the pulse oximeter off his finger.

RN2 'Lie nice and still.'

(Observation session 5, consultant anaesthesiologist)

Here, although both nurse and two anaesthesiologists are present, it is the senior anaesthesiologist who does all the talking. Only when the patient has regained strength, and the anaesthesiologist diverts his attention to the patient-controlled analgesia machine, does the nurse enter the conversation.

Handover to Recovery Staff

The handovers we observed took place in amongst many other activities. In the first extract in the box below, the anaesthesiologist is mixing and giving an intravenous antibiotic, writing on the prescription chart and chatting to the nurse as well as passing on relevant clinical information. Many different members of staff were transiently involved in the care of patients in the recovery area, including porters, operating department practitioners, nurses and surgeons and as such, there is considerable movement in and out of this space. There were thus a number of obstacles to, and distractions from, the business of safely handing over the care of the patient recovering from anaesthesia.

Within this study, 'handing over' achieved three objectives: it offered an opportunity to convey the anaesthetist's knowledge of the patient's perioperative care to the receiving nurse in order to facilitate the patient's ongoing care; it marked the transition of responsibility from one professional to the other and it provided an 'audit point' in care to review what has been done and plan for further management. The length and information content of the anaesthetists' handovers we witnessed varied with the complexity of the patient's condition and operation. However, they were typically brief, and concerned with the patient's preoperative state, operation performed, analgesics given in the operating theatre and any problems encountered. An element of familiarity was also seen – anaesthetists often referring to 'my usual' – a combination of anaesthetic drugs and techniques they favoured, which they expected the recovery staff to know. While a brief handover might be expected for a straightforward case, we also observed instances where quite complex problems encountered during anaesthesia– for instance, an unexpected prolonged drop in oxygen saturation just before removal of a breathing tube – were almost glossed over.

The location and timing of the transfer of responsibility varied considerably and did not always coincide with the point of transfer of knowledge described above. The transfer of knowledge did not in itself oblige the nurse to accept responsibility for the patient if he or she considered the knowledge in some way incomplete. How this was determined seemed to depend not on any written protocol or procedure but rather on an informal and unspoken arrangement shaped by mutual trust and experience. Thus, in the second extract the nurse is initially reluctant to accept sole responsibility for the patient, doing so only when the laryngeal mask airway has been removed and the patient is more alert.

Both extracts show a significant feature of recovery handovers, the use of the word 'happy'. The anaesthesiologist asking the nurse if he or she was 'OK' or, more commonly, 'happy', was the usual way of completing the handover. 'Happy' in this context related both to the clinical condition of the patient and the professional relationship between anaesthetist and nurse. In most instances, the reply would be affirmative. Sometimes, though, as in the second extract above, the nurse was clearly not willing for the anaesthetist to go. However, here, as elsewhere, direct contradiction was avoided; her reply, 'You can go but I'd like someone around', was interpreted, as she intended, by the anaesthetist as an indication that he should stay. This he did, until the patient woke up, and his second enquiry ('OK?') was met with agreement. In this extract there is also apparently overt criticism of the anaesthesiologist's behaviour regarding the reusing of a partially used bag of intravenous fluid. However, it is clear from the tone of the dialogue that the two individuals knew each other well and that this was a serious point made in a light-hearted manner. Finally, handover is also used to check that all the actions necessary for the patient's transition back to the ward have been completed (as in the second extract when the nurse asks if postoperative medications and fluids have been prescribed).

Extracts from Observation Transcripts of Handovers in the Recovery Room

1

A4 and ODP2 begin to wheel the patient to Recovery, O1 takes over the foot end of the bed. ODP2 hands the antibiotics to A4. The way out of theatre is a bit cluttered, they bump into another bed on the way to Recovery. In Recovery RN4 (nurse) goes to the head of the patient. She jokes to A4 about the researcher 'oh no, you've got that person following you around'. A4 prepares the antibiotic whilst handing over to RN4.

A4   'Lady, 87... left DHS [dynamic hip screw]. Couldn't get a good sats trace [shaking the antibiotic]. Long history of pulmonary fibrosis.'

A4 hangs the antibiotic, looks closely at it. RN4 looks at the monitor.

RN4   'It was 98% a minute ago.'

A4   'Her sats are absolutely fine, I'm sure.'

A4 is writing on the prescription chart, waiting for the antibiotic to infuse. A4 puts the second antibiotic up.

A4   'She's to have a cup of tea when she gets to the ward.' A4 sits down.

A4   'So, you off out tonight?' (to RN4)

The antibiotic has finished infusing, A4 reattaches the part used bag of fluids, he squeezes all the fluid to the top expelling the air then inserts the giving set.

RN4   'Ooh, you shouldn't do that.'

A4   'Well, I had to give the antibiotics. You happy?'

RN4   'Ecstatic.'

A4 and the researcher leave the recovery room.

(Observation session 4, senior house officer)

2

The patient is transferred to Recovery, A5 lifts and supports the chin as the patient is wheeled to Recovery. A5 hands over to RN5

A5   '12 of morphine, 50 Voltarol PR, fit and well, gas induction, difficult veins ...'

RN5   'Written up for Oramorph? … What about fluid?'

A5   'That's just to go through …'

There are noises coming from the patient which sound like a cross between a loud exhalation and a whine.

RN5   'All right Daniel, open your mouth.'

A5 waits by the patient's side. The LMA moves in the patient's mouth.

A5   'He's just toying with it now.'

RN5   'This is the one who took hours to wake up last time.'

A5   'Are you happy?'

RN5   'I would rather someone was about, you can go but I'd like someone around.'

A5 stays.

10.50

LM is removed by RN5. Daniel coughs and rubs his nose.

RN5 bandages the cannula in.

A5   'OK?'

RN5   'Yeah.'

A5   'I'll just check he is written up for morphine … he should just need that one bag of fluid.'

(Observation session 18, senior house officer)

Discussion

Our recovery room observations revealed a dynamic, rapidly changing environment where staff must care for patients in a risky state often under considerable time pressure. Anaesthetists' handovers were typically brief and took place amidst a range of other activities which compete for the receiving nurse's attention. However, the transfer of information did not automatically lead to transfer of professional responsibility for the patient. How, and at what point, this occurred depended on individual informal negotiation between nurse and anaesthetist and appeared to rely on mutual trust, and balancing differing expectations and power in the relationship (Strauss et al. 1963). The handover also provided an opportunity to review the patient's care and plan further actions, but this too had to be delicately handled as the anaesthetist's practice is being 'laid bare' during the transfer of information.

We deliberately chose an ethnographic approach to build up a detailed picture of anaesthetic practice and knowledge which made sense to the participants. The methods used are ideally suited to situations where such rich detail is required and they provide analyses that are exploratory and descriptive rather than quantifying or measuring behaviour. In this study, our analysis was further enhanced by the range of perspectives within the team – two sociologists with interests both in health and the sociology of science and knowledge, a former anaesthetic nurse and an anaesthesiologist. Qualitative research is sometimes criticized as subjective, because it relies on the researcher to act as the research instrument (in contrast to experimental science which may involve 'objective' measurement tools). To guard against potential bias, qualitative researchers take pains to systematically reflect on and be honest with themselves throughout the course of the research about their own views and feelings and how these might impact on data collection and interpretation.

We identified a number of types of 'talk work' in anaesthetic practice. There was teaching talk, stories (especially what we termed 'atrocity stories' or cautionary tales from experience) and the repetitive, soothing words or phrases forming the communication routines of induction and emergence illustrated above. None of these communication activities are formally taught. In particular, the functions or indeed presence of such talk between the professionals in the anaesthesia team at each of these points is seldom articulated or commented on directly by anaesthesiologists. Communication routines are rooted in tacit knowledge contained in the workplace and are evident in the minimal verbal communication and stock words or phrases are used that gloss or 'stand in' for a series of assumptions and shared knowledge about patient status. Thus collective expertise usually passes unnoticed, un-remarked upon by staff who simply learn by osmosis to 'talk the talk'.

In previous research, Hindmarsh and Pilnick (2002, p. 148) used conversational analysis (a more structured approach to analysing naturally occurring talk) to explore how talk is structured and the moment-to-moment organization of the anaesthetic team interaction. They suggested that talk directed to the patient (e.g., during induction) is principally used as a resource by the anaesthetic team to organize their work. To them, talk 'simultaneously makes features of an individual's work visible and available to their colleagues'. For us, understanding anaesthetic talk is part of understanding the interplay of explicit and tacit knowledge of anaesthetic practice. Expertise in anaesthesia, as in other fields of practice, rests on the successful relationship between these different forms of knowledge. There is 'explicit' knowledge, which is capable of being written down, codified and communicated in textbooks and journals and set out in examination syllabuses. There is also 'tacit' knowledge, defined as 'knowledge that has not been (and perhaps cannot be) formulated explicitly and therefore cannot be stored or transferred entirely by impersonal means' (MacKenzie and Spinardi 1995, p. 45). It is typically acquired via demonstration followed by practice. Our work has begun to unravel the relationship between formal knowledge and the knowledge born of experience in expert anaesthetic practice. Formal training in communication skills is to be welcomed but we would suggest that a substantial amount of teaching and learning of these skills goes on almost unrecognized during the kinds of interactions we have documented. The danger of course is that if safe, effective care depends on the understanding of informal, idiosyncratic procedures and communicative devices, then staff who are not familiar with them pose a threat. These may include locum and agency staff and those from overseas or otherwise different working cultures.

There does not seem to be a great deal in the research literature on how relationships between members of the interprofessional team are negotiated. In the context of handovers, there is a substantial body of research on nurse-to-nurse handovers (Kerr 2002, Manias and Street 2000, Sherlock 1995), and some recent interest in handovers between doctors (Horn et al. 2004, Solet et al. 2005), but little work exploring interprofessional handover. Our data suggest that nurses may sometimes be manoeuvred into taking the responsibility for setting the boundaries of doctors' safe practice – for instance in saying when they consider the anaesthetist can safely leave the patient and return to the operating theatre – and this may prevent them from effectively voicing concerns about safety. Paradoxically, they do appear to influence medical practice, though not in the explicit fashion one would expect in a fully developed 'safety culture', but instead in variable, informal, and less visible ways. Handovers provide an opportunity to check progress and review care. Manias and Street (2000) have suggested that nurse-to-nurse handovers (observed in an intensive care unit) act to maintain conformity of practice, as a nurse's work during the previous shift is under scrutiny by the colleague relieving her or him. Typically, intraoperative problems were underplayed in the handovers we observed. This may simply be because few of them lead to problems in the recovery room, but we suggest that anaesthetists' practice may be similarly exposed to the recovery nurses' subtle and implicit judgement of what constitutes an acceptable clinical standard. Whatever the circumstances, the handover process must still be conducted to the satisfaction of both parties, and take place in such a way that neither party 'loses face' so that future encounters are not jeopardized (Goffman 1967). One characteristic of safety-sensitive organizations is that everyone, no matter how junior they are, feels free to voice concerns about safety (Sexton et al. 2000, Smith et al. 2006b). In the context of anaesthetic practice this has to be done using coded language and without confrontation. This informal, implicit approach goes against the standardized approaches to handover in safety critical industries (Arora and Johnson 2006, Patterson et al. 2004).

Conclusion

Approaches to improving care relying on protocol and standardization are widely promoted as ways of enhancing patient safety. We argue that, unless the tacit and implicit cultural factors underlying interprofessional working and communication in the operating theatre are taken into account, such approaches will not achieve their potential. In research terms, future work might usefully explore the effect of different styles of communication on patient anxiety, patient satisfaction, anaesthetic team performance and markers of patient safety.

Key to Extended Transcript Extracts

A	Anaesthetist
O	Orderly or porter
ODP	Operating department assistant
RN	Recovery room nurse
N	Surgical nurse
S	Surgeon
LM/LMA	Laryngeal mask airway (airway management device)
PCA	Patient-controlled analgesia machine

Names, where given, have been changed.

References

Arora, V. and Johnson, J. (2006) A model for building a standardized hand-off protocol. *Joint Commission Journal on Quality and Patient Safety* 32, 646–55.

Atkinson, P., Coffey, A., Delamont, S., Lofland, J. and Lofland, L. (eds) (2001) *Handbook of Ethnography*. London: Sage Publications.

Goffman, E. (1967) *Interaction Ritual: Essays on Face to Face Behavior*. New York: Doubleday.

Goodwin, D., Pope, C., Mort, M., and Smith, A. (2005) Access, boundaries and their effects: Legitimate participation in anaesthesia. *Sociology of Health and Illness* 27, 855–71.

Harms, C., Young, J.R., Amsler, F., Zettler, C., Scheidegger, D. and Kindler, C.H. (2004) Improving anesthesiologists' communication skills. *Anaesthesia* 59, 166–72.

Hindmarsh, J. and Pilnick, A. (2002) The tacit order of teamwork: Collaboration and embodied conduct in anaesthesia. *Sociological Quarterly* 43, 139–64.

Horn, J., Bell, M.D.D. and Moss, E. (2004) Handover of responsibility for the anaesthetised patient – opinion and practice. *Anaesthesia* 59, 658–63.

Kerr, M.P. (2002) A qualitative study of shift handover practice and function from a socio-technical perspective. *Journal of Advanced Nursing* 37, 125–34.

Kopp, V.J. and Shafer, A. (2000) Anesthesiologists and perioperative communication. *Anesthesiology* 93, 548–55.

MacKenzie, D. and Spinardi, G. (1995) Tacit knowledge, weapons design and the uninvention of nuclear weapons. *American Journal of Sociology* 101, 44–99.

Manias, E. and Street, A. (2000) The handover: Uncovering the hidden practices of nurses. *Intensive and Critical Care Nursing* 16, 373–83.

Miles, M.B. and Huberman, A.M. (1994) *Qualitative Data Analysis. An Expanded Sourcebook*, 2nd edition. Thousand Oaks, CA: Sage Publications.

Mort, M., Goodwin, D., Smith, A.F. and Pope C. (2005) Safe asleep? Human-machine relations in medical practice. *Social Science and Medicine* 61, 2027–37.

Patterson, E.S., Roth, E.M., Woods, D.D., Chow, R. and Gomes, J.O. (2004) Handoff strategies in settings with high consequences for failure: Lessons for health care operations. *International Journal of Quality in Health Care* 16, 125–32.

Pope, C. (2005) Conducting ethnography in medical settings. *Medical Education* 39, 1180–7.

Pope, C., Ziebland, S. and Mays, N. (2000) Analysing qualitative data. *British Medical Journal* 320, 114–16.

Pope, C., Smith, A., Goodwin, D. and Mort, M. (2003) Passing on tacit knowledge in anaesthesia: A qualitative study. *Medical Education* 37, 650–5.

Savage, J. (2000) Ethnography and health care. *British Medical Journal* 321, 1400–1402.

Sexton, J.B., Thomas, E.J. and Helmreich, R.L. (2000) Error, stress and teamwork in medicine and aviation: Cross sectional surveys. *British Medical Journal* 320, 745–9.

Sherlock, C. (1995) The patient handover: A study of its form, function and efficiency. *Nursing Standard* 9, 33–6.

Silverman, D. (2001) *Interpreting Qualitative Data: Methods for Analysing Talk, Text and Interaction*, 2nd edition. London: Sage Publications.

Smith, A.F. (2007) Reaching the parts that are hard to reach: Expanding the scope of professional education in anaesthesia. *British Journal of Anaesthesia* 99, 453–6.

Smith, A.F. and Shelly, M.P. (1999) Communication skills for anesthesiologists. *Canadian Journal of Anesthesia* 46, 1082–8.

Smith, A.F., Goodwin, D., Mort, M. and Pope, C. (2003a) Expertise in practice: An ethnographic study exploring acquisition and use of knowledge in anaesthesia. *British Journal of Anaesthesia* 91, 319–28.

Smith, A., Mort, M., Goodwin, D. and Pope, C. (2003b) Making monitoring 'work': Human-machine interaction and patient safety in anaesthesia. *Anaesthesia* 58, 1070–8.

Smith, A.F., Pope, C., Goodwin, D. and Mort, M. (2005) Communication between anesthesiologists, patients and the anesthesia team: A descriptive study of induction and emergence. *Canadian Journal of Anesthesia* 52, 915–20.

Smith, A.F., Goodwin, D., Mort, M. and Pope, C. (2006a) Adverse events in anaesthetic practice: Qualitative study of definition, discussion and reporting. *British Journal of Anaesthesia* 96, 715–21.

Smith, A., Pope, C., Goodwin, D. and Mort, M. (2006b) What defines expertise in regional anaesthesia? An observational analysis of practice. *British Journal of Anaesthesia* 97, 401–407.

Smith, A.F., Pope, C., Goodwin, D. and Mort, M. (2008) Interprofessional handover and patient safety in anaesthesia: Observational study of handovers in the recovery room. *British Journal of Anaesthesia* 101, 332–337.

Solet, D.J., Norvell, J.M., Rutan, G.H. and Frankel, R.M. (2005) Lost in translation: Challenges and opportunities in physician-to-physician communication in patient handoffs. *Academic Medicine* 80, 1094–9.

Strauss, A., Schatzman, L., Ehrlich, D., Bucher, R. and Sabshin, M. (1963) The hospital and its negotiated order. In E. Freidson (ed.) *The Hospital in Modern Society*. New York: Free Press.

PART III
Observation of Theatre Teams

Chapter 16

An Empiric Study of Surgical Team Behaviours, Patient Outcomes, and a Programme Based on its Results

Eric Thomas, Karen Mazzocco, Suzanne Graham, Diana Petitti, Kenneth Fong, Doug Bonacum, John Brookey, Robert Lasky and Bryan Sexton

Introduction

As one of five principles for creating safe systems of healthcare delivery, the Institute of Medicine (IOM) report on medical error (Kohn et al. 2000) concluded that healthcare organizations need to 'promote effective team functioning.' Their recommendation for promoting team behaviour was based primarily upon qualitative research methodologies and approaches such as root cause analyses. In the airline industry, research linking effective team functioning to flight safety led to specific training in teamwork that was subsequently associated with improvements in safety. Healthcare settings involving high risk of harm such as labour and delivery (Sexton et al. 2006b), critical care (Pronovost et al. forthcoming) and especially surgery (Makary et al. 2006a, Sexton et al. 2006c) share many of the same fundamental elements of the airline industry, where people are working with other people in a high-tech and high risk work environment. Research suggests the need for improved teamwork and communication in neonatal intensive care (Falck et al. 2003, Halamek et al. 2000, Thomas et al. 2006) emergency departments (Morey et al. 2002) the operating room (Carthey et al. 2003, Makary et al. 2006b), trauma resuscitation (Santora et al. 1996, Sugrue et al. 1995, Xiao et al. 1996) and among residents of all disciplines (Sutcliffe et al. 2004).

Nevertheless, very little quantitative research has assessed the relationship between team behaviours and outcomes in healthcare. Despite a significant amount of rhetoric around teamwork, team training and the impact of communication breakdowns, the evidence that directly links the interpersonal interactions of caregivers to the outcomes of their patients has not been well documented. For example, two recent reviews concluded that no studies have shown that team training can improve teamwork and the quality of care (Baker et al. 2005, Salas et al. 2006) and a cluster randomized trial of team training for labour and delivery teams did not find significant changes in process of care or outcome measures (Nielsen et al. 2007). Knowledge about how to improve team behaviour appears to be in its infancy. We conducted and have published the results of study to determine whether patients of surgical teams who exhibited good teamwork had better outcomes than patients of teams with poor teamwork (Mazzocco et al. 2008). We summarize this study's methods and findings and go on to describe how the data from the study were used to develop and implement a multi-institutional programme to improve surgical teamwork.

Methods

This study was conducted in the operating rooms of two medical centres and two ambulatory surgical centres affiliated with the Kaiser Foundation Health Plan in the USA. It involved structured observation of personnel (surgeons, anaesthesiology providers, nurses, technicians and others) doing surgical procedures at the four sites during the period from March to August, 2005 and assessment of 30-day post-surgical outcomes (by retrospective chart review) of patients whose surgical team had been observed.

Observed providers consented in writing to be observed. We approached 149 physicians, registered nurses, operating room technicians and nurse anaesthetists; 19 (12.7 percent) declined to participate. Provider consent was first sought after presentation of information about the project at a regular meeting of the provider group. Some provider groups (surgeons, MD anaesthesiologists and Certified Registered Nurse Anaesthetists) voted at the information meeting to participate universally, although 2 of 44 of the physicians attending the informational meeting declined in spite of this group vote. Seventeen of 69 (25 percent) nurses and technicians attending the informational meeting initially declined to participate in the study but some of these providers consented to have specific procedures observed when they were asked at the time the procedure was selected. Providers who did not attend the informational meetings were asked whether or not they consented to participate in having specific procedures observed but the consent rate by provider was not tracked for these individuals. Patients were observed if they did not opt out of observation after being informed of the study during their pre-operative visit (29 patients opted out of the study). The study sample size of 300 surgical cases was chosen based on resource and time availability. A statistical power analysis done *a priori* based on the sample size showed that the study had a power of 0.95 to detect a correlation of 0.20 or more between a rating of team behaviour on a four-point scale and rating of outcome on a five-point scale using a two-tailed statistical test. The study was reviewed and approved by the Kaiser Permanente Institutional Review Board for protection of human subjects.

Observers and Training

Observers of the surgical procedures were all registered nurses. Standardization of observations and calibration between observers was achieved in a training session given at the Johns Hopkins University Quality and Safety Research Group. Training of four registered nurse observers included an overview of behavioural observation and peri-operative teamwork, and a series of calibration exercises whereby observers watched video clips of team behaviours, rated the frequency with which the behaviours occurred on the data collection form used in the study, and then debriefed the exercise to discuss discrepancies and verbally justify their ratings. This iterative process involved observing, rating and debriefing five videos, during which time the real-time calibration level of the observers was calculated and shared with the observers using a within group measure of inter-rater agreement (RWG) (James et al. 1984), requiring a .70 cut-off for acceptable agreement.

Behavioural Markers

The study defined team function based on behavioural markers (Klampfer et al. 2001). Behavioural markers are observable, non-technical behaviours that have been demonstrated empirically to contribute to performance in work environments, including the airline industry (Sexton et al. 2000) and healthcare (Thomas et al. 2004). Behavioural marker data were collected using a standard instrument adapted for this study (Thomas et al. 2006).

The instrument used in this study assessed the following six behaviour domains: briefing, information sharing, inquiry, assertion, vigilance and awareness, and contingency management. Operational definitions for behaviours in each domain are given in Table 16.1 (Mazzocco et al. 2008). For each domain, the observer gave the surgical team a score from 0 to 4 on how often the specified behaviours related to that domain were observed. A score of 0 was given if the behaviours were never observed; 1 if the behaviours were observed rarely; 2 if there were isolated examples of the behaviour; 3 if the behaviours were observed intermittently; and 4 if behaviours were observed frequently throughout the observation period. For each domain, separate team scores were assigned for the induction, intra-operative and hand-off (transition to the next level of care) phases of the procedure.

Selection of Procedures for Observation

Procedures were selected for observation on the morning of the surgery based on consent of all team members to be observed, compatibility with the operational needs of the surgical suite, anticipated length of the procedure and availability of the observer. Each selected procedure was observed by one observer, who joined the team to begin observation when the patient was brought to the operating room. Observation ended when the patient was taken out of the operating room and handed off to the next level of care.

Table 16.1   Description of domains behavioural markers of team behaviour assessed by the observers

Behavioural Marker Domain	Description
Used in univariate analysis and calculation of Behavioural Marker Risk Index	
Briefing	Situation/relevant background shared; patient, procedure, site/side identified; plans are stated; questions asked; ongoing monitoring and communication encouraged
Information sharing	Information is shared; intentions are stated; mutual respect is evident; social conversations are appropriate
Inquiry	Asks for input and other relevant information
Vigilance and awareness	Tasks are prioritized; attention is focused; patient/equipment monitoring is maintained; tunnel vision is avoided; red flags are identified
Not used in univariate analysis calculation of Behavioural Marker Risk Index	
Assertion	The members of the team are speaking up with their observations and recommendations during critical times
Contingency management	Relevant risks are identified; back-up plans are made and executed

Adjustment Variables and Outcomes

The American Society of Anesthesiologists (ASA) score assigned by the anaesthesiologist was recorded. The ASA score subjectively categorizes patients into five sub-groups by preoperative physical fitness and appear in Table 16.2 (Mazzocco et al. 2008).

The ASA score was devised in 1941 by the ASA as a statistical tool for retrospective analysis of hospital records and has been revised periodically (Walker 2002). In nine patients, the ASA score was not recorded in either the medical record or on the observation sheet. In these cases, an anaesthesiologist independent of the study reviewed information on patient characteristics obtained from the medical record review and assigned an ASA score.

The surgical procedures were classified as low, medium or high risk for post-operative complications according to American College of Cardiology and American Heart Association guidelines (Eagle et al. 2002). Low risk procedures included biopsy, excision of mass, hernia repair and laparoscopic cholecystectomy;

Table 16.2   Definitions of measures: patient risk of complications (American Society of Anesthesiologists – ASA – classification), procedure risk (American College of Cardiologists – ACC-score) and outcome (outcome score)

Measure	Definition	Example
ASA patient classification		
I	Completely healthy patient	A fit patient
II	Patient with mild systemic disease	Essential hypertension, mild diabetes without end organ damage
III	Patient with severe systemic disease that is not incapacitating	Angina, moderate to severe COPD[†]
IV	Patient with incapacitating disease that is a constant threat to life	Advanced COPD, cardiac failure
V	A moribund patient who is not expected to live 24 hours with or without surgery	Ruptured aortic aneurysm, massive pulmonary embolism
ACC/AHA procedure risk[*]		
Low	Low risk of non –cardiac complications	Biopsy, excision of mass, hernia repair, laparoscopic cholecystectomy
Medium	Medium risk of non-cardiac complications	Mastectomy, thoracotomy, thyroidectomy, exploratory laparotomy
High	High risk of non-cardiac complications	Repair of abdominal aortic aneurysm
Outcome score		
1	No complications	
2	One or more indicators of potential harm	
3	Minor complication	
4	Major complication	
5	Death or permanent disability	

[*]   Procedures listed as examples for the ACC/AHA procedure risk accounted for 85 percent of all procedures observed in this study.

[†]   Chronic Obstructive Pulmonary Disease.

medium risk included open laparotomy, carotid endarterectomy and thyroidectomy; and high risk included aortic aneurysm repair and femoral popliteal bypass. The 30-day outcome of each observed procedure was determined by medical record review using a standard instrument. The medical record reviewer was blinded to the behavioural risk index. Each reviewer had a list of common surgical complications (see the Appendix to this chapter) and these complications and other significant outcomes were grouped into five outcome categories: (1) no complications; (2) one or more indicators of potential harm (change in procedure; intubation/reintubation/ BiPap in PACU; non-routine X-ray intra-operative or in PACU; intra-op epinephrine or norepinephrine use; post op Troponin level > 0.5; change anaesthetic during surgery; consult requested in Post Anaesthetic Care Unit (PACU); path report normal or unrelated to diagnosis; and insertion of arterial or central venous line during surgery.); (3) minor complication characterized by one of the following: prolonged, unplanned operative time (e.g., greater than 1.5 × expected time); post-operative transfer to a higher level of care; unplanned return to surgery (within 72 hours); and unplanned ventilatory support for greater than 24 hours or more post-operatively; (4) major intra- or post-operative complication characterized by: prolonged, unplanned operative time (e.g., greater than 1.5 × expected time); post-operative transfer to a higher level of care; unplanned return to surgery (within 72 hours); unplanned ventilatory support for greater than 24 hours or more post-operatively (i.e., inability to extubate); unplanned emergency intervention by the surgical team or code team; and (5) death or permanent disability.

Behaviour Risk Index

For each procedure/team, the behavioural marker data were summarized using a single score, the Behavioural Marker Risk Index (BMRI), following the approach used by researchers studying group interactions in high risk environments (Dietrich and Childress 2004). Based on inspection of the univariate behavioural marker data, the markers assertion and contingency management were excluded from the BMRI because they were rarely observed in these generally low risk procedures done on mostly low and intermediate risk patients.

The BMRI calculates the percent of ratings of behaviour made during the procedure that were less frequent than a rating of 3, or intermittent. BMRI was calculated by assigning a value of 1 if the observer rating for the domain was 0 (behaviour never observed) or 1 (behaviour rarely observed) or 2 (isolated or minimal observation of the behaviour). These values were summed across all phases of surgery for the four behavioural marker domains and then divided by the total number of domains/phases in which an observation was made. The BMRI thus had a range from 0.0 to 1.0 where values closer to 0.0 indicated more frequent observations of team behaviour. Those closer to 1.0 indicated less frequent observations of team behaviour (or as the label implies, 'riskier' team behaviour). The valence of the BMRI means that positive correlations of the BMRI with the patient outcome score reflect an association of failure to observe 'good team behaviour' with worse outcomes.

Analysis

Patient characteristics were summarized using means, counts and percent distributions as appropriate to the distribution of the variable.

For descriptive analysis, patient outcomes were categorized into two categories – 'complications or death' or 'no complications or death.' The first category included patients with both major and minor complications in addition to deaths. The second category included patients with one or more indicators of potential harm in addition to no complications. For each operative phase and BMRI domain, the increased odds of having complications or death associated with lower scores for team behaviour (0–2) were estimated by calculating odds ratios (OR) and 95 percent confidence intervals (CI). Multiple logistic regressions were calculated to assess the independence of the associations of the BMRI domains with outcome after taking into account the ASA patient risk score. Two-way interactions involving the BMRI domains with the ASA patient risk were considered but were not significantly (p>0.20) related to the outcome and not included in the final adjusted models.

Similar unadjusted and adjusted odds ratios and 95 percent confidence intervals were calculated by logistic regressions with the BMRI as the predictor variable, the ASA patient risk score as the covariate adjusted for in the adjusted model, and 'complications or death' as the predicted outcome. Finally, we used the logistic regression model to calculate the predicted relationship between the BMRI and the OR for complications and death. Statistical analyses were conducted using SPSS version 14.0.

Results

Observer calibration was achieved to a RWG of 0.9 for the two main observers and a RWG calibration of 0.85 for all observers at the conclusion of training. A total of 300 patients/procedures were observed. The medical records for seven patients could not be located, so their observational data was excluded from the analysis. Table 16.3, reproduced from the prior publication (Mazzocco et al. 2008), shows characteristics of the 293 observed patients and procedures included in the analysis. The patients were mostly middle-aged. The gender and race/ethnicity distribution were generally representative of Kaiser Permanente members undergoing general surgery procedures at the participating hospitals. The patients were mostly low and medium risk; there were no patients in the ASA category V and only five in the ASA high risk category. All but four of the procedures were ACC/AHA low or intermediate risk. More than one-half of the procedures had 'no complications' as the outcome rating. Three patients had an outcome of death or disability. In

Table 16.3   Characteristics of 293 patients and procedures

Characteristics	N	%
Age range		
18–34	44	(15)
35–49	64	(22)
50–74	145	(49)
75+	40	(14)
Race/ethnicity		
Asian/Pacific Islander	10	(3)
African American	26	(9)
Hispanic	49	(17)
Non-Hispanic white	188	(64)
Missing	20	(7)
Gender		
Female	174	(59)
Male	119	(41)
ASA classification		
I	47	(16)
II	155	(53)
III	86	(29)
IV	5	(2)
V	0	(0)
ACC/AHA procedure risk		
Low	233	(80)
Medium	56	(19)
High	4	(1)
Outcome		
No complications	158	(54)

Table 16.3   *Concluded*

Characteristics	N	%
One or more indicators of potential harm	71	(24)
Minor complication	48	(16)
Major complication	13	(4)
Death or disability	3	(1)
Behavioural Marker Risk Index categorical ranges		
0.00–0.24	83	(28)
0.25–0.49	136	(46)
0.50–0.74	56	(19)
0.75–1.00	18	(6)

about 25 percent of procedures, the BMRI was more than 0.50 indicating a high proportion of operative phases and domains with infrequent observation of good team behaviours.

Table 16.4 (Mazzocco et al. 2008) shows, for each operative phase (induction, intra-operative, hand-off) and behavioural marker domain, the behavioural marker scores after dichotomizing them into categories of less frequent (0–2) or more frequent (3–4) observation of 'good' team behaviours along with the percentage of more frequent observation of good team behaviours. The table also shows the number and percentage of patients/procedures with a complication (major or minor) or death according to these scores by operative phase and behavioural marker domain along with the ORs and 95 percent CIs for complication or death for patients/procedures with scores indicating less frequent observation of 'good' team behavior. Because the referent in this analysis is patients with scores indicating more frequent observation of 'good' team behaviours, an OR above 1.0 indicates an association of less frequent team behaviors with poorer outcome.

For most of the phases and domains, good team behaviours were observed frequently or always (scores 3–4) in a substantial percentage of procedures; however, for none of the phases or domains were good teams behaviours observed frequently or always, all of the time.

The ORs for complication or death were greater than 1.0 when team behaviours were observed less frequently (scores 0–2) in all operative phases and behavioral domains except the briefing domain of the intra-operative phase and the vigilance domain of the hand-off domain. The OR estimates for complication or death excluded 1.0 in association with low scores for the information sharing domain of the intra-operative phase (OR 2.45; 95 percent CI 1.36–4.42) and for the briefing

Table 16.4　Description of behavioural markers scores by operative phase, number and percentage of procedures with complication or death, and odds ratios (OR) and 95 per cent confidence intervals (CI) for complication or death for less frequent observation of 'good' team behaviours

Operative Phase and Behavioral Marker Domain	Score	Teams/ Procedures		Major or Minor Complications or Death			
		N	% of Total	n	(%)	OR*	95% C.I.
Induction Phase							
Briefing	0-2†	71		20	(28)	1.59	(0.86-2.93)
	3-4‡	222	(76)	44	(20)	referent	--
Information sharing	0-2†	48		12	(25)	1.24	(0.60-2.55)
	3-4‡	145	(84)	52	(21)	referent	--
Inquiry score	0-2†	118		28	(24)	1.20	(0.69-2.10)
	3-4‡	175	(60)	36	(21)	referent	--
Vigilance	0-2†	38		13	(34)	2.08	(0.99-4.35)
	3-4‡	255	(87)	51	(20)	referent	--
		N	% of Total	n	(%)	OR*	95% C.I.
Intraoperative Phase							
Briefing	0-2†	258		56	(20)	0.94	(0.40-2.17)
	3-4‡	35	(12)	8	(23)	referent	--
Information sharing	0-2†	76		26	(34)	2.45	(1.36-4.42)
	3-4‡	217	(74)	38	(18)	referent	--
Inquiry	0-2†	145		34	(23)	1.20	(0.69-2.10)
	3-4‡	147	(50)	30	(20)	referent	--
Vigilance	0-2†	89		23	(26)	1.39	(0.77-2.49)
	3-4‡	204	(70)	41	(80)	referent	--

and information sharing domains of the hand-off phase (OR 2.34; 95 percent CI 1.23–4.46 and OR 2.21; 95 percent CI 1/18–4.16, respectively). The elevated OR for complication or death was close to 1.0 in association with a low score for the vigilance domain of the induction phase (OR 2.08; 95 percent CI 0.99–4.35). There were no significant findings for the remaining behavioural markers.

Table 16.4 *Concluded*

		N	% of Total	n	(%)	OR*	95% C.I.
Handoff Phase							
Briefing	0-2†	54		19	(35)	2.34	(1.23-4.46)
	3-4‡	239	(82)	45	(19)	referent	--
Information sharing	0-2†	59		20	(34)	2.21	(1.18-4.16)
	3-4‡	234	(80)	44	(19)	referent	--
Inquiry	0-2†	175		43	(25)	1.50	(0.84-2.70)
	3-4‡	118	(40)	21	(18)	referent	--
Vigilance	0-2†	84		18	(21)	0.97	(0.52-1.79)
	3-4‡	209	(71)	46	(22)	referent	--

*　　Odds ratio for a major or minor complication or death in teams with score of 0–2 for markers of team behavior relative to score of 3-4 for markers of team behaviors

† scores of 0-2 indicate that markers of 'good' team behavior were never or rarely observed or there was isolated or minimal observation of the behaviors

‡ scores of 3-4 indicate that markers of 'good' team behavior were observed often or always

Table 16.5 (Mazzocco et al. 2008) shows the results of the logistic regression models using the BMRI and ASA as predictors and surgical outcome as the dependent variable. Odds ratios greater than 1.0 indicate an association of less frequently observed 'good' behaviour with poorer outcome. The BMRI was significantly associated with any complication or death after adjusting for ASA score (adjusted OR 4.82, 95 percent CI 1.30, 17.87). In other words, when teamwork behaviours were relatively infrequent during surgical procedures, patients were more likely to experience death or a major complication.

Table 16.5　The association of the Behavioural Marker Risk Index with post-operative complications and death

	Unadjusted Odds Ratio	95% C.I. on the unadjusted OR	p-value (Wald test)	Adjusted# Odds Ratio	95% C.I. on the adjusted OR	p-value* (Wald test)
Risk factor						
BMRI	5.61	1.53, 20.54	0.009	4.82	1.30, 17.87	0.019
ASA	1.59	1.06, 2.38	0.024	1.51	1.00, 2.27	0.049

Figure 16.1 (Mazzocco et al. 2008) graphically shows the positive association between the BMRI (with a higher score indicating fewer instances of teamwork behaviour) and poorer patient outcome as predicted by our logistic regression model.

Discussion

Principal Findings and Conclusions from the Published Study

We found that patients whose surgical teams exhibited less teamwork behaviours were at higher risk for death or complications, even after adjusting for ASA risk category. We believed that was an important addition to the international conversation on teamwork in healthcare, providing quantitative evidence of a direct link between teamwork during the surgical case and subsequent patient outcome. This discussion reiterates the strengths and limitations of the prior study (Mazzocco et al. 2008) and expands our previous publication by an in-depth discussion of previous research and by describing team training programmes that followed this study.

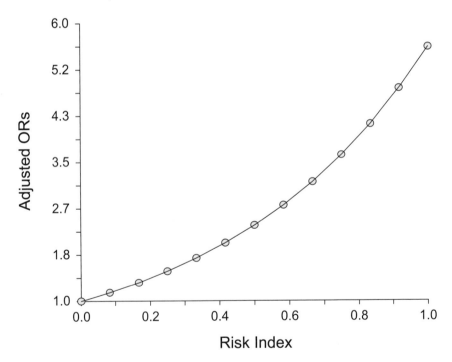

Figure 16.1 The predicted relationship between Behavioral Marker Risk Index and post-operative complications and death

Strengths and Limitations

Our study had several strengths. It was conducted in a community setting that is likely to be representative of surgical procedures. A variety of procedures were observed and the teams were diverse. The outcomes were ascertained with the reviewer blinded to the team behaviour scores. Behavioural markers have been applied to healthcare settings such as neonatal resuscitation (Thomas et al. 2006), and this study builds on that work. We modified the behavioural markers and the observation tool to apply to the operating room environment and used the same calibration techniques for our nurse observers as those used in prior studies. Continuous communication among the observers throughout the study ensured a sustained level of inter-rater reliability.

The study has some important limitations. First, the study was observational and we did not establish a cause and effect relationship between good team behaviour and better outcome. Second, it is not possible to conclude which behaviours are most important or whether their influence varies by operative stage (induction, etc.). Developing an intervention solely based on these findings would not be straightforward. Third, to obtain cooperation in conducting the study, we had to protect the identities of the members of the team and we were thus not able to describe team characteristics (e.g., training, experience) in detail. Research, including an extensive qualitative analysis based on observer comments, is ongoing with these data. Fourth, some of our analyses, notably our grouping of the outcomes into a dichotomous variable, were conducted post-hoc.

Comparisons to Other Research

Previous studies of operating room teams have focused on characteristics of surgeons such as 'individual excellence' (McDonald et al. 1995) and technical competence (Gawande et al. 2003). They have also examined the impact of major and minor human failures upon patient outcomes; Carthey et al. (2003) conducted qualitative analyses of major system features that influence team performance and patient safety (Davenport et al. 2007, Greenberg et al. 2007) and performed retrospective reviews of malpractice claims files (Gawande et al. 2003). Our methods and results complement and extend this literature in several ways. For example, we used direct observation of procedures and then used different study personnel to prospectively collect patient outcome data. This addresses limitations of malpractice claims file analyses such as hindsight bias (knowledge of the bad outcome can bias reviewers to rate teamwork as lower) and sole reliance on the documents in claims files to make judgements about complicated and dynamic team behaviours. Compared to Carthey et al (2003) we studied a more generalizable and common group of surgical procedures, thus extending their findings to other types of surgeries. Greenberg et al. studied the entire spectrum of surgical care, not just intra-operative care, and identified communication breakdowns during surgeon communication with other caregivers (Greenberg et al. 2007). They recommended defined triggers that mandate communication with an attending surgeon; structured hand-offs and transfer protocols; and standard use of read-backs. Our work complements these studies by specifying the intra-operative team behaviours (briefings, information sharing, inquiry and vigilance) that should be useful in preventing negative outcomes. Finally, a recent study reported a significant correlation between subjective ratings of teamwork with postoperative morbidity (Davenport et al. 2007), a finding which lends more support to our conclusions.

Implications and Future Directions

Development of interventions based on changing teamwork behaviour and their evaluation is a logical next step for research in this arena. Our study provides general support for development of team training programmes for surgical teams. Such programmes should be rigorously tested because they will require significant investments of time and money; some studies in other areas have found only marginal benefit for patients (Nielsen et al. 2007).

We believe that there are two broad lines of research that should be pursued and that will ultimately converge in the form of effective team training programmes. First, research should focus on implementation and evaluation of training programmes. There is already a large body of knowledge that can inform the content of such programmes (Baker et al. 2005, Clancy and Tornberg 2007). These may focus on relatively specific processes of care, like neonatal resuscitation (Thomas et al. 2006); they may try to address multiple processes within a site of care like labour and delivery (Nielsen et al. 2007); or there are training programmes (like TeamSTEPPS) which may be applicable across many locations, processes and disciplines (Clancy and Tornberg 2007). However, given the inconclusive results of initial evaluations of such programmes, it is clear that there is a need for a second line of research which asks more fundamental questions about the relationships between specific team behaviours and specific tasks carried out by providers (Undre et al. 2006, Yule et al. 2006). Such knowledge should result in training that teaches behaviours which are more likely to improve quality. This would include studies that draw upon the 'basic sciences' of safety (Brennan et al. 2005). For example, human factors experts can perform task analyses to determine exactly which behaviours might be most useful for specific tasks, and cognitive psychologists can help link teamwork to prevention of mental slips and mistakes.

At Kaiser Permanente we are implementing a comprehensive surgical safety programme (described below) which is an example of how these two lines of research can inform the development and implementation of team training programmes. At the University of Texas we have developed a team training curriculum for the Neonatal Resuscitation Program which increases the frequency of team behaviours during simulated resuscitations (Thomas et al. 2007).

The Kaiser programme was a direct outgrowth of the research described above and is described in more detail below.

From Science to Execution – Implementation of a Highly Reliable Surgical Team Programme at Kaiser Permanente

The primary driver of the research described above was to develop strategies to continually improve the safety of the care that we provide to our patients. The secondary driver was to answer the question of whether or not the communication and teamwork demonstrated by the surgical team had an impact on surgical outcomes. Prior to performing this research our patient safety strategy for the peri-operative area had focused on education and training related to human factors, communication and teamwork and implementation of structured pre-operative briefings. Based on this work, a pilot project was performed in the operating rooms of one of our Southern California hospitals. The overarching purpose of the project was to improve safety by enhancing teamwork, collaboration and communication among team members in the peri-operative setting.

The pilot consisted of providing education and training in human factors and communication and teamwork to the entire peri-operative staff. Following the educational programme, a steering committee was formed and a structured pre-operative briefing (including script) was developed. The hospital used four different indicators of safety culture to measure the programme's success: occurrence of wrong site/wrong procedures, attitudinal survey data, near-miss reporting and turnover data. Several areas of significant improvement were noted. The most notable result was reducing verification injuries to zero within a year; additionally, there was a 19 percent increase in employee satisfaction and a 16 percent decrease in nurse turnover; and the safety climate in the operating room increased from 'good' to 'outstanding' after implementation of the pilot study. Although this pilot programme was successful and has sustained itself as an ongoing programme at the one hospital, the efforts to spread the programme to other hospitals were not successful. One of the major concerns expressed by leadership and clinicians was that the data did not demonstrate that the effort put into communication and teamwork and pre-operative briefings made a difference to surgical outcomes.

The evidence base provided by the Highly Reliable Surgical Team (HRST) research project discussed above, coupled with the outcomes of the pilot programme, provided us with a much stronger case for requiring a highly reliable surgical programme in all of our hospitals. The HRST research project also had a qualitative component (narratives of observations provided by the observers) that allowed us to provide leadership and clinicians with information related to potential threats to patient safety that existed within our system. The primary 'threats' included: interruptions and distractions; inadequate briefing and/or time out; incomplete or no transfer of information during transfer of patient, shift change or break; equipment and material problems including malfunctioning equipment, potential operator error and incomplete or wrong supplies and equipment for the task at hand; lack of respectful interactions among surgical team members; and interdepartmental coordination and communication challenges. These qualitative data enriched the quantitative findings, and armed with these data, we were able to convince both leadership and clinicians that improved communication and teamwork including pre-operative briefings would not only improve attitudes but also improve the safety of the surgical care that we provide to our patients. When the data were presented to executive and physician leadership, the consensus was that the combination of the evidence presented a compelling argument for a mandated programme.

The information from the research was presented at our initial expert surgical groups that were charged with developing the programme, clinicians who had previously been sceptical and concerned that strategies such as pre-operative briefings would do nothing but slow down procedure start time began to discuss how, in fact, interventions could potentially end up saving time.

Once the pilots were initiated we began to receive 'stories' from clinicians. An early story shared by a surgeon at a meeting of surgical leaders related to how, during a briefing, it was discovered that the team did not have all the equipment that was needed for the procedure. The surgeon indicated that in the past, not having the correct equipment was in many cases not discovered until a point when the operation was underway. The surgeon went on to say that when missing equipment was not identified early on this not only led to delays in the procedure and increased operating time but also potentially impacted the safety of the patient.

In 2007, in conjunction with peri-operative leadership, the Northern California regional leadership required all 19 of the Northern California medical centres to initiate the Highly Reliable Surgical Team Program. Expert groups consisting of surgeons, anaesthesiologists and nurse managers met to develop the programme and in the spring of 2007 a regional surgical summit was held. Peri-operative teams from each medical centre attended. The summit opened with sharing of the results from the research project along with the current state of surgical safety in Northern California (e.g., days in-between surgical events, our medical malpractice experience). Education and training during the summit related to human factors, communication and teamwork, and the importance of the highly reliable surgical team programme. Participants were provided with all of the tools necessary to initiate the programme at their individual medical centres. The expectations for 2007 required that each hospital develop and implement the infrastructure and processes necessary to support highly reliable surgical teams. The four requirements for each medical centre were:

1. Develop and implement a surgical safety committee that would lead the programme.
2. Implement scripted peri-operative briefings where all members of the team had a speaking role. A whiteboard with all team members' names was also required.
3. Educate and train the entire peri-operative team in human factors/ communication and teamwork – every medical centre closed the operating rooms for 2–3 hours for this training. The training included

presenting national, regional, and medical centre specific data related to surgical safety and set the 'burning platform' as to why this programme was important. Additionally, experts in the area of communication and teamwork discussed the importance and fundamentals of human factors, communication, and teamwork. The session ended with planning for how to implement the programme in every operating room for every specialty. Additional elements such as debriefings and 'glitch books' were discussed as potential additional programme elements.

4. Institute regular observation audits to ensure that the briefings were taking place and all required elements were included. One of the lessons from our research was the importance of observation by someone not directly involved with the procedure. Often, behaviours in the OR are the reality in which the surgical team works and, digressing from the appropriate or required way of doing things is not recognized. By doing the observational audits and reviewing these with the teams and OR leadership, we are able to point out how the teams can improve the communication and teamwork.

The success of the surgical summit exceeded our expectations. Teams remained after the summit to work on plans for implementation in their medical centres. Formal evaluations indicated that 100 percent of the participants found the programme had met its goals and 96 percent felt that the programme met expectations. More convincing evaluations, however, were the anecdotal comments noting that the summit had moved people to take further action to improve surgical safety. Completion of the process requirements outlined above was monitored and quarterly reports were submitted to the medical centre executive committee and regional leadership. All medical centres met the requirement that these four elements be in place by the end of 2007. In addition to the above process measures an outcome measure of days in-between verification injuries was also utilized. The days in-between events related to verification has substantially increased since the inception of the programme. In the latter part of 2007, the requirements were further refined to make the briefings pre-induction, thereby including the patient in the process (when appropriate). The Surgical Care Improvement Project safety checks (Bratzler and Hunt 2006) were added to the briefing checklist to enhance reliable protection from infection, Venous Thromboembolism (VTE) and Miocardial Infarction (MI).

Building on the successes achieved in 2007, the programme was expanded in 2008. Each one of the elements required the input from a multidisciplinary expert team whose job was to research current literature, define recommended practices, perform small test of change and develop tools/playbooks to guide the change in practice. The additional elements included:

1. Refinement and monitoring of the surgical briefing and debriefing to build communication, teamwork and eliminate verification events – this included use of the script; team engagement; and leadership of the surgeon.

2. Administration of the Safety Attitude Questionnaires (Sexton et al. 2006a) to measure the culture of safety and teamwork at each medical centre.
3. Continued monitoring of the Surgical Care Improvement Project (SCIP) bundles.
4. Implementation of peri-operative practice changes that will eliminate retained foreign bodies (RFO).
5. Implementation of a briefing protocol specific to intraocular lens implants (IOL) to prevent wrong lens implants in all settings where cataracts are performed. Establish a protocol to eliminate wrong side thoracentesis procedures in all settings.
6. Provide a second surgical summit in the fall to celebrate successes and inspire the operative teams to continue to sustain the programme.

In conclusion, the quantitative and qualitative data from our research project were critical to get buy-in and inform the design and implementation of our Highly Reliable Surgical Team programme. The key contributors to the success of this programme have been:

1. Immediate utilization of the Highly Reliable Surgical Team research to develop and implement the programme in all operating rooms in the 19 hospitals of the Northern California Region of Kaiser Permanente.
2. Strong executive and physician leadership.
3. Provision of tools and project management to the medical centres.
4. Independent observational audits of the surgical briefing by staff who are not members of the peri-operative team.
5. Regular dialogue and communication with the peri-operative nursing directors and managers.
6. Development of a surgical safety scorecard measuring compliance rate with the SCIP bundles, briefing elements of script, engagement and leadership and listing of surgical never events by facilities.

Future work will expand and refine these efforts for both surgical and non-surgical teams.

References

Baker, D.P., Gustafson, S., Beaubien, J.M., Salas, E. and Barach, P. (2005) Medical team training programs in health care. Advances in patient safety: From research to implementation. In K. Henriksen, J.B. Battles, E.S. Marks and D.I. Lewin (eds) *Vol. 4, Programs, Tools and Products*. AHRQ Publication No. 05-0021-2. Rockville, MD: AHRQ.

Bratzler, D.W. and Hunt D.R. (2006) The surgical infection prevention and surgical care improvement projects: National initiatives to improve outcomes for patients having surgery. *Clinical Infectious Diseases* 43, 3, 322–30.

Brennan, T.A., Gawande, A., Thomas, E. and Studdart, D. (2005) Accidental deaths, saved lives, and improved quality. *New England Journal of Medicine* 353, 1405–409.

Carthey, J., de Leval, M.R., Wright, D.J., Farewell, V.T. and Reason, J.T. (2003) Behavioral markers of surgical excellence. *Safety Science* 41, 409–25.

Clancy, C.M. and Tornberg, D.N. (2007) TeamSTEPPS: Assuring optimal teamwork in clinical settings. *American Journal of Medical Quality* 22, 214–17.

Davenport, D.L., Henderson, W.G., Mosca, C.L., Khuri, S. and Mentzer Jr, R. (2007) Risk-adjusted morbidity in teaching hospital correlates with reported levels of communication and collaboration on surgical teams but not with scale measures of teamwork climate, safety climate, or working conditions. *Journal of the American College of Surgery* 205(6), 778–84.

Dietrich, R. and Childress, T.M. (eds) (2004) *Group Interaction in High Risk Environments*. Aldershot: Ashgate.

Eagle, K.A., Berger, P.B., Calkins, H. et al. (2002) ACC/AHA guideline update for perioperative cardiovascular evaluation for noncardiac surgery – executive summary: A report of the American College of Cardiology/American Heart Association Task Force on Practice Guidelines (Committee to Update the 1996 Guidelines on Perioperative Cardiovascular Evaluation for Noncardiac Surgery). *Journal of the American College of Cardiology* 39, 542–53.

Falck, A.J., Escobedo, M.B., Baillargeon, J.G., Villard, L.G. and Gunkel, J.H. (2003) Proficiency of pediatric residents in performing neonatal endotracheal intubation. *Pediatrics* 112, 1242–7.

Gawande, A., Zinner, M.J., Studdert, D.M. and Brennan, T.A. (2003) Analysis of errors reported by surgeons at three teaching hospitals. *Surgery* 133, 614–21.

Greenberg, C.C., Regenbogen, S.E., Studdert, D.M., Lipsitz, S.R., Rogers, S.O., Zinner, M.J. and Gawande, A.A. (2007) Patterns of communication breakdowns resulting in injury to surgical patients. *Journal of the American College of Surgery* 204, 533–40.

Halamek, L.P., Kaegi, D.M., Gaba, D.M., Sowb, Y.A., Smith, B.C., Smith, B.E. and Howard, S.K. (2000) Time for a new paradigm in pediatric medical education: Teaching neonatal resuscitation in a simulated delivery room environment. *Pediatrics* 106, E45.

James, L.R., Demaree, P and Wolf, G. (1984) Estimating within-group interrater reliability with and without response bias. *Journal of Applied Psychology* 69, 85–98.

Klampfer, B., Flin, R., Helmreich, R.L. et al. (2001) Enhancing performance in high risk environments: Recommendations for the use of behavioral markers. Presented at the Behavioural Markers Workshop sponsored by the Daimler-Benz Stiftung GIHRE-Kolleg, Swissair Training Center, Zurich, 5–6 July.

Kohn, L.T., Corrigan, J.M. and Donaldson, M.D. (eds) (2000) *To Err Is Human*. Washington DC: National Academy Press.

Makary, M.A., Sexton, J.B., Freischlag, J.A., Millman, E.A., Pryor, D. Holzmueller, C. and Pronovost, P. (2006a) Patient safety in surgery. *Annals of Surgery* 243(5), 628–35.

Makary, M.A., Sexton, J., Freischlag, J., Holzmueller, C., Millman, E., Rowen, L. and Pronovost, P. (2006b) Operating room teamwork among physicians and nurses: Teamwork in the eye of the beholder. *Journal of the American College of Surgery* 202(5), 746–52.

Mazzocco K, Petitti, D.B., Fong, K.T. et al. (2008) Surgical team behaviors and patient outcomes. *American Journal of Surgery* [doi: 10.1016/j.amjsurg.2008.03.002].

McDonald, J., Orlick, T. and Letts, M. (1995) Mental readiness in surgeons and its links to performance excellence in surgery. *Journal of Pediatric Orthopedics* 15(5), 691–7.

Morey, J.C., Simon, R., Jay, G.D., Wears, R.L., Salisbury, M., Dukes, K.A. and Berns, S.D. (2002) Error reduction and performance improvement in the emergency department through formal teamwork training: Evaluation results of the MedTeams project. *Health Services Research* 37, 1553–81.

Nielsen, P.E., Goldman, M.B., Shapiro, D.E. and Sachs, B.P. (2007) Effects of teamwork training on adverse outcomes and process of care in labor and delivery: A randomized controlled trial. *Obstetrics and Gynecology* 109, 48–55.

Pronovost, P.J. et al. (forthcoming) A multi-faceted intervention to reduce catheter-related blood stream infections in Michigan intensive care units. *New England Journal of Medicine*.

Salas, E., Wilson, K.A., Burke, C.S. and Wightman, D.C. (2006) Does crew resource management work? An update, an extension, and some critical needs. *Human Factors* 48(2), 392–412.

Santora, T.A., Trooskin, S.Z., Blank, C.A., Clarke, J.R. and Schinco, M.A. (1996) Video assessment of trauma response: Adherence to ATLS protocols. *American Journal of Emergency Medicine* 14(6), 564–9.

Sexton, J.B., Thomas, E.J. and Helmreich, R.L. (2000) Error, stress, and teamwork in medicine and aviation: Cross sectional surveys. *British Medical Journal* 320, 745–9.

Sexton, J.B., Helmreich, R.L, Neilands, T.B., Rown, K., Vella, K, Boyden, J. Roberts, P.R., Thomas, E.J. (2006a) The Safety Attitudes Questionnaire: Psychometric Properties, Benchmarking Data, and Emerging Research. *BMC Health Services Research* 6, 44.

Sexton, J.B., Holzmueller, C.G., Pronovost, P.J., Thomas, E.J., McFerran, S., Nunes, J., Thompson, D.A., Knight, A.P., Penning, D.H. and Fox, H.E. (2006b) Variation in caregiver perceptions of teamwork climate in labor and delivery units. *Journal of Perinatology* 26, 463–70.

Sexton, J.B., Makary, M.A., Tersigni, A.R., Pryor, D., Hendrich, A., Thomas, E.J., Holzmueller, C.G., Knight, A.P., Wu, Y. and Pronovost, P.J. (2006c) Teamwork in the operating room: Frontline perspectives among hospitals and operating room personnel. *Anesthesiology* 105, 877–84.

Sugrue, M., Seger, M., Kerridge, R., Sloane, D. and Deane, S. (1995) A prospective study of the performance of the trauma team leader. *Journal of Trauma* 38(1), 79–82.

Sutcliffe, K.M., Lewton, E. and Rosenthal, M.M. (2004) Communication failures: An insidious contributor to medical mishaps. *Academic Medicine* 79, 186–94.

Thomas, E.J., Sexton, J.B. and Helmreich, R.L. (2004) Translating teamwork behaviors from aviation to healthcare: Development of behavioral markers for neonatal resuscitation. *Quality and Safety in Health Care* 13, S1, 57–64.

Thomas, E.J., Sexton, J.B., Lasky, R.E., Helmreich, R.L., Crandell, S. and Tyson, J. (2006) Teamwork and quality during neonatal care in the delivery room. *Journal of Perinatology* 26, 163–9.

Thomas, E.J., Taggart, B., Crandell, S., Lasky, R.E., Williams, A.L., Love, L.J., Sexton, J.B., Tyson, J.E. and Helmreich, R.L. (2007) Teaching teamwork during the neonatal resuscitation program: A randomized trial. *Journal of Perinatology* 27, 409–14.

Undre, S., Healey, A.N., Darzi, A., Vincent, C.A. (2006) Observational assessment of surgical teamwork: A feasibility study. *World Journal of Surgery* 30, 1774–83.

Walker, R. (2002) ASA and CEPOD scoring. *Update in Anaesthesia* [serial online] 14(5), 1-1. Available at: <http://www.nda.ox.ac.uk/wfsa/html/u14/u1405_01.htm> [accessed August 2006].

Xiao, Y, Hunter, W.A., Mackenzie, C.F., Jefferies, N.J. and Horst, R.L. (1996) Task complexity in emergency medical care and its implications for team coordination. LOTAS Group. Level One Trauma Anesthesia Simulation. *Human Factors* 38(4), 636–45.

Yule, S., Flin, R., Paterson-Brown, S., Maran, N. and Rowley, D. (2006) Development of a rating system for surgeons' non-technical skills. *Medical Education* 40, 1098–104.

Appendix: List of Potential Complications Referred to by Data Abstractors when Reviewing Medical Records

This list was not all-inclusive – abstractors recorded additional complications as indicated. Complications were grouped into outcome categories based upon the impact on subsequent care and harm to patients.

1. Accidental puncture or laceration.
2. Surgical burn (heat-producing equipment, chemical).
3. Adverse drug reaction.
4. Wrong patient/procedure/site/side/device.

5. Retention of foreign object.
6. Transfusion reaction.
7. Pressure ulcers.
8. Peripheral nerve damage/short-term neurological deficits.
9. Complications of anaesthesia (anaesthetic medication error, reaction or endotracheal tube misplacement, regional anaesthetic complications, broken teeth).
10. Iatrogenic pneumothorax.
11. Pneumonia.
12. Selected post-operative infections (ICD-9 CM codes 9993 or 00662).
13. Post-operative haemorrhage or haematoma.
14. Post-operative pulmonary embolus or DVT (deep vein thrombosis).
15. Post-operative DIC (disseminating intravascular coagulopathy).
16. Post-operative respiratory failure (acute).
17. Post-operative sepsis.
18. Postoperative wound dehiscence.
19. Post-operative fracture (excluding unrelated post-operative falls).
20. Post-operative physiologic/metabolic derangement.
21. Post-operative cardiac arrest.
22. Post-operative hemodynamic instability.
23. Myocardial infarction.
24. CVA.
25. Other undesired outcome, not otherwise specified (e.g., excessive and prolonged pain, unanticipated restriction in range of motion, musculoskeletal injury).

Chapter 17

Counting Silence: Complexities in the Evaluation of Team Communication

Lorelei Lingard, Sarah Whyte, Glenn Regehr and Fauzia Gardezi

Purpose

Many in the domain of surgical performance research have developed tools to objectively evaluate team communication. Our own tool has been used to describe communication failure patterns in the context of a pre-operative team briefing intervention in four urban teaching hospitals. Using examples from this research programme, this chapter explores a critical problem in the objective evaluation of team communication: how do we 'count' silence? Because it is relatively easy to document 'presence' (communications that can be directly observed), our conventional approaches are not well equipped to deal with 'absence' (communicative silences). Yet silence abounds in the operating room, and a comprehensive accounting of team communication must grapple with the meanings of silence, including both its functional and problematic dimensions. Drawing on theories of discourse and power, this chapter will describe recurrent patterns of silence in the operating room, consider the actions and relations that these silences embody and discuss their implications for sophisticated evaluation of the communicative behaviour of operating room teams.

Background

Communication has been a dominant focus in the study of operating room (OR) team performance. This focus has emerged largely in response to evidence suggesting that preventable adverse events happen at unacceptably high rates in the surgical setting, and that ineffective or insufficient communication among team members is often a contributing factor (Kohn et al. 2000, Helmreich 2000, Helmreich and Davies 1994, Joint Commission on Accreditation of Healthcare Organizations 2003). However, despite the general agreement that ineffective communication threatens patient safety, until recently there was little evidence regarding what specific team communication practices and attitudes compromise safety, what methods might effectively change these patterns, or how the outcomes of such changes might be measured.

Researchers studying OR team performance have sought to address this deficit by developing tools that include in their purview the objective evaluation of team communication (Salas et al. 2007, Undre et al. 2007). Our recent research in the OR has elaborated a theory of interprofessional team communication that describes tension catalysts, reveals interpretive patterns, and classifies recurrent failures (Lingard et al. 2002c, 2002b, 2004). This work suggests clear directions for educational interventions aimed at improving the status quo of OR communication practices (Lingard et al. 2005). Assessing the effectiveness of such interventions requires appropriate measures of team communication. The challenge in creating such measures is to provide analytical traction while continuing to reflect the complex, often subtle and evolving nature of team communication.

Our Communication Failures Tool

To address this measurement need, we developed a theory-based instrument that reflected the findings of our observational research (Lingard et al. 2006). The instrument is a checklist of types of communication failure and their outcomes based on our classification of 'communication failure' in the OR, framed by rhetorical theory (Lingard et al. 2004). Four communication failure types are tracked by the instrument: occasion, content, purpose and audience (see Table 17.1). 'Occasion' involves communication problems related to time and space. For instance, a common timing problem is the surgeon's request for a special piece of equipment at the moment of need, rather than before the procedure commences (assuming the need for the equipment could be foreseen). 'Content' failures consist of communicative exchanges that contain incomplete or inaccurate information, such as a nurse's inaccurate announcement that a patient was positive for hepatitis C. The 'Purpose' category includes situations in which questions are asked but not answered, prompting repeated and increasingly urgent requests. Finally, 'Audience' captures the problem of communication that excludes a key individual, such as conversations between anaesthesia and surgery about the operative plan that have implications for nursing work but do not include a nursing representative. The observational instrument also captures consequences of the communication failure that are immediately visible to the observer, including delay, inefficiency, team tension, resource waste and procedural error. We use the tool in our research programme to measure the effect of a team communication intervention (a team briefing) on overall communication failure rates at the level of procedure (Lingard et al. 2008).

We have found that this communication failures tool has worked well from the perspective of describing the overall quality of team communication over the course of a procedure. It has demonstrated reasonable inter-rater reliability in assessing the relative rate of communication failures displayed per procedure, in classifying the type of failure observed, and in identifying the consequences of that failure for the team's functioning. Its ability to distinguish failure-rich

Table 17.1 Definitions of types of communicative failure with illustrative examples and notes

Failure	Definition	Illustrative example and *analytical note*
Occasion Failures	Problems in the situation or context of the communicative event	The staff surgeon asks the anaesthesiologist whether the antibiotics have been administered. At the point of this question, the procedure has been underway for over an hour. *Since antibiotics are optimally given within 30 minutes of incision, the timing of this inquiry is ineffective both as a prompt and a as safety redundancy measure.*
Content Failures	Insufficiency or inaccuracy apparent in the information being transferred	As the case is set up, the anaesthesia fellow asks the staff surgeon if the patient has an ICU (intensive care unit) bed. The staff surgeon replies that the 'bed is probably not needed, and there isn't likely one available anyway, so we'll just go ahead'. *Relevant information is missing and questions are left unresolved: has an ICU bed been requested, and what will the plan be if the patient does need critical care and an ICU bed is not available? [Note: this example was classified as both a content and a purpose failure]*
Audience Failures	Gaps in the composition of the group engaged in the communication	The nurses and anaesthesiologist discuss how the patient should be positioned for surgery without the participation of a surgical representative. *Surgeons have particular positioning needs, so they should be participants in this discussion. Decisions made in their absence occasionally lead to renewed discussions and repositioning upon their arrival.*
Purpose Failures	Communicative events in which purpose is unclear, not achieved, or inappropriate	During a living donor liver resection, the nurses discuss whether ice is needed in the basin they are preparing for the liver. Neither knows. No further discussion ensues. *The purpose of this communication – to find out if ice is required – is not achieved. No plan to achieve it is articulated.*

Reprinted from Lingard et al. (2004)

from failure-sparse procedures has prompted us to use it in our current research (Lingard et al. 2006).

A particular strength of this approach to assessing communication is that it provides the opportunity to assess OR team communication performance not by single summative snapshots but rather by assembled records that can be used to construct a multifaceted communication 'profile' over time. Our theoretical work in this domain has demonstrated that team communication is rarely straightforwardly 'good' or 'bad', suggesting that measures need to be structured to pick up patterns that surface across a series of exchanges. Therefore, the tool requires observers to intuit links and attribute motives in the context of the multifocal, overlapping and evolving nature of communication events. We have discussed elsewhere (Lingard et al. 2006) the balance between reliability and ecological validity in such interpretive assessment efforts. Notwithstanding this delicate balance, we have consciously sought a sophisticated accounting of team communication that grapples with communication events within an evolving social context of discourse, rather than assigning them *a priori* meaning. Attending to this balance, our tool allows the assessment process to acknowledge and represent these complexities rather than eliding them.

The Challenge of Silence

Our tool is similar to other communication evaluation instruments in its predominant focus on 'presence' – communication exchanges that can be seen and heard. For instance, audience failures are evident through the presence of communication events from which at least one relevant team member is visibly absent. Timing failures are evident through the presence of a request for antibiotics 30 minutes *after* the surgical incision. Content failures are evident when incorrect information is communicated by one team member and then corrected by another, or when a later exchange reveals that only part of the relevant information had been transferred.

In using the tool to assess >1500 surgical procedures over the past four years, an intriguing challenge has emerged: how to account for the meanings of silence? While observers track the *presence* of communication events, these presences reveal salient *absences* in the communication event. In this regard, the audience category highlights the absence of a team member; the timing category highlights the absence of proactive communication earlier in the case; the content category highlights absent information (or the absence of a mechanism for providing and correcting information); and the purpose category highlights an absence of resolution. Each of these absences manifests itself as a form of silence in our data, often visible through the categories of the evaluation tool but not always straightforwardly captured by them. All the examples which follow are derived from field note excerpts in the study database. They have been selected for their commonness, that is, their representation of situations that recur. They have been altered for presentation in two ways: their details have been changed to preserve anonymity, and they have been turned into succinct narratives for efficient presentation.

Consider the following example of the relationship between the 'presence' and 'absence' of communication, between speech and silence as recounted in an observer's field notes:

> The circulating nurse and scrub nurse are doing their count near the end of the case. The surgical resident requests '4-0 Vicryl please' from the scrub nurse.

The nurse's back is to him, and she doesn't immediately respond. The resident requests again with a slightly louder voice: 'Can I get a 4-0 Vicryl please?' The scrub nurse still does not respond. The surgical resident raises his eyebrow at the junior resident across the table from him. A few moments later, the count is completed. The scrub nurse repeats '4-0 Vicryl', handing the suture. The resident takes it, appears irritated, sighing loudly and shaking his head.

What is the meaning of the nurse's silence? A number of interpretations are possible, with different implications for the categorization of this exchange as a communication failure or not. One interpretation is that the silence has no purpose, because it is not a 'response' to the request. This is plausible if the request has not been heard because the nurse's attention is focused on the counting protocol. An observer taking this interpretive stance would categorize this exchange as 'purpose not achieved', given that the resident makes three attempts before getting a response. Alternatively, the nurse may have heard the request, and the non-response reflects her prioritizing of the counting activity and subordinating the suture request in her own task management. Taking this approach, we might categorize this as a 'content' problem, using the argument that an explicit indication of this prioritizing might avoid the resident's growing irritation at the non-response. Also possible is that the request has been heard, and the prioritizing of nursing tasks has happened, but the nurse's silence carries an additional purpose of indirectly delaying the incision closure until the count is complete. She may purposefully avoid explicit articulation of this purpose: her silence may, in effect, be a conflict-avoidance mechanism. Taking this approach, we might characterize the resident's original request as a timing failure, reflecting that the request is made at an inopportune time. Each interpretation of the silence casts a different light on the communication exchange, the communicative expertise of the team members, and the nature of any failure that might be coded.

A slight shift in the social context of this event could radically change how it unfolds. Imagine that the suture request in this instance comes from a staff person rather than a resident and that the counting scrub nurse is a less assertive staff member. Then, we might see the suture request responded to more immediately, and we would not capture a purpose failure – all would appear to go smoothly. In this case, however, the responsiveness might itself be the failure – reminding us that absence of communication, silence, is not necessarily always problematic. Sometimes communication progresses very smoothly towards a dangerous outcome.

This example powerfully illustrates the theoretical premise that silence is not the absence of communicative meaning; rather, silence can be purposeful and meaningful, a complex mode of communicative participation (Glenn 2004, Saville-Troike 1985). While some silences reflect linguistic conventions, such as turn taking in conversational speech, other silences contain propositional content – that is, they are 'communicative acts' (Glenn 2004, Saville-Troike 2003). Silence may also be a socially constructed response, as suggested by studies of the communicative constraints on subordinated groups such as nurses (Manias and Street 2001, Riley and Manias 2005, Gillespie et al. 2008, Bradbury-Jones et al. 2007). Thus, silences are meaningful in the sense that people often use silence to communicate, and silences tell us about social structures and power relations. The relationship of silence to power is not straightforward, however. Foucault points out that this relationship is highly ambiguous, as silence functions both as a shelter from power and a shelter for power (Brown 2005). Thus, understanding what silence does – what attitudes it advertises, what purposes it enacts, what relations it reflects – can be a thorny issue for the 'objective' observer of team communication.

Analysing Silence

The purpose and content categories of our instrument yield the most examples of silence. This section describes the kinds of silence that are prominent within these categories, illustrating the complexity of interpretation using examples from our failures database. One researcher reviewed our entire failures database for instances of 'silence' from these two coding categories. Many of these instances had undergone group discussion in regular analytical meetings of the observation team over the course of the study. Both field notes and reflective notes were reviewed.

Silences that Emerge in the Purpose Category

Failures documented in the purpose category often require the most observer interpretation. A purpose – and its lack of resolution – may not be visible in the way that, for example, a surgeon's absence from a discussion about patient positioning is visible (audience failure). We persistently struggle with the attribution of intent that is required to ascertain whether a purpose failure has occurred, particularly when silence is a factor and we have previously described our efforts to achieve good inter-rater reliability among trained observers using this team communication evaluation tool (Lingard et al. 2006). Our report discussed the delicate balancing act between authenticity/ecological validity and reliability/objective quantification. In particular, while the tool's overall reliability was good, we reported low inter-rater reliability for purpose failures (kappa coefficient 0.33).

For instance, in our first published description of the purpose failure category, we used the following example:

> During a living donor liver resection, one nurse approaches another and they discuss whether ice is needed in the basin they are preparing for the liver. Neither knows. No further discussion ensues.

In order to categorize this exchange as a purpose failure, the observer must infer that the exchange is originated by the first nurse with the purpose of resolving the question of whether ice is required. (The attribution of a purpose invariably requires ruling out other possibilities with a range of legitimacy; for instance, this exchange could be more social than functional, and the initiating nurse may have an implicit plan that she's checking through discussion.) Since the nurses in this exchange neither come to a resolution of the question nor articulate a plan to resolve it by some other means, the exchange is coded as having failed to achieve its intended purpose. The lack of ongoing communication – their conversation trails off into silence, and they both eventually drift away to other tasks – is the source of the failure. This interpretation is supported later in the observation: when the liver is removed, the basin still has no ice, and, upon the surgeon's exclamation that ice is necessary, the nurses scramble to find some.

In the purpose failure category, silence recurrently manifests itself as apparent non-responsiveness following questions or requests. Rarely, a team member will explicitly comment on the silence. Sometimes their comment simply points to the non-responsiveness as problematic and serves to resolve it:

> The circulating nurse, who is new to the room, relieving someone on break, says to the scrub nurse: 'How many sets of sponges did you have?' (The circulating nurse speaks loudly; the scrub nurse is soft spoken.) The staff surgeon picks up on this exchange and asks: 'What are you missing?' Neither nurse responds to his question. The circulating nurse leaves the theatre and checks something with the earlier circulating nurse, then returns to the room. The staff surgeon says, 'You're not answering the question. Are you missing something?' The circulating nurse says there is no issue.

In this case, the nurses' silence in response to the staff surgeon's question may be because they do not have the answer; additionally, it may reflect a territory issue, in that the sponge count is nursing's domain, and the standard practice is for nurses to take the lead in communicating any emergent count issues to other team members, not for others to enquire about them out of turn.

The infrequent cases when team members share their interpretation of the meaning of non-responsive silences can be quite instructive to observers:

> The surgical resident indirectly requests another instrument, noting 'I guess you guys don't have a Belfour.' The circulating nurse goes out into corridor and returns, announcing, 'I have a Belfour here if you want me to open it.' There is no response, as the surgeons continue talking to one another. Over the next 15 seconds, the scrub nurses (preceptor and student) ask four more times if the surgeons want the Belfour; their questions are never asked loudly and they get no response. The medical student appears to hear but doesn't say anything. The circulating nurse comments: 'They want to ignore us. So they're not going to get

the Belfour then.' She puts the Belfour on the cart. There's no further mention of the Belfour during the case.

In this instance, the circulating nurse attributes to the surgeons' silence a purpose: 'They want to ignore us'. The field notes suggest an alternative explanation that the nurses' questions are not heard by the surgical team.

In cases where there is no explicit comment on the silence by team members, silence may be interpreted as a signal that a 'public' request or question has not been understood as directed at a particular listener. Recurrently in our data, such 'public' announcements or requests are followed by silence:

> The staff surgeon noted loudly, without looking at anyone in particular: 'So we'll maybe give this guy a couple of doses of post-operative antibiotics'. There is no immediate response from anyone present, although the staff anaesthetist looks up, seems to register what the staff surgeon has said, pauses in her work, but does not respond. A couple of minutes later, the junior surgical resident asks, 'What did you say about postoperative antibiotics?' There is no response from the staff surgeon. The question remains unresolved.

In this case, the staff anaesthetist's body language suggests that she hears the request, but she apparently decides not to respond. Her silence could mean that she interprets the request as directed at the surgical resident rather than herself, an interpretation supported by the junior resident's later uptake of the issue. Alternatively, however, such silence in the context of a request or statement may be suggestive of team members handling sensitive issues indirectly and non-verbally. A study of team members' perceptions of roles and responsibilities regarding antibiotic administration in the operating room found that surgeons may be reluctant to directly ask anaesthetists to administer antibiotics, and that anaesthetists may resent such requests to administer drugs that have been ordered by another physician on the team (Tan et al. 2006). In such contexts, communicative exchanges may involve indirect and implicit discursive 'moves' as both members avoid explicitly engaging on topics associated with interprofessional tension.

What other team members make of – and intend by – such silences in their communicative exchanges is often ambiguous. This is particularly true when the recipient of a question or request is clear and circumstances suggest that they have indeed heard the communication:

> The staff surgeon says loudly without taking his eyes from the surgical field: 'Almost certainly we're going to need a flexible sigmoidoscope and Dr Black [urologist].' The circulating nurse responds, using the staff surgeon's first name, 'When, Larry?' There is no response from the staff surgeon, who continues working. The nurse goes to call central processing to get the equipment sent up, after which she pages the urologist.

This silence is quite pointed, given that it breaks off a direct communication exchange. We could arguably code this as a purpose failure, because the nurse's purpose of ascertaining the timing of these emergent needs is not explicitly resolved. However, the silence seems to act as a resolution itself, judging by the nurse's decision to act immediately to track down both the equipment and the urologist. It may be that she interprets the surgeon's silence to mean that the same situation that prompted his requests is requiring his full attention at the moment, and therefore the need is immediate. Particularly if the urologist's assistance was not predicted, then the need is likely to be urgent. Alternately, it may be that the surgeon does not have an answer to the nurse's query of 'When?', and so he chooses to remain silent until the answer reveals itself. Or, the silence may reflect the surgeon's concentration on the surgery and signal that the timing is not appropriate for questions. Finally, it may be that the surgeon hears the question and thinks it not worthy of response: the tacit message of the silence being, 'If I'm asking now, then I need it now.' In fact, in our observations we have seen surgeons articulate this very response when nurses have pressed them for an answer in the face of similar silences. In such situations, the silence carries tacit messages about power relations, and the nurses' decision to press for an answer or interpret the silence illustrates the complex relational dance at work in the tacit layers of team communication exchanges.

One way in which nurses demonstrate their expertise is by knowing implicitly when something is urgent. In fact, explicit queries about urgency can both advertise lack of situational awareness and produce frustration in other team members. Consider the following example:

> Surgeons need suction. I [the observer] can see blood and fluid pooling up on the laporoscopic video screen. For some reason another case cart has to be brought in with another suction tip. It's been some time since original request when suction finally arrives.
>
> SN: 'Do you still need the suction?'
>
> Surgeons (frustrated): 'Yes! We do!'

In such cases, silent assumptions and action are preferable to an explicit question.

Silences that Emerge in the Content Category

The other common pattern of silence visible to the research observer revolves around the failure to communicate relevant information. This kind of failure was documented as a subtype of the Content code on our instrument. The most common of these is instances in which team members do not update one another on the status of outstanding issues:

> At 8:38am, the staff anaesthetist is looking for the patient card to stamp some paperwork. The circulating nurse doesn't know where it is. They look in a few places. There's no further discussion. At 9:04am, the anaesthetist still can't find the patient card and asks the circulating nurse again. She can't find it either. The anaesthetist suggests, 'Maybe it's in the linens.' No plan is articulated for resolving this issue. At 9:42am, the anaesthetist asks the circulating nurse, 'Did you find it [the patient card]? No?' The nurse replies, 'Yes.' The anaesthetist perks up: 'Where?' The circulating nurse responds, 'In all the stuff. Once I tidy, I usually find things.' (Observer's note: I didn't see when the circulating nurse found the card, but it is evident from this exchange that she hadn't thought to tell the anaesthetist, who had been looking for it.)

In such instances, it is difficult to determine whether team members have forgotten to relay the information or whether they have decided it is not important enough to bother. Particularly in cases where an issue is not yet resolved, team members appear to decide not to update their colleagues, instead staying silent until they have something definitive to report:

> At 9:28am, an issue arises with the light supply for the laparascopic equipment. The circulating nurse plays with the monitor lines; the surgical resident tries to give her instructions. She goes to call the charge nurse for help. She doesn't announce that she's doing this. The surgical resident suggests that they should try turning the machine off and then on again. The circulating nurse tells him that the charge nurse is on her way.

> The charge nurse arrives and the surgical resident addresses her by first name and asks for 'the usual cord that doesn't drop down?' The charge nurse replies: 'Unfortunately there are not always enough of the nice cords.' Then the charge nurse calls the vendor hotline. She doesn't announce what she's doing. The surgical resident says, 'I'm sorry, can you in the meantime try turning everything off and on again?' The circulating nurse answers, 'Sure', but it sounds like she's working hard to sound pleasant. Surgical resident offers, 'I think we need a new cord.' Now clearly frustrated, the circulating nurse says, 'I've called for one.' The charge nurse continues to try things suggested by the vendor on the phone. Shortly, the circulating nurse reports: 'The new cord is here.' The problem seems to be resolved though, so the cord is not used.

A key issue in this example is that requests and suggestions go unacknowledged. In conversation with the observer, the nurse interprets this as producing a kind of invisibility around her efforts:

When I come, and I'm not usually here, I don't know anything, and I don't have any credibility. They [surgeons] only want to talk to [charge nurse]. And when she says the exact same thing I did, they listen to her. And then I'm [CN waves as though trying to get recognition].

Another issue, however, is that throughout the example, the nurses do not announce what they are doing to resolve the monitor issue. The question is whether these silences constitute content failures; that is, if team members decide not to comprehensively update while they are en route to a solution to an identified problem, is this a communication failure or communication efficiency? Observers struggle to ascertain the threshold at which these bits of 'relevant information missing' become problematic, creating a patchwork of silence that undermines the team's efforts overall.

One hint that silence is problematic in such communicative chains is the insertion of a new communicator into the exchange to fill the 'gap' created by the silence:

The staff surgeon asks 'Can we have a peanut [small sponge]?' There is no response. The scrub nurse looks around. Directing his comment to the scrub nurse and using her name, the staff surgeon says, 'Just tell us when you have the peanut, Jill.' The scrub nurse shakes her head, 'no'. There is a pause. The staff surgeon calls for the circulating nurse: 'I need a peanut.' Later in the case, the staff surgeon indicates to the scrub nurse, 'Make sure you have [??] vessel loops up, Jill.' The scrub nurse says nothing. The circulating nurse goes and gets some.

The scrub nurse's silence in this example produces two immediate effects: the staff surgeon correctly interprets her silence to mean that the peanut is not immediately available, and then, following her head shake, he draws the circulating nurse into the exchange to ensure that the peanut will be retrieved. Later in the case, the scrub nurse again is silent when she might choose to confirm the availability of vessel loops, and the circulating nurse again steps in to the exchange. This exchange is trickier to assess, since the scrub nurse's silence might emerge from her knowledge that the circulating nurse standing nearby has heard the request for vessel loops and will comply with it. However, the observer notes from this case document that 'there's rising tension from [this] series of exchanges', suggesting that the silences interfere with team relations even if they do not interfere with the straightforward transfer of information and fulfilment of procedural tasks.

Content failures like these, where silence is related to a 'quiet' team member, often present themselves in a cluster of problematic exchanges, none of which themselves seem to justify a coding of 'communication failure' but the accumulation of which suggests the detrimental effects of silence on the team.

The most senior nurse in the room, who is in the circulating role, was very quiet. This seemed to hinder resolution of problems. For example, when the staff surgeon runs into trouble with the screen (11:22am), he asks a series of questions (Can you manually adjust white balance? Let's try again. Can you adjust the colour?). The circulating nurse hears and acts on these questions but never articulates or announces her actions. She eventually goes to call for help; this time she announces that she has called. The OR-coordinator arrives and then the PSA. OR-coordinator leaves. PSA arrives, [fiddles] with controls for a while (though it seems he doesn't have any solutions). The staff surgeon finally asks again: 'Are we getting another tower?' The circulating nurse pages a second PSA, returns and asks this PSA if there's another in the office. The circulating nurse disappears without indicating that she's going. Second PSA arrives and mumbles about being in six rooms, can't hear the pages. The staff surgeon asks the first PSA about the resolution. PSA1 says they can bring another or turn this one off and on again. They try turning off and on, with no success. Third screen arrives (a second was rolled in earlier but nobody pointed it out). PSA1 and the circulating nurse (who is now back in the room) set up new screen at 11:30am.

Observer notes: This seems to be primarily a style problem. Neither staff surgeon nor (especially) circulating nurse speaks very assertively in naming and navigating the situation. There seems to be less communication than needed for efficient resolution of the problem. I've also recorded this as a 'content' failure to capture that element of the exchange. Relevant information seems lacking (for example, status of attempt to fix the problem, plan to fix the problem, opinions about what should be done).

As this observer notes, the silences in this communication exchange seem attributable to personal 'style': some team members are more 'quiet' than others. In fact, volume and degree of communicative involvement – particularly the consistent patterning of who speaks more loudly and who speaks more quietly in the OR – is a function of social structures and power relationships, not only an issue of personal preference.

Degree of communicative involvement can be a cultural – as well as a personal – pattern. Survey research by Sexton et al. (2000) suggests that surgical culture discourages questioning and cross-checking across the team's hierarchical layers, which can create an involvement where team members are more likely to speak when spoken to than to offer comments or questions. Examples in the field notes suggest that this culture persists, particularly in instances where a volunteered question or comment reveals ignorance or mis-assumptions:

As the surgeons close, the anaesthetist asks if they still have to do a stoma. The staff surgeon replies: 'We're not doing a stoma today doctor. We're taking away the stoma. He came in with one and he's leaving without it.'

The anaesthetist's question reveals his ignorance of the surgical procedure and wins him public ridicule, confirming that it would have been prudent to keep quiet. Medical sociological studies of uncertainty (Fox 1957, Lingard et al. 2002a) draw attention to the tacit prohibitions against advertising what one does not know, and this cultural value likely shapes patterns of silence in an interprofessional and hierarchical environment such as the OR.

A third pattern of silences emerges in the Content failures category: team exchanges in which barely concealed conflict or anger simmers persistently but is never addressed. The following field note excerpt illustrates the issue of silence and tacit conflict:

> I think that the failures scale underestimated the communication problems for this case. There was a sense that the scrub nurse, the student scrub nurse, and the circulating nurse (this was a more novice circulating nurse; the senior circulating nurse from the preceding case was out of the room for much of this one) were not being effective at handing equipment or solving problems. I was aware of this, but the room remained quite quiet, and I was only able to document the issues in three failures. At the end of the procedure, the surgical fellow told me that she 'was boiling inside' for the whole case. 'Usually they're at least paying attention. Today, it was like, "Hello! We're operating here". I worry, based on the fellow's comment, that my observational skills weren't sharp enough today – but I also think that the surgeons internalized their frustration, so it was difficult to capture it through communication records.

This example crystallizes the issue of tacit communication. Although the room was silent for much of the case, the observer could sense the conflict and tension in the room, a sense confirmed by the fellow's comments. Such lurking tensions can pose grave difficulties for effective collaboration, yet they are difficult to capture in terms of a rating of explicit communication.

Uncategorized Silences

We have focused so far on the kinds of silences that our evaluative tool does manage to capture to some degree. While these examples illustrate the complexity of interpretation in assigning meanings to silence, another set of examples also require consideration: those for which our tool offers little or no basis for documentation. For example, in some observed cases there is no evidence on which to ascribe meaning to silence – just a description that there is no talk among team members: 'The case proceeds uneventfully but there is no talk at all between professions before the case begins.' Is this silence problematic? Certainly we have seen cases where such interprofessional silence is problematic, but we have also seen instances that suggest a team's non-verbal fluency. In one case, a nurse suggested pride in such silent team fluidity, announcing cheerfully to the team, 'Let's see if we can do the whole case without talking'; in another case a surgeon noted to the observer, 'Did you catch all of that non-verbal communication?' Instances of complete silence present such ambiguity that we cannot confidently assign them a category in our evaluative tool; therefore, if they are problematic, they are lost from the communication failures database. And, because our field note descriptions of complete silence are so lean, we are equally unable to satisfactorily capture their productive functions.

Summary and Implications

Our approach to evaluating team communication is based on the premise of assessing communication within its social context, interpreting rather than eliding the richness of communicative events that emerge, overlap, evolve, echo, resolve, abort or die away. Within such complex discursive webs, we have faced the challenge of addressing the relationships between communicative presence and absence – between speech and silence. This chapter is a preliminary description of that challenge, not in an attempt to offer conclusions or gain closure, but rather to interrogate and open up this complexity in communicative performance data.

This chapter foregrounds issues of interpretation rather than risking the perils of taking a literal approach to language: silences are meaningful but ambiguously so, and we have laid out our interpretive logic based on the rhetorical framework underpinning our evaluation tool. Our framework of audience, content, occasion and purpose is a way of categorizing communication failures that draws our attention to certain forms of communicative presence: an untimely instrument request, for instance, or a repeated question that rises in urgency. As we have described, in attending to the presence of such speech events, our attention is also drawn to the silences intertwined with them: the absence of an earlier, more proactive request or the absence of a response to the repeated question. In fact, our framework may impose a useful structure that helps render such silences 'visible' when they might otherwise escape observer's evaluative attention, particularly in relation to two areas of our framework (purpose and content) where silences tend to recur. However, we acknowledge that other patterns of silence do not so readily surface within our framework, and further critical attention needs to be paid to delineating the interpretive challenges associated with these.

The examples we consider illustrate that silence is neither straightforwardly 'good' nor straightforwardly 'bad'. Silence *can* reflect a lack of communication – an absence or gap in the chain of communication, such as when a request is not heard by a team member. But silence can also function as a communicative act that implies support, willingness to assist, inviting another to speak, keeping the peace, or pausing to reflect. And it can function as the operationalization of power relations, such as when a team member is 'silenced' by another's speech or the silence in the OR environment is oppressive, suggestive of unvoiced emotions running beneath the surface.

Because silence is often a communicative act, an important part of team members' communicative expertise is their ability to interpret and use silence. For instance, expert nurses possess a form of situation awareness that allows them to distinguish the right moment to interrupt the surgeon's silent concentration with questions. Similarly, decisions about what, when and how much to update on 'in-progress' issues likely involve a weighing of the desire for clarity and the prohibition against 'cluttering up' an already complex communicative environment with low-value messages such as 'ultrasound hasn't called back yet'.

Understanding silence as more than communicative absence requires the assignment of meaning based on social and ecological cues: a complex but necessary endeavour if we are to achieve an authentic and ecologically valid assessment of communicative performance. As we account for silence in the evaluation of communication failures as an outcome in a team briefing intervention, there are two key interpretive dangers. We can underestimate communication failures by not accounting for silences at all or by misreading them as productive when they are not, or we can overestimate communication problems by misreading silences as problematic when they are not. Further, we can distort the distribution of failure types by forcing an assignment of meaning in a particular direction, such as interpreting all requests-without-responses as purpose failures when in fact silence may send a tacit message that resolves the question's purpose. In our own work, we have used spontaneous interviews whenever possible to judge the meanings of silences for which contextual cues are ambiguous or lacking; however, this is not always a viable technique for performance assessment.

Silence is intimately linked to speech in complex communicative environments like the operating room. While the evaluation of a team's communicative performance traditionally focuses on what observers can see and objectively label, we need to pay attention to the interplay of speech and silence and articulate our logical frameworks for assigning meaning to silence. 'Counting silence' is a complicated but necessary business for performance evaluation for safer surgery: silence can promote safety when team members 'count to ten' and think before acting, and it can undermine safety when team members fail to cross-check and respond to one another's questions. We hope that our reflection on the patterns of silence as they emerge within the rhetorical framework of our evaluation tool will prompt surgical performance researchers to consider the problem of silence, towards carefully theorized and situated accounts of its role in teamwork.

References

Bradbury-Jones, C., Sambrook, S. and Irvine, F. (2007) Power and empowerment in nursing: A fourth theoretical approach. *Journal of Advanced Nursing* 62(2), 258–66.

Brown, W. (2005) Freedom's silences. In *Edgework: Critical Essays on Knowledge and Politics* (pp. 83–96). Princeton, NJ: Princeton University Press.

Fox, R. (1957) Training for certainty. In R.K. Merton, G. Reader and P.L. Kendall (eds) *The Student Physician*. Cambridge, MA: Harvard University Press.

Gillespie, B.M., Wallis, M. and Chaboyer, W. (2008) Operating theater culture: Implications for nurse retention. *Western Journal of Nursing Research* 30(2), 259–77.

Glenn, C. (2004) *Unspoken: A Rhetoric of Silence.* Carbondale, IL: Southern Illinois University Press.

Helmreich, R.L. (2000) On error management: Lessons from aviation. *British Medical Journal* 320(7237), 781–5.

Helmreich, R.L. and Davies, J.M. (1994) Team performance in the operating room. In M.S. Bogner (ed.) *Human Error in Medicine* (pp. 225–53). Hillside, NJ: Erlbaum.

Joint Commission on Accreditation of Healthcare Organizations (2003) Sentinel event statistics. 24 June. Available from: <http://www.jointcommission.org/SentinelEvents/SentinelEventAlert/sea_29.htm> [last accessed March 2009].

Kohn, L.T., Corrigan, J.M., and Donaldson, M.S. (eds) (2000) *To Err is Human: Building a Safer Health System.* Washington, DC: National Academy Press.

Lingard, L., Espin, S., Rubin, B., Whyte, S., Colmenares, M., Baker, G.R., Doran, D., Grober, E., Orser, B., Bohnen, J. and Reznick, R. (2005) Getting teams to talk: Development and pilot implementation of a checklist to promote safer operating room communication. *Quality and Safety in Health Care* 14, 340–6.

Lingard, L., Espin, S., Whyte, S., Regehr, G., Baker, R., Orser, B., Doran, D., Reznick, R., Bohnen, J. and Grober, E. (2004) Communication failures in the operating room: An observational classification of recurrent types and outcomes. *Quality and Safety in Healthcare* 13, 330–4.

Lingard, L., Garwood, K., Schryer, C., and Spafford, M. (2002a) A certain art of uncertainty: Case presentation and the development of professional identity. *Social Science and Medicine* 56, 603–17.

Lingard, L., Regehr, G., Orser, B., Reznick, R., Baker, G.R., Doran, D., Espin, S., Bohnen, J. and Whyte, S. (2008) Team talk: Preoperative briefings among surgeons, nurses and anesthetists reduce communication failures. *Archives of Surgery* 143(1), 12–17.

Lingard, L., Regehr, G., Whyte, S., Reznick, R., Bohnen, J., Baker, G.R., Espin, S., Doran, D., Orser, B. and Grober, E. (2006) A theory-based instrument to evaluate team communication in the operating room: Balancing measurement authenticity and reliability. *Quality and Safety in Health Care* 15, 422–6.

Lingard, L., Reznick, R., DeVito, I. and Espin, S. (2002b) Forming professional identities on the healthcare team: Discursive constructions of the 'other' in the operating room. *Medical Education* 36(8), 728–34.

Lingard, L., Reznick, R., Espin, S., DeVito, I. and Regehr, G. (2002c) Team communication in the operating room: Talk patterns, sites of tension and implications for novices. *Academic Medicine* 77(3), 37–42.

Manias, E. and Street, A. (2001) Nurse-doctor interactions during critical care ward rounds. *Journal of Clinical Nursing* 10, 442–50.

Riley, R. and Manias, E. (2005) Rethinking theatre in modern operating rooms. *Nursing Inquiry* 12, 2–9.

Salas, E., Rosen, M.A., Burke, C.S., Nicholson, D. and Howse, W.R. (2007) Markers for enhancing team cognition in complex environments: The power of team performance diagnosis. *Aviation Space and Environmental Medicine* 78(5 Suppl), B77–85.

Saville-Troike, M. (1985) The place of silence in an integrated theory of communication. In D. Tannen and M. Saville-Troike (eds) *Perspectives on Silence*. Norwood, NJ: Ablex Publishing Corporation.

Saville-Troike, M. (2003) *The Ethnography of Communication: An Introduction.* 3rd edition. Malden, MA: Blackwell Publishing.

Sexton, B.J., Thomas, E.J. and Helmreich, R.I. (2000) Error, stress and teamwork in medicine and aviation: Cross sectional surveys. *British Medical Journal* 320, 745–9.

Tan, J., Naik, V. and Lingard, L. (2006) Exploring obstacles to proper timing of prophylactic antibiotics for surgical site infections. *Quality and Safety in Health Care* 15(1), 32–8.

Undre, S., Sevdalis, N., Healey, A.N., Darzi, A. and Vincent, C.A. (2007) Observational Teamwork Assessment for Surgery (OTAS): Refinement and application in urological surgery. *World Journal of Surgery* 31(7), 1373–81.

Chapter 18

Observing Team Problem Solving and Communication in Critical Incidents

Gesine Hofinger and Cornelius Buerschaper

Introduction

Although a relatively recent research area, we are beginning to understand the significance of human factors for patient safety, especially the role of interpersonal skills (e.g., Fletcher et al. 2003, Kohn et al. 1999) and the importance of non-technical skills on technical outcome factors (Mishra et al. 2008, Reader et al. 2006).

Many efforts to improve non-technical skills have been made in different domains; for example the crew resource management training (CRM) in aviation, and adaptations in healthcare. CRM training was designed to strengthen team-related skills for decision-making in critical situations and to enhance safety during routine situations (Cannon-Bowers et al. 1995, Jensen 1995, Merrit and Helmreich 1997, Wiener et al. 1993). In unexpected situations, standard operating procedures (SOPs) do not help so then crews need to actively solve problems. Thus, the idea of CRM includes problem-solving and team skills or, rather, communication and teamwork are seen as means for good decision-making in the cockpit. One concept that combines communication, teamwork and problem solving is that of 'shared mental models' (Cannon-Bowers and Salas 2001, Klimoski and Mohammed 1994, Schöbel and Kleindienst 2001).

Sharing mental models is critical for team problem solving because it is the process by which problem solving becomes a team activity. 'Problem solving' is a thinking process that integrates perception and processing of relevant clues from the environment (like a sudden drop in a patient's blood pressure), the development of a plan and the decision for one option. Being a thinking process it can be observed *only* by observing speech acts accompanying thought ('thinking aloud') or overt behaviour. This is true for team members as well as for researchers. So, team problem solving can only occur if people share relevant thoughts using explicit communication.

Shared mental models enable members of a team to gain a shared understanding of the task and to cooperate accordingly. The shared understanding of the problem allows all the participants in the operation to remain 'in the loop'. Team research has highlighted the importance of shared mental models for team performance (Entin and Serfaty 1999, Orasanu 1990, Stout et al. 1999).

As we see it, healthcare has willingly adopted the idea of training for team-related skills in medically critical situations (Davies 2001, Glavin and Maran 2003, Howard et al. 1992, Risser et al. 1999, Thomas et al. 2004), without putting much emphasis on the process of problem solving. Good decision-making on the other hand is a result of adequate problem solving. There is a long-standing tradition of problem-solving research in psychology (e.g., Dörner 1996, Frensch and Funke 1995), but little of that has been translated into the field of healthcare.

Research into CRM courses shows that some training programmes lead to measurable results and some do not. In spite of the diversity of results, we can conclude that CRM training in general has proven to be useful in terms of changing behaviour and values, and that it can improve the efficiency of teams (Morey et al. 2002, Salas et al. 2001, 2006). Yet what we do not seem to fully understand is how improved communication skills in teams and improved decision-making interact.

One pre-requisite of evaluating CRM training programmes is the development of tools for measuring behaviour. The use of behavioural markers is now a widely accepted approach in aviation (Häusler et al. 2004, Transportation 1998) where in many countries the evaluation of CRM skills has become part of the licence check (e.g., Joint Aviation Authorities 2006). Also in healthcare, over the last decade many research groups have developed sets of behavioural markers for team-related skills (e.g., Carthey et al. 2003, Fletcher et al. 2004, Gaba et al. 1998, Thomas et al. 2004, Undre et al. 2007, Yule et al. 2006). The behaviours covered are similar; communication, team leadership and decision-making are always part of the set.

Thus, it seems possible to measure CRM performance in terms of the team showing certain classes of behaviour more or less adequately. But there is still a lack of knowledge about what actually happens while a healthcare team is solving problems, e.g., in an incident in the operating room (OR). How do they approach the problem? How do they find a decision? Do they negotiate goals and plans? Do they actively build shared mental models by talking about their perception of the problem?

Being psychologists interested in action and in problem solving we carried out, together with anaesthetists, an observational study on problem solving in critical incidents in the OR. We aimed to understand the process of problem solving in a team, so we developed two tools for the observation and evaluation: one for problem solving in the team and a very specific behavioural marker system for communication in defined critical incidents. The observational study was part of a research project on the development and evaluation of training of problem solving which was funded by the German Federal Ministry of Education and Research. Here, we report only our approach to observing problem solving and communication in the OR.

Observing Problem Solving and Communication in Anaesthesia

Concept

Good problem solving skills are essential for team members in dynamic, high risk domains such as the OR. Since this is especially true during unexpected events we focussed on observing critical incidents within the OR.

Communication is an essential part of team problem solving and is also important for the creation of a cooperative team atmosphere, for the maintenance of professional identity, and the exchange of information to coordinate routine activities (St Pierre et al. 2007). But in critical situations like incidents during an operation, communication must, above all, serve to establish and maintain a shared understanding and coordinate behaviour; the other functions of communication become secondary (a cooperative team atmosphere, e.g., must be established *before* an incident).

When incidents in the OR occur – at least in the German hospital system – the anaesthesiologists are often responsible for coordinating the overall situation. This includes conferring with the surgeons, but also with the anaesthesia assistants, whose integration is essential. Additionally, contact must be maintained with superiors, the laboratory, the blood bank, and the intensive care unit. Anaesthesiologists plan their own behaviour and organize the team. Thus, they have a central function for the problem solving processes in the system OR. For this reason, the study presented here focuses on anaesthesiologists.

As said above, little is known about the communication behaviour in the OR. Analogously to many studies of cockpit communication (e.g., Dietrich and von Meltzer 2003, Sexton and Helmreich 2000), some studies of communication in operations (e.g., Grommes 2000) have focused on the structures of language and their potential to distort communication (linguistic approach). The other approach to communication in the cockpit, the socio-psychological approach, has rarely been pursued for operations (but see Coiera and Tombs 1998). This approach understands communication as a behaviour correlate of specific attitudes, personality traits, etc. and correlates it with the team's achievement: 'It investigates which communicative patterns contribute to effective teamwork.' (Silberstein 2001, p. 5)

Behaviour during incidents in the operating theatre is difficult to investigate, because (at least in Germany) there are no recordings of all events in all operations, in contrast to the cockpit voice recorder and 'black box' in aviation. Field observations would be uneconomical due to the low frequency of critical incidents. Furthermore, in real crisis situations, the presence of an observer may be a distraction.

For this reason, the study presented here captured on video and analysed incidents processed in the anaesthesia simulator. In the setting used for this study, the surgical side of the simulator is not realized so the surgeons and nursing staff simply play a role. The nursing staff's field of activity during anaesthesia is also only partially represented. The specialized field of activity for the anaesthesiologists is thus more realistic than for the other occupation groups. Since the content of the communication is determined by specialist activity, in this study we investigated only the anaesthesiologists' communication, not that of the surgeons or the nursing staff.

Anaesthesia simulators, like most flight simulators, are high fidelity simulators. These offer the advantage of allowing a relatively standardized way of observing how incidents are dealt with. Complete standardization is not possible, because the behaviour of the anaesthesiologists influences the further course of the incident. The analysis of such scenarios thus faces the same problems as does problem-solving research with highly complex computer-simulated scenarios (see Dörner et al. 1983).

Behaviour in simulator scenarios can already deviate from real operation situations because, in calm beginning phases, the participants are more prepared for critical events during an operation. Additionally, at least at the beginning, the participants are aware that they are in an observation situation. For this reason, utterances that often occur in calm phases of real operations, like jokes, lessons, and private conversation (Pettinari 1988), are rarely heard. Despite these limitations, physiologically and as an operation setting for anaesthesiologists, the simulator is at least apparently valid. In the scenarios we used (cf. Section 2.3), the anaesthesiologists exhibited a high degree of involvement which was confirmed in self reports (St Pierre et al. 2004). This high degree of the participants' involvement during 'hot phases' of the scenario suggests that here they used their customary communication strategies, especially to coordinate with the nursing staff and surgeons.

Research Questions

The study presented here investigated how anaesthesiologists in critical situations in the simulator communicate with their nursing staff and the surgeons. The focus of the investigation is on the analysis of the anaesthesiologists' utterances arose during the processed scenarios, focussing on communication. This includes the organization of behaviour and the coordination of the team: establishing shared mental models, conveying and requesting information, defining goals, planning, deciding, control, conflict management, reflection, etc. Special attention is paid to the interaction with the surgeons. Here, we pursued three issues:

Description of the Communication (Exploratory, Descriptive Question) Since there are so few studies of communication in operations, we first investigated what general kinds of utterances arise in the processed scenarios. A focus is on communication related to problem solving.

We were also particularly interested in finding out whether clinical experience, gender or the kind of scenario had an influence on the kinds of utterance.

Connection between the Categories of Communication and the Quality of Medical Management (Hypothesis-testing and Exploratory Question)   The results of human factors research in other occupational fields permits us to deduce the hypothesis that the quality of medical management is connected with communication. We therefore ask: how does the communication behaviour of anaesthesiologists differ under good and bad medical management in the scenarios?

Quality of Communication in Critical Situations (Exploratory Question, Normative Approach)   During the scenario's critical situations, the communication was evaluated in terms of previously formulated behavioural expectations (behavioural markers): did the anaesthesiologists exhibit the type of communication behaviour that psychological and medical experts would expect in a team problem-solving process?

Method

Data Background: The Training Study 'Human Factors in Anaesthesia'

With cooperation between the Simulator Centre of the Anaesthesia Clinic at Erlangen University Clinic and the Institute for Theoretical Psychology, a curriculum for physicians training for their specialization, 'Human Factors in Anaesthesia', was developed (St Pierre et al. 2004). This combined previously introduced simulator training for crisis management and psychological training modules on specific human factors topics. The psychological trainers are also involved in the feedback about the processing of anaesthesiological crisis scenarios in the simulator. For the first module, 'communication and cooperation in the OR', three scenarios were developed that made specific demands on team problem solving and communication while dealing with incidents. This made it possible to evaluate not only the medical competence of the participants, but also their team-related problem-solving competence. Thus, the desirable integration of non-technical abilities (e.g., communication in an interdisciplinary team) and specialized procedures (e.g., stabilizing blood pressure) was achieved.

The first module of the curriculum was evaluated in an experimental design with a test group and a control group. The control group received a lecture on human factors in anaesthesia instead of the training unit. They worked through the same simulator scenarios. For a more detailed presentation of the study and of the training evaluation, (see St Pierre et al. 2004). The scenarios both groups worked through in the course of training were used for the evaluations presented here, because few differences were to be expected within the training (any differences are highlighted in this chapter).

Sample

The participants in the study were 34 interns at the University Clinic for Anaesthesiology in Erlangen. This was a random sample, except that women and men were distributed evenly between the two groups and among the training sessions. Because the sample was small, the participating women worked through Scenario 2 whenever possible. This means that the effects of sex and scenarios are confounded, but recognizable. Despite the partly chance allotment, it was possible to obtain homogeneous partial samples, with the exception that the individual scenarios were differently filled in terms of the sex and experience of the participants. Clinical experience ranged from one to six years with a mean of 3.3 years. Men and women did not significantly differ in their mean length of clinical or in simulator experience.

Table 18.1   Sample of the sample

	Men	Women	Total sample
N	22	12	34
Years of clinical experience	3.4	3.1	3.3
Proportion of participants with simulator experience	68%	42%	59%
Scenario 1	11	1	12
Scenario 2	1	10	11
Scenario 3	10	1	11

Scenarios Used

For the training programme, the following scenarios were developed so as to make specific demands not only on the management of a medical incident, but also on problem solving and communication in the team. Each scenario (detailed below) was designed to take 30 minutes (the actual duration of the scenarios ranged from 16 to 42 minutes).

The training programme's three scenarios were each worked through by one participant, each supported by a real nurse. Simulator staff assumed the role of the surgeon, sometimes supported by a participant. The scenarios are based on a script that calls for fairly standardized communication from the instructed role-players in predetermined critical situations. For example, after a drop in blood pressure, the surgeon asks one of the anaesthesiologists whether he or she 'isn't managing back there'. If the participant ignores the question, the script prescribes as the surgeon's 'answer strategy' that he or she 'exert verbal pressure'. But if the anaesthesiologist communicates a problem, the script instructs to offer cooperation.

The participants judged all three scenarios to be adequately realistic and to be stressful. On a five-step Likert scale (1 = very realistic, 5 = not realistic at all), the means for evaluated realism were between 1.8 and 2.55 (n.s.); on a ten-step Likert scale (1 = boredom, 10 = overburdening), the stress caused by the scenario was reported as between 5.3 and 7.6 (n.s.). While extreme stress would deteriorate participants' ability to problem solve whereas boredom would mean that they did not experience a critical situation (but instead routine), the medium stress levels reported seems to indicate that participants were challenged but not working at their limit.

Scenario 1: Laparoscopic Cholecystectomy with Volume Deficiency Reaction and Air Embolism

In a laparoscopic cholecystectomy, the abdominal cavity is filled with CO_2 gas to provide the surgeon with better visibility. If the abdomen is inflated too much, less blood can flow back from the abdomen to the heart, resulting in lower blood pressure and a faster pulse. This is the first complication in the scenario. After the therapy, which requires close communication between the surgeon and the anaesthesiologist, operative inattention leads to bleeding in the abdominal cavity. CO_2 gas flows into the bloodstream and results in an air embolism. The anaesthesiologist must recognize this situation, which is acutely life-threatening for the patient, and plan the therapy, in which the surgeon must be integrated. The therapy consists in administering medications that stabilize circulation and, if appropriate, changing the operating procedure, organizing transesophageal ultrasound and transfer to the intensive care unit (ICU).

Scenario 2: Occluded Perforated Abdominal Aorta Aneurysm

This clinical picture is an aneurysm of the main artery in the upper abdomen (acute intense pain). The aneurysm tears or bursts, resulting in a life-threatening situation. This is the situation in this case.

The anaesthesiologist must rapidly coordinate the operating procedure in close discussion with the surgeon and the nursing staff and attempt to stabilize circulation with the aid of providing volume (blood, infusions) and medications supporting circulation (catecholamines). Special communicative demands arise if clamping off is too fast or if the surgeon opens the aorta. In the end, the patient should be sent to the intensive care ward in a stable state.

Scenario 3: Lung Embolism after Speculum Examination of the Knee in the Recovery Room

This scenario is about a postoperative complication resulting from vascular congestion. The clinical picture develops suddenly when the bloodstream carries a blood clot (thrombus) into the lung, where it blocks a blood vessel. Thus, a section of the lung is no longer supplied with blood, and no gas exchange occurs here. The blood backs up to the heart and the heart muscle is acutely overburdened, resulting in circulatory failure and intense pain.

The anaesthesiologist is called to a patient (who has had a knee operation) as an emergency and must familiarize him or herself with the situation, collect the necessary information and then organize the therapy. Treatment includes firstly, applying medications that support circulation, anaesthesia and respiration and thereafter, medications that reduce blood clotting. But, the use of such a thrombolytic after surgery must be discussed with the surgeon. For the severity of the embolism and the state of therapy to be judged, a number of specialists must be brought in and their judgements discussed.

Observation Evaluation Tools

The analysis of the scenarios is based on the methods of evaluation described in the following:

- a system of categories, 'problem solving in a team'
- behavioural markers for specific communication behaviours
- experts' judgement of medical management.

A Tool for Observing Problem Solving in the Anaesthesia Team

A system of categories, 'problem solving in a team', was developed to categorize everything uttered in each scenario. It comprises 24 categories organised into five 'overarching categories' labelled: (i) formal characteristics of the statement, (ii) organization of activity, (iii) relation the team and of processes, (iv) conflict management and (v) other. The development of the system was oriented toward the phases of action organization, as developed by Dörner (1996), and toward considerations emerging from research on solving complex problems in groups (e.g., Stempfle and Badke-Schaub 2002, 2003). It was supplemented by inductive category formation on the basis of video data from the anaesthesia simulator. Every remark was classified on the formal level and in one of the other four overarching categories. Randomness-corrected observer agreement on these categorizations reached 61 percent–80 percent (Cohen's Kappa). Table 18.2 shows the overarching and subsidiary categories.

Behavioural Markers for Specific Communication Behaviour

Behavioural markers for communication were developed. Behavioural markers are behaviour patterns whose presence in a stream of behaviour indicates certain skills. For the present evaluations, anaesthesiologists and psychologists developed a set of behavioural expectations based on the scenario scripts. Studies using

Table 18.2   Category system 'Problem solving in a team'

Overarching category	Categories
Formal characteristics	Question, statement, directive/order, other New unit of activity, addressing the surgeon on own initiative
Organization of activity	Information gathering, model formation, conveying information (facts), decision, explanation of own activity, commentary on activity, conveying problem and situation, conveying problem and situation with model, redundance, control, confirming understanding, hypothesis, anticipation, goal, plan
Relation to team and process	Utterances related to team and relationship, process organization Reflection/emotional utterances/own feelings[a]
Conflict management	Offer to engage in conflict;[b] anaesthesiologist: objective, escalating, ignoring, de-escalating
Other	

a   Because pure utterances of reflection were not expected, these categories were bundled together.

b   This is the only category that considers the surgeon's utterances, because a conflict always arises from interaction. All utterances that could be considered offers to engage in conflict were counted.

behavioural markers often report low inter-rater reliability, but for our project, which aims to evaluate a training programme, a high concordance between observers was essential. So, we decided to formulate a set of very specific markers. They describe communicative behaviour required to solve a scenario optimally, for example the insistence on a slow de-clamping in the aorta aneurysm scenario. A list of behaviour-oriented observable items was developed that operationalizes the necessary communication competencies.

The demands of each scenario were different, so 16 to 22 different markers were defined for each scenario. Two observers judged the presence of each marker in each person in the scenario (possible answers: yes, no, not applicable). The randomness-corrected observer agreement here was 82 percent (Cohen's Kappa). This shows that it is easier to achieve good inter-rater reliability using more specific markers (but of course, the marker set has to be defined for every scenario that is evaluated). Examples for the behavioural markers used are shown in Table 18.3.

Experts' Judgement of Medical Management

Two anaesthesia experts also independently judged the medical management of the scenarios. The experts were not aware that the videos were being evaluated in

Table 18.3   Examples of behavioural markers for evaluating communication in the scenarios used

	Critical situation in accordance with script	Behavioural marker
Scenario 1	*Before the OP*	Gives the OK for the OP only after his/her own preparations are completed
	Changed position (head raised, feet lowered)	Anaesthesiologist conveys concern to the surgeon early Anaesthesiologist asks for a change of position/release of pressure
Scenario 2	*Cut*	Requests rapid clamping or conveys problem Asks the surgeon to report
	Clamping	Intermediate briefing with nurse Improvement of circulation conveyed to surgeon
Scenario 3	*Anaesthesiologist enters recovery room*	Anaesthesiologist asks nurse what has happened Responsible superior is informed
	Surgeon rejects heparin	Anaesthesiologist remains objective Anaesthesiologist conveys reasons (acute danger to patient, life takes priority over knee … vital problem)

accordance with the aforementioned tools. Differing observations were discussed until agreement was achieved (communicative validation, e.g., Bauer and Gaskell 2000). For each phase of each scenario, a system was used in which points were given for quality of therapy, diagnostics, and, where applicable, monitoring. Each item could be scored from 0 to 2 points (bad to very good), which resulted in scores between 16 and 24 points for the scenarios. Table 18.4 shows the eight evaluation items for Scenario 1.

Some Results

As studies on problem solving or the analysis of thinking processes in the medical field are rare (but see Gaba 1992), we started with explorative questions. We were able to formulate hypotheses concerning the field of communication. We would like to highlight some of the findings of our analysis that helped us improve our training programmes. In short:

Table 18.4   Items for evaluating medical management (Scenario 1)

Acute phase 1 (pneumoperitoneum with circulatory reaction)			Acute phase 2 (discr. venous bleeding)	Acute phase 3 (air embolism)			
Anaesthesia introduced (0–2Pt)	Differential diagnose (0–2Pt)	Therapy (0–2Pt)	Therapy (0–2Pt)	Diag. standard (0–2Pt)	Diag. advanced (0–2Pt)	Therapy circulation (0–2Pt)	Therapy breathing (0–2Pt)

- Anaesthetists talked more often than they expected they would across all scenarios.
- Almost half of all utterances help pacing or establishing shared mental models.
- We found nearly no explicit addressing of the team.
- There was nearly no talking about aims and plans (of more than one step).
- There were very few real questions.
- We found a high correlation (.56) between the quality of clinical management and communication measured with the behavioural markers.

In reporting some results, we will give the explorative questions that lead us in the analysis followed by the answer.

Description of Communication

Amount and Type of Utterances

How much do the participants talk, and what kind of remarks do they make? The anaesthesiologists spoke more during the scenarios than even they themselves expected: in preliminary talks, the intention to investigate communication during operations was repeatedly belittled as senseless on the grounds that there is little speaking during an operation (which also contradicts our observations of operations). There was a mean of 228 utterances per person; with an average scenario duration of 28 minutes, that is 8.2 utterances per minute. The sample showed no difference between men and women in the amount spoken. Utterances in the form of orders – an average of 25.4 per scenario – account for almost a tenth of all utterances. There were 31.3 questions asked per scenario. In terms of content, it should be considered that the proportion of genuine questions is much lower, because many directives are clothed in the form of a question ('Would you hold the bag?'). Table 18.5 shows the distribution of these formal categories in the scenarios.

The formal categories showed no significant differences between the scenarios, sexes, or experience – nor any interaction between the factors. This finding is surprising, because it seems to mean that anaesthesiologists in the simulator

Table 18.5   Formal characteristics of utterances in the scenarios

Category	Question	Directive/ order	Statement/ utterance	Other/ filler phrases	*Utterances total*
Mean	31.6	25.5	162.5	8.2	*227.9*
Minimum	10	2	89	0	*126*
Maximum	75	62	349	26	*433*

utter a certain number of utterances of a specific kind. This should be further investigated.

Proportion of Utterances Aiming at Team Coordination and the Establishment of a Shared Mental Model

How much of what is said relates to the coordination of team activity and the establishment of shared mental models? Here we looked at the categories: *conveying information; thinking out loud; conveying problems (facts only); conveying problems with an explanation or model; explanation of one's own activity; redundancy; confirming understanding; addressing the surgeon (anaesthesiologist's initiative).*

An essential factor in successful problem solving is establishing shared mental models. This process cannot be completely observed, but there are utterances that explicitly suggest the intention of improving a shared mental model (e.g., *confirming understanding; explanation of one's own activity*) and some that can help the other team members in 'pacing' (e.g., *thinking aloud; conveying information*). The importance of these tasks for problem solving is reflected in the frequency of such utterances: the anaesthesiologist says something that can contribute to team coordination a mean of 108 times per scenario, almost four times per minute. This corresponds, in the mean, to almost half of all utterances (47 percent). But a mean of only 18 utterances were explicitly related to establishing shared mental models (*conveying problems with explanation; explanation of one's own activity; confirming understanding*). Table 18.6 shows the distribution among categories that we regard as helpful in or as aiming directly at constructing shared mental models. As with the categories of action organization, there are enormous individual differences. The frequency of *redundance* seems to indicate the anaesthesiologist's intense safety awareness.

In these categories, we found there are no differences in relation to experience or sex.

Table 18.6   **Utterances related to team coordination and shared mental models**

Category	Mean	Minimum	Maximum
Conveying information	16.6	4	42
Thinking out loud	14.0	1	68
Conveying problems (facts)	22.4	5	49
Addressing surgeon on own initiative	9.4	0	34
Conveying problems with explanation	4.7	0	11
Explanation of own activity	7.5	0	15
Confirming understanding	5.8	0	16
Redundance	27.8	2	49
Total	*111.3*	*49*	*203*

Utterances Concerning the Team and the Team Problem-solving Process

How much of what is said relates to the team and the process of working together? We counted the categories: *reflection or emotional utterance*; *references to relationships*; *process*.

A large part of the speaking is devoted to coordinating activity (especially with the nurse); but very few utterances are directly related to the team. In the scenarios, only the relationship to the surgeon was thematized, usually to draw boundaries (in the sense of 'Don't interfere with my work, I don't try to tell you what to do, either'), seldom to underscore the shared team task (e.g., 'Now we have to manage this together'). Reflection on the problem-solving process was bundled together with utterances of one's own emotional state (e.g., 'Here I'm not so sure, either...'), because we expected (and found) few self-reflective utterances in the sense of strategy evaluation. Utterances related to the work process ('Let's do this now one step at a time') accounted for a mean proportion of 5 percent; this is less than one would expect for 'good team achievement' (see Table 18.7).

Interestingly, there was virtually no communication about goals or plans (less than 1 percent of all utterances). This may be due to the pressure of the situation, or it could indicate a learning need for team problem solving. The individual differences are substantial in the categories of team and problem-solving process, but women and men do not significantly differ in their use of these categories ($p=.360$, $t=.93$; $df=32$). Nor do experience or the scenario type lead to significant differences in these categories ($F=2.04$; $p=.15$; and $F=0.17$; $p=.84$).

Table 18.7   Utterances related to the team and the problem-solving process

Category	Thematization of the relationship	Reflection/ emotional utterances	Process	*Total*
Mean	5.5	2.9	12.2	*20.5*
Minimum	0	0	1	*4*
Maximum	22	10	32	*47*

Quality of Communication in Critical Situations

Quality of Communication as Evaluated by the Behavioural Markers

How well do the participants fulfil the expectations concerning good communication that we formulated as behavioural markers? The number of behavioural markers confirmed in the utterances of each participant showed a rather weak performance. In fact, only 58 percent of the expected behaviours were shown (with an inter-rater reliability of 83 percent). For example, in 61 percent of all scenarios, the anaesthetists did not explicitly seek agreement with the surgeon (we also repeatedly found this in OR observations) before important steps in the process.

Clinical Experience and Quality of Communication

What role does clinical experience play in the quality of communication? Based on our observations in the OR, we expected that senior anaesthetists would not necessarily perform better because simply working longer in the setting 'hospital' does not seem to imply learning more about good communication. This was exactly what we found when looking at the behavioural markers.

Communication Skills and the Quality of Medical Problem Solving

Based on the literature on human factors, we expected a substantial correlation between the evaluation of medical management and the quality of communication, as captured in the behavioural markers. We found a surprisingly high correlation of $r=.57$ ($p=.001$; $t=3.77$; $df=31$; see Figure 18.1). Those doctors who communicated most adequately also performed best.

Interestingly, the quality of medical management is not connected with the total number of things said ($r=-.08$; $p>.1$). Talking a lot during a medical crisis is not useful in itself; what is important is the quality of communication.

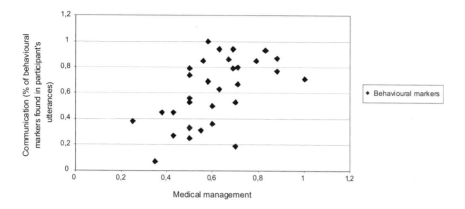

Figure 18.1   Connection between medical management and the quality of communication

The Influence of Establishing Shared Mental Models on the Quality of Medical Management

Is there a connection between the quality of medical management and the establishment of shared mental models, as found in the categories *spontaneously addressing the surgeon*; *confirming understanding*; *conveying problems with explanation*; *explanation of one's own activity*? For the entire 'package' of variables relevant to this question, correlation is zero ($r=.09$; $p>.1$). Because the literature (see above) postulates the importance of the establishment of shared mental models – a judgement we share – we examined the individual correlations. In our scenarios, utterances directed primarily to the nursing staff (*confirming understanding*; *explanation of one's own activity*) did not significantly contribute to effectiveness of the doctor's problem solving ($r=.20$; $p>.1$ and $r=.09$; $p>.1$). Nevertheless, this kind of utterance remains important for patient safety. The case is different for *conveying problems with explanation*, a behaviour usually directed at the surgeon; here, the assumed importance of a shared understanding of the situation is found ($r=.25$; $p=.045$). Telling a problem *and* giving explanations allows the team partner to think along the same lines.

Discussion and Outlook

The findings presented in this chapter suggest that it is possible to investigate and analyse the content of the communication of anaesthesiologists in (simulated) critical situations. Substantial portions of spoken communication serve the problem-solving regulation of activity and the coordination of the team.

Several factors limit this approach. First, despite the similarity of the setting, an incident in the simulator differs emotionally and medically from an incident in an actual operation – the genuine danger and the genuine support are both lacking. Second, communication during an operation is not solely verbal – coordination of actions is also achieved implicitly often by gesture and especially by expressions of the eyes, which impress observers with their differentiation. Nevertheless, the spoken word is indispensable and essential for common activity on the basis of shared mental models, including during an operation.

What can be deduced from the presented results for specialized training and advanced training? First, we can confirm that communication is indeed important for managing incidents in anaesthesiology. The high correlation between the quality of medical management and the quality of communication permits us to conclude that good communication alone cannot, of course, produce a good physician, but it helps in finding strategies for successful problem-solving activity in critical, i.e., medically dangerous, situations. Expressed negatively: poor communication prevents, among other things, the securing of adequate support in medically overchallenging situations. Also of course, (medical) overburdening favours poor communication.

But anaesthesiologists' abilities to express problem solving and team coordination in communication differ very widely. There is a marked need for improvement. The behaviour data thus support the need to include more non-technical skills in professional and advanced training as seen in the literature presented in the introduction. The observing tools presented here need to be developed further. Currently we are involved in a small study on team management in the emergency department. The aim is to find out how teams in emergency rooms organize and how they communicate in order to solve complex problems. We will test our observation tool for team problem solving in the emergency room setting to investigate whether observation in a multi-player context can be achieved with sufficient accuracy.

The communication data permit the deduction of the following training contents: *explicit formation of shared mental models* (especially relating to the future development of the situation) and organisation of action (stages of the problem-solving process).

References

Bauer, M. and Gaskell, G. (eds) (2000) *Qualitative Researching with Text, Image and Sound: A Practical Handbook for Social Research*. London: Sage.

Cannon-Bowers, J.A. and Salas, E. (2001) Reflections on shared cognition. *Journal of Organizational Behavior* 22, 195–202.

Cannon-Bowers, J.A., Tannenbaum, S.I., Salas, E. and Volpe, C.E. (1995) Defining team competencies and establishing team training requirements. In R. Guzzo and E. Salas (eds), *Team Effectiveness and Decision Making in Organizations* (pp. 330–80). San Francisco: Jossey-Bass.

Carthey, J., de Levala, M.R., Wright, D.J., Farewell, V.T. and Reason, J.T. (2003) Behavioural markers of surgical excellence. *Safety Science* 41(5), 409–25.

Coiera, E. and Tombs, V. (1998) Communication behaviors in a hospital setting: An observational study. *British Medical Journal* 316, 673–6.

Davies, J. (2001) Medical applications of crew resource management. In E. Salas, C. Bowers and E. Edens (eds), *Improving Teamwork in Oranizations. Application of Resource Management Training* (pp. 265–81). Mahwah: Lawrence Erlbaum.

Dietrich, R. and von Meltzer, T. (eds) (2003) Communication in high risk environments. *Linguistische Berichte*, special issue 12. Hamburg: Buske.

Dörner, D. (1996) *The Logic of Failure. Recognizing and Avoiding Error in Complex Situations*. New York: Metropolitan Books.

Dörner, D., Reither, F. and Stäudel, T. (1983) *Lohhausen. Über den Umgang mit Komplexität und Unbestmmtheit [On Dealing with Complexity and Uncertainty]*. Bern: Huber.

Entin, E. and Serfaty, D. (1999) Adaptive team coordination. *Human Factors* 41(2), 312–25.

Fletcher, G., Flin, R., McGeorge, P., Glavin, R., Maran, N. and Patey, R. (2003) Anaesthetists' Non-Technical Skills (ANTS): Evaluation of a behavioural marker system. *British Journal of Anaesthesia* 90(5), 580–8.

Fletcher, G., Flin, R., McGeorge, P., Glavin, R., Maran, N. and Patey, R. (2004) Rating non-technical skills: Developing a behavioural marker system for use in anaesthesia. *Cognition, Technology and Work* 6, 165–71.

Frensch, P.A. and Funke, J. (eds) (1995) *Complex Problem Solving: The European Perspective*. Hillsdale, NJ: Lawrence Erlbaum Associate.

Gaba, D.M. (1992) Dynamic decision-making in anesthesiology: Cognitive models and training approaches. In D. Evans and V. Patel (eds) *Advanced Models of Cognition for Medical Training and Practice* (pp. 122–47). Berlin: Springer.

Gaba, D.M., Howard, S.K., Flanagan, B., Smith, B.E., Fish, K.J. and Botney, R. (1998) Assessment of clinical performance during simulated crises using both technical and behavioral ratings. *Anesthesiology* 89(1), 8–18.

Glavin, R.J. and Maran, N.J. (2003) Integrating human factors into the medical curriculum. *Medical Education* 37 (November, Suppl 1), 59–64.

Grommes, P. (2000) Contributing to coherence: An empirical study on OR-team-communication. In M. Minnick-Fox, A. Williams and E. Kaiser (eds), *Proceedings of the 24th Penn Linguistics Colloquium*, U. Penn Working Papers in Linguistics, 7.1. Philadelphia, PA: University of Pennsylvania.

Häusler, R., Klampfer, B., Amacher, A. and Naef, W. (2004) Behavioral markers in analyzing team performance of cockpit crews. In R. Dietrich and T.M. Childress (eds), *Group Interaction in High Risk Environments*. Aldershot: Ashgate.

Howard, S.K., Gaba, D.M., Fish, K.J., Yang, G. and Sarnquist, F.H. (1992) Anesthesia crisis resource management training: Teaching anesthesiologists to handle critical incidents. *Aviation, Space and Environmental Medicine* 63(9), 763–70.

Jensen, R. (1995) *Pilot Judgement and Crew Resource Management*. Aldershot: Ashgate.

Joint Aviation Authorities (2006) JAR-OPS 1.965 (Appendix). *JAR-FCL-1*. Available at: <http://www.jaa.nl/publications/jars/607069.pdf> [last accessed March 2009].

Klimoski, R. and Mohammed, S. (1994) Team mental model: Construct or metaphor. *Journal of Management* 20(2), 403–37.

Kohn, L., Corrigan, J. and Donaldson, M. (eds) (1999) To err is human: Building a safer health system. *Committee on Quality of Health Care in America, Institute of Medicine (IOM)*. Washington DC: National Academy Press.

Merrit, A.C. and Helmreich, R.L. (1997) CRM: I hate it, what is it? (Error, stress, culture). *Proceedings of the Orient Airlines Association Air Safety Seminar*. Jakarta, Indonesia, April 23, 1996 (pp. 123–34). Manila: Orient Airlines Association. Available at: <http://homepage.psy.utexas.edu/homepage/group/HelmreichLAB/> [last accessed March 2009]..

Mishra, A., Catpole, K., Dale, T. and McCulloch, P. (2008) The influence of non-technical performance on technical outcome in laparoscopic cholecystectomy. *Surgical Endoscopy* 22(1), 68–73.

Morey, J.C., Simon, R., Jay, G.D., Wears, R.L., Salisbury, M., Dukes, K.A., et al. (2002) Error reduction and performance improvement in the emergency department through formal teamwork training: Evaluation results of the MedTeams project. *Health Services Research* 37(6), 1553–81.

Orasanu, J. (1990) *Shared Mental Models and Crew Performance*. Princeton, NJ: Princeton University, Cognitive Sciences Laboratory.

Pettinari, C.J. (1988) *Task, Talk, and Text in the Operating Room: A Study in Medical Discourse*. Norwood, NJ: Ablex Publishing.

Reader, T., Flin, R., Lauche, K. and Cuthbertson, B.H. (2006) Non-technical skills in the intensive care unit. *British Journal of Anaesthesia* 96(5), 551–99.

Risser, D.T., Rice, M.M., Salisbury, M.L., Simon, R., Jay, G.D. and Berns, S.D. (1999) The potential for improved teamwork to reduce medical errors in the emergency department. *The MedTeams Research Consortium. Annals of Emergency Medicine* 34(3), 373–83.

Salas, E., Burke, C.S., Bowers, C.A. and Wilson, K.A. (2001) Team training in the skies: Does crew resource management (CRM) training work? *Human Factors* 43(4), 641–74.

Salas, E., Wilson, K.A., Burke, C.S. and Wightman, D.C. (2006) Does crew resource management training work? An update, an extension, and some critical needs. *Human Factors* 48(2), 392–412.

Schöbel, M., and Kleindienst, C. (2001) The psychology of team interaction. *Acta Neurochirurgica* suppl 78, 33–8.

Sexton, J.B., and Helmreich, R.L. (2000). Analyzing cockpit communications: The links between language, performance, error, and workload. *Human Performance in Extreme Environments* 5(1), 63–8.

Silberstein, D. (2001) *Final Report of the Subproject 'Initiating Team Resources under High Cognitive Workload'*. Berlin: Technische Universität.

St Pierre, M., Hofinger, G., Buerschaper, C., Grapengeter, M., Harms, H., Breuer, G., et al. (2004) Simulator-based modular human factor training in anesthesiology. Concept and results of the module 'Communication and Team Cooperation'. *Anaesthesist* 53(2), 144–52.

St Pierre, M., Hofinger, G. and Buerschaper, C. (2007) *Crisis Management in Acute Care Settings: Human Factors and Team Psychology in a High Stakes Environment*. New York: Springer.

Stempfle, J.J. and Badke-Schaub, P. (2002) Kommunikation und Problemlösen in Gruppen: eine Prozessanalyse [Communication and problem solving in groups: A process analysis]. *Gruppendynamik und Organisationsberatung [Group Dynamics and Organizational Consultancy]* 33(1), 57–81.

Stempfle, J.J. and Badke-Schaub, P. (2003) Eine integrative Theorie des Problemlösens in Gruppen I: Problemlöseprozess und Problemlöseerfolg [An integrative theory of problem solving in groups I: Problem solving process and problem solving success]. *Gruppendynamik und Organisationsberatung [Group Dynamics and Organizational Consultancy]* 35(4), 335–58.

Stout, R., Cannon-Bowers, J.A., Salas, E. and Milanovich, D. (1999) Planning, shared mental models, and coordinated performance: An empirical link is established. *Human Factors* 41(61–71).

Thomas, E.J., Sexton, J.B. and Helmreich, R.L. (2004) Translating teamwork behaviors from aviation to healthcare: Development of behavioural markers for neonatal resuscitation. *Quality of Safety in Health Care* 13 (suppl 1), 57–64.

Transportation, U.S.D. (1998) *Crew Resource Management Training, AC No: 120-51C*. Advisory Circular (AC). Available at: <http://www.crm-devel.org/resources/ac/ac120_51c.htm> [last accessed November 2008].

Undre, S., Koutantji, M., Sevdalis, N., Gautama, S., Selvapatt, N., Williams, S., Sains, P., McCulloch, P., Darzi, A. and Vincent, C. (2007) Multidisciplinary crisis simulations: The way forward for training surgical teams. *World Journal of Surgery* 31(9), 1843–53.

Wiener, E.L., Kanki, B. and Helmreich, B. (eds) (1993) *Cockpit Resource Management*. San Diego: Academic Press.

Yule, S., Flin, R., Paterson-Brown, S., Maran, N. and Rowley, D. (2006) Development of a rating system for surgeons' non-technical skills. *Medical Education* 40(11), 1098–104.

Chapter 19

Observing Failures in Successful Orthopaedic Surgery

Ken Catchpole

Introduction

It is becoming increasingly recognized from accidents in a range of high-risk industries that small and recurrent failures, deriving from or predisposed by deficiencies in system function, can accumulate to create a catastrophic event (Fennell 1998, Gaba 1989, Helmreich 1994, Kennedy 2001, Lawton and Ward 2005). Surgery sits at the apex of the healthcare service, which makes it ideal for understanding both human error and the systemic properties that predispose error, since the sources of problems observed inside the operating theatre can often be attributed to deficient elements of the system. Success depends upon the pre-operative work-up, team coordination and appropriate equipment (Cook and Woods 1996), and also requires an organization and culture which support the progress of the patient through their treatment, and the activities of the team in the operating theatre (Kirklin et al. 1992). A sequence of human factors studies in paediatric cardiac surgery based on the structured post-hoc analysis of free-form notes made by expert observers found that seemingly innocuous intra-operative problems could accumulate to affect the outcome for the patients (de Leval et al. 2000b) and were more likely to create a serious risk in longer, more complex operations (Catchpole et al. 2006). Given that cardiac paediatric surgery is complex, high risk and relatively rare, it may not be representative of most operations, so we sought to identify properties of surgical systems that predispose errors in a routine, higher volume, lower risk surgery.

Observing small, recurrent problems in the operating theatre makes it possible to identify prospectively latent failures within the system which are regularly mitigated for, but occasionally cause harm. This prospective identification of weak points in the system has three important advantages; it is resistant to hindsight bias, which often afflicts the response to catastrophic failure (Berlin 2000, Fischhoff 1975, Woods and Cook 1999); it can help to build defences before adverse events occur (Carthey et al. 2001, Cook and Woods 1994); and by rectifying frequent problems, it may also improve the efficiency of surgery. We built on previous attempts to study systemic threats to patient safety (Helmreich 2000, Kaplan et al. 1998, Vincent et al. 1998), by attempting to identify the common causes of a larger number of observable problems. For our work in paediatric cardiac surgery, we had previously developed an analysis technique referred to as the *failure source model* (Catchpole et al. 2006, Catchpole et al. 2008), which provided a weighting network for each failure based on the source of the problems, and allowed systematic distinction between human errors in the operating theatre and aspects of the patient, task, environment (which included equipment and workspace), organization and culture that predisposed those errors before the operation. This made it possible to develop a profile of the different systemic contributions to problems during the course of an operation, reinforcing the view that human errors might be avoided and providing a semi-objective evaluation of where the most frequently encountered systemic problems lay.

Total knee replacement (TKR) surgery is an elective and proceduralized operation usually involving two surgeons, an anaesthetist, a scrub nurse, a circulating nurse and an anaesthetic nurse. There are two basic types; the first insertion of a knee prosethetic, known as a primary TKR (Table 19.1); and the replacement of an existing prosthetic, known as a TKR revision. This latter operation is less frequent, more complex, more unpredictable, higher risk and requires a larger array of instruments than a primary TKR.

We aimed to:

- confirm that the escalation from small problems to serious risk was influenced by complexity;
- examine further the collection of human errors and systemic predisposition of error; and
- apply the failure source model technique to reinforce the view that errors in surgery are avoidable by systemic redesign.

By comparing the results of two observers – one with a human factors background and experience in the operating theatre; the other who had previously worked in the operating theatre and had training in human factors – in multiple TKR cases, it was also possible to explore the reliability of this semi-quantitative, free-form observational technique.

Case and Team Mix

Fourteen cases carried out under one consultant orthopaedic surgeon were studied by dual observers in a single operating theatre at a large UK hospital. The first surgeon was always the consultant or his specialist registrar. All 18 operations featured the same anaesthetist, and the scrub nurse and circulating nurses came from a pool of four individuals who regularly interchanged roles. This meant that while the team composition was not always identical, operations usually featured the same individuals, often in the same roles. Ten operations were TKR operations and four were revisions of a TKR. Prosthetic implants from a range of manufacturers were studied. Mean operative duration was 107.8 mins (95 percent

Table 19.1   Phases of a typical primary total knee replacement operation

Key phases in the total knee replacement operation
The total knee replacement operation replaces damaged and painful knee joints with a completely artificial joint prosthesis.

1. The patient is anaesthetized in the anaesthetic room which adjoins the operating theatre.
2. The patient is transferred to operating table in the operating theatre.
3. The treatment site is cleaned, and a tourniquet is applied to the thigh to be treated.
4. The first incision is made, and carried to the knee capsule.
5. The knee is dislocated, and an intra-medullary rod inserted to fix the femoral cutting block.
6. The femur is cut distally with an oscillating saw. Following appropriate sizing, a second cutting block is used to make anterior posterior and chamfer cuts.
7. The tibial cut is made following alignment with the lower leg, and configuration of the tibial cutting block.
8. Trial tibial and femoral prostheses are used to test the fit and confirm sizing of the implant.
9. The patella is re-surfaced if required.
10. Cement is prepared and applied to tibial and femoral prosthetic components, which are firmly seated. The leg is again checked for fit.
11. Once the cement has cured, the wound is washed and closed.
12. The tourniquet is removed, tourniquet time is recorded, and the patient is transferred to the recovery suite.

C.I. ± 26.3), and mean tourniquet time was 115.6 mins (95 percent C.I. ± 17.2). The patients ranged from 60 to 84 years of age. All operations were successful, and no observed failure was deemed worthy of further investigation either by the individuals involved, or by the hospital.

Method for Identifying Minor and Major Failures

To prepare for the observations, ten similar cases were studied by both researchers before data collection began, and a task analysis and procedural-based error-capture checklists were produced for TKR operations (Catchpole et al. 2005). This checklist allowed structured error-capture observations, and included over 100 items and 17 time-marker events. However, since they did not capture all the salient events, it was also necessary during data collection to make detailed notes of activities and communications, which produced descriptions of events in theatre and the time and sequence in which those events occurred. In all 14 cases a video recording was made of the operating theatre from two views, one at the head of the table, looking toward the surgical field from behind the anaesthetist, and one on the left-hand side of the patient, utilizing a wide-angle lens to record the scrub nurse, surgeons and surgical field, and the anaesthetist

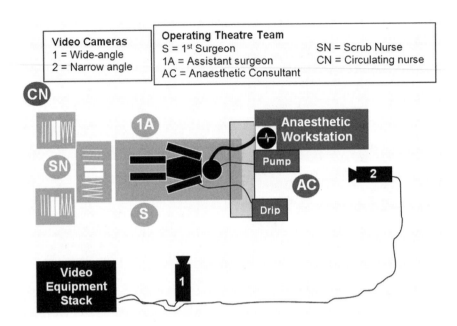

Figure 19.1   Video equipment configuration for orthopaedic surgery

Source: Catchpole et al. (2005)

(Figure 19.1). Other relevant data were recorded, including operative duration (first incision to final closing suture), tourniquet time and the composition of the surgical team. For the purposes of the study, risk was classified at levels; low risk for primary TKR procedures,and high risk for TKR revisions. One operation was a TKR revision, but was classed at low risk as it involved only the removal of the existing prosthesis. Another operation was a primary knee replacement, but was classed as high risk as it required instruments, prostheses and techniques used in revision operations.

Events were selected for analysis if they were judged to have increased the duration or difficulty of the operation, increased the risk to the patient, or increased the demand for resources. They were all categorized individually as minor failures. A major failure category was reserved for events which were approaching an incident or accident (see Box 19.1). Where major failures or unusual or complex minor failures occurred, brief reviews were conducted with relevant theatre team members at a convenient time following the operation to ensure that the supporting specialist information had been recorded. Video evidence was used to check the results of the observers. Minor failures were grouped into 20 types previously defined for paediatric cardiac surgery (Catchpole et al. 2006) (Table 19.2).

Table 19.2   Descriptions and examples of minor failure types

Failure	Description and example
Absence	Lack of personnel when required. Example: circulating nurse is absent when scrub nurse needs more suture material.
Coordination/ communication failure	Failures in task coordination and communication between individuals. Example: surgeon asks for the drill, but the scrub nurse is busy doing something else.
Decision-related surgical error	Surgeon fails to make the appropriate decision. Example: the surgeon finds the tibial cut is sloping, after the assistant surgeon has repeatedly expressed his concern.
Distraction	Disturbance from external sources not related to current case during a critical period. Examples: (i) telephone rings in theatre; (ii) another nurse enters theatre and distracts the scrub nurse.
Equipment/ workspace management failure	Failures in the organization of workspace and equipment. Examples: (i) the surgeon tries to use the saw, but it is not plugged in; (ii) x-rays are displayed the wrong way round.
Equipment configuration failure	Failure to use or operate equipment appropriately. Example: (i) intra-medullary rod not inserted far enough into femur; (ii) cutting block moves as pins are hammered in.
Equipment failure	Inter-operative equipment failure. Examples: (i) sutures break; (ii) tibial tray is bent when it comes to being used.
Expertise/skill failure	Failures associated with lack of expertise or skill in trainees. Example: (i) assistant surgeon does not know how to use the bone saw correctly; (ii) not enough cement is applied to the prosthetic.
External resource failure	Failures in elements of the external organization to provide equipment or human resources. Examples: (i) piece of equipment is missing from the standard set; (ii) correct pins unavailable from prosthetic manufacturer.
Patient-sourced procedural difficulties	Features of the patient that make the planned procedure more challenging to carry out than would be expected from the pre-operative diagnosis. Example: (i) patient apnoeic, requiring re-intubation (ii) not enough femur left to make box cuts.
Planning failure	Failure to anticipate or discuss future task requirements. Example: surgeon consults patient notes after the start of the operation.

Table 19.2   *Concluded*

Failure	Description and example
Pre-operative diagnosis failure	Failure to provide accurate diagnosis prior to operation. Example: surgical team have decided upon an implant from one manufacturer, but the x-rays show the previous implant to be from another manufacturer.
Procedure-related error	Procedural errors by surgeon, assistant surgeon, anaesthetist, scrub nurse, or circulating nurse. Examples: (i) surgeon forgets to plug the intra-medullary hole (ii) cement mixing time is not recorded.
Psychomotor error (general)	Handling errors. Example: surgeon drops prosthesis while applying cement.
Psychomotor-related surgical error	Technical manipulation errors by surgeon. Examples: (i) assistant surgeon gets forceps tangled in sutures; (ii) assistant surgeon hits finger of surgeon with hammer.
Resource management	Failures in the organization of available people or things in the operating theatre. Example: surgeon leaves assistant surgeon to close without confirming ability to do so.
Safety consciousness	Failures to observe basic elements of patient safety. Examples: (i) mask is not fitted on entry to theatre; (ii) surgeon does not have eye protection while making bone cuts.
Team conflict	Team members have differing opinions, or give conflicting commands, that are not resolved. Example: scrub nurse and assistant surgeon argue over procedural requirements.
Unintended effects on patient	Unplanned problems arising with the patient as a result of the treatment. Example: blood pressure increases unexpectedly after bag of fluids is changed.
Vigilance/awareness failure	Failures to notice immediately important aspects of the task or the patient's condition. Example: anaesthetist does not notice a drop in blood pressure.

Minor Failures

The two observers found 327 minor failures in the study, varying between 10 and 50 in each operation, with a mean of 23.3 per operation (95 percent C.I. ± 7.82). The number of minor failures in an operation showed a moderate relationship with duration ($rho(14)=0.678$, $p<0.01$) and tourniquet time ($rho(14)=0.788$, $p<0.005$).

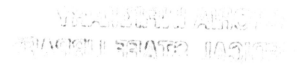

There was also an effect of operative risk on the number of failures encountered in each operation, with an independent samples t-test assuming unequal variances showing significantly more minor failures in high risk operations ($t(3.6)$=-6.53, $p<0.005$), though the small number of TKR revisions limits the confidence of this relationship.

One operation was considered to have contained a major failure sequence where the tibial cut was misaligned (see Box 19.1). Though this was identified and resolved by making further tibial cuts, it was considered a major failure because

A 66 year old male was anaesthetised and prepared for a primary total knee replacement operation. The surgeon was already aware that the knee was in an advanced state of wear, and might require additional prosthetic components usually required only for second stage TKR revisions, so the corresponding instrument trays and prostheses were kept on standby. The sales representative for the prosthetic manufacturer was present for the operation, as was normal for TKR revisions, to assist in the selection and configuration of the implants. On this occasion, the surgeon also chose to use a new computer navigation device that was on trial from the prosthetic manufacturer. This was normally used for standard primary TKR operations, and had not previously been used by the team for this type of operation.

Though the surgical team were all experienced and familiar with one another, early in the operation the scrub nurse showed signs of uncertainty both about the use of the computer equipment, and the surgical direction being taken. The sales representative offered his support to the scrub nurse, but his advice conflicted with instructions from the surgeon, and the scrub nurse became confused about what was required next. At the same time, the surgeon was struggling to operate the computer navigation system, becoming increasingly frustrated with it. The sales rep also tried to support the surgeon, but was unable to support both scrub nurse and surgeon at once. He was also trying to coach a second sales representative at the same time. There was a high level of conversational noise in the operating theatre.

As the operation progressed, the scrub nurse began to unpack several extra trays of instruments required for the additional implants, with help from the sales rep. While the rep was outside the theatre, the surgeon removed one of the navigation sensors, and on his return the rep expressed concern that this may have upset the calibration of the navigation system. A few minutes later, the assistant surgeon became concerned about the tibial cut that had been made. The surgeon and sales rep dismissed his concerns and instead teased him for being overly anxious. In the following minutes there were a number of other confused exchanges between the sales rep, the scrub nurse and the surgeon. Sixty three minutes after the start operation the surgeon noticed that the tibial plateau had not been cut properly and was on a slope. The operating theatre went silent. The assistant surgeon then confirmed that this was his earlier concern, and appropriate cuts are made to rectify the problem. Following a number of further co-ordination difficulties, the operation was eventually completed after 126 minutes.

Box 19.1   Description of a major failure

it demonstrated a substantial deviation from the normal operative course which had a direct affect on the patient as it required the removal of more bone than was intended. This event was indirectly precipitated by a number of other issues, including uncertainty, high workload, task requirements, non-technical errors and the introduction of new technology into the operating theatre. This event occurred in the higher risk operation, and also had the greatest number of minor failures in any operation observed.

The 327 failures were classed by 20 failure types, and the average number observed per operation is shown in Figure 19.2. Approximately half the minor failures observed were distributed among three failure types, reflecting either aspects of theatre culture and environment, or the more difficult elements of the equipment and procedure. Distractions were the most numerous failure, accounting for nearly twice the number of the next most frequently observed failure. The greatest distracters were communication devices, including 16 wrong numbers or calls for people not in the theatre, 26 other non-case-related telephone calls (case-related calls were excluded from the data), 10 mobile phone calls and 9

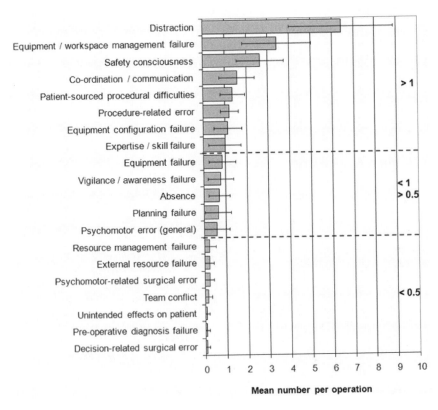

Figure 19.2   Mean number of minor failures per operation by type

instances of bleepers/pagers sounding in theatre. The demands for intra-operative teaching, as well as the presence of newspapers and other non-case-related reading material during the operation, also contributed to this high level of distraction. Several instances were observed where these distractions coincided with parts of the procedure particularly susceptible to interference, such as equipment counts and timing of bone cement curing.

The demands to organize, prepare and exchange different pieces of equipment (jigs, drill bits, saw blades, cutting blocks, implants) during the operation is reflected in the high number of equipment and workspace management failures where equipment was needed and was not immediately available (such as finding the drill not plugged into the air line when attempting to use it), or where it was placed in a physical configuration that compromised the operation of the equipment (such as tangled diathermy wires). There were also more than 40 instances suggesting reduced safety consciousness, mostly relating to mask discipline – failures to wear masks appropriately at all times – in theatre, but also including one event where the scrub nurse left the theatre and returned while still scrubbed. Coordination and communication problems were frequent, suggesting problems either in the distribution of important information within the surgical team, or to the timely execution of procedural sequences requiring interaction between individuals. Procedure-related errors, expertise/skill failures and equipment configuration failures also reflect the close-coupling of procedures, equipment and expertise in this type of surgery. In particular, less experienced surgeons and scrub nurses suffered expertise or skill failures because of tightly coupled tasks, especially in the more demanding TKR revision surgery. Failures in equipment, vigilance/awareness failures and absences that had an impact on the operation were not as frequent, but still occurred in over half the operations. However, technical skill-based issues including decision-related error, diagnosis failures and psychomotor errors were considerably less frequent, along with more undesirable elements of the operation, notably unintended effects on the patient, and team conflicts.

Applying the Failure Source Model

As failures sometimes reflect individual errors, failures in group processes, threats outside theatre that affected events in theatre, or combinations of all three, the failure source model (Figure 19.3) was applied. This allowed the description of events in terms of the number and types of failures that could be observed, and the systemic threats and human errors that they represented. Equipment, workspace and resource threats and organizational/cultural threats were associated with four different minor failure types each. Task threats were associated with eight different minor failure types and patient threats were associated with three minor failure types. Technical errors were associated with five different minor failure types and non-technical errors were associated with nine different types of minor failure. As it was not always possible to observe the specific source of the failure in

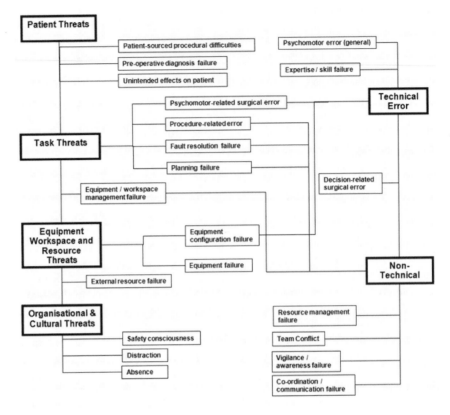

Figure 19.3   Failure source model which links observable minor failures (small boxes) and common systemic causes (large boxes)

every case, the model assumed that all potential sources had contributed in equal proportions. Applying this failure source model allowed the generation of a threat and error profile for each operation (Vincent et al. 2004) which was used in the final systems analyses.

From the failure source model it was possible to estimate the rates of systemic threats and human errors. Figure 19.4, top panel, shows the mean failure rates in terms of threat type within each operation divided by the length of the operations. Cultural and organizational threats were the most frequently encountered, and are more frequent in higher risk operations. Task threats and equipment threats occur at approximately the same rate, regardless of risk, with patient threats the least frequent. This general pattern would be expected given the process and equipment driven nature of the TKR surgery where patients are relatively invariant. Figure 19.4, bottom panel, shows the minor failure data treated in a similar way to estimate human error rates. As might be expected, error rates were higher for high risk operations. Also, non-technical errors, occurring once every 10–15 mins, were

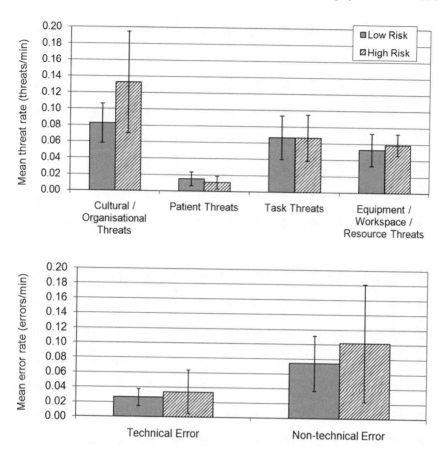

Figure 19.4 Mean rates of threats (top panel) and errors (bottom panel), with 95 percent confidence intervals

considerably more frequent than technical errors, which occurred only once every 30–50 mins, though the latter appear to be less variable between operations.

Comparison Between Dual Observers

All operations were dual-observed to examine the agreement between observers with two very different backgrounds. Observer 1 was a human factors practitioner, experienced in observational methods in the operating theatre, human performance measurement and the evaluation of non-technical skills. Observer 2 was a research scientist with prior experience of working in operating theatres and with some prior knowledge of non-technical skills, but no specific human factors or observer training. The 17 time markers anchored to specific points in the primary TKR operations allowed an assessment of the level of understanding that the observers had of the basic stages of the operation. Correlation between time markers in the ten dual-observed primary TKR operations was almost perfect (rho(151)=0.998, p<0.001). Although all 17 times were not always recorded in each operation, this suggests that both observers were in close agreement about when each stage of the operation occurred. Of the 327 different failures recorded in the dual-observer operations, 72 were recorded by both observers, 193 were recorded by observer one only, and 62 were recorded by observer two only. Overlap between observations was often low, accounting for between 0 percent and 42 percent of the total number of failures observed in each operation.

A Bland-Altman plot (Bland and Altman 1986) was used to examine inter-observer agreement, and can be found in Figure 19.5. Observer one generally saw the same or twice as many failures as Observer two. There were three outliers where the number of failures noted by Observer one was considerably more than the number noted by Observer two. One was the computer-navigated operation, which was a technique unfamiliar to Observer two. The other two outliers show a floor effect, where the number of intra-operative failures was generally small. One outlier was found in the operation with the lowest number of failures, where Observer two did not see any failures independently, while in the other outlying operation there was no overlap between observations, suggesting that both observers had a different focus of attention. This might be expected in operations where the number of intra-operative failures was small. Though both observers

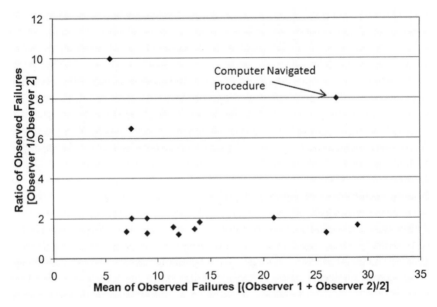

Figure 19.5   Bland-Altman plot for agreement between two observers

viewed events differently, and both under-reported the total number of observable intra-operative failures, both demonstrated a good understanding of the process and the observations from both remained similarly proportional across the range of operations viewed. Thus, though different in absolute terms, judgement between operations was consistent between observers.

While each individual observer did not observe all intra-operative failures, there was general consensus between the observers about the success of each operation. Both were able to identify a considerable number of failures, with the small overlap between observations suggesting differences in experience and focus of attention between observers. Intra-observer reliability might be improved by the explicit definition of salient events, and the present study could undoubtedly inform a comprehensive approach to the structured observation of pre-defined intra-operative failures. However, given the unpredictable nature of errors and the importance of understanding the context in which they happen, explicit tools are unlikely to be sufficient. Rather, we would strongly advocate the value of implicit error capture conducted by experienced observers, which should then utilize a structured assessment protocol. Since the human factors practitioner with experience in surgery was able to observe nearly twice as many failures as the observer with surgical experience but little human factors training, it is also clear that observation by non-medically trained observers is vital for identifying and reducing medical errors. Understanding the threats and errors encountered by surgical teams in this way makes possible the diagnosis of these important but often neglected events.

Discussion

Intra-operative events that resulted in small increases in the duration or difficulty of the operation, risks to the patient, or demands for resources were frequent, and varied considerably between operations. Distractions, equipment management problems, safety consciousness and coordination and communication problems were the most frequently occurring types of failure. Decision-making and diagnostic errors were the least frequent type of failure, reflecting the skill and competence with which the individuals studied carried out the technical demands of their tasks (or possibly a failure of the observers to detect failures in these areas). The variability in the number of failures, given that the team varied so little, suggests that these failures must have their source in variable systemic conditions. Higher risk operations were more likely to include a greater number of errors than lower risk operations, and though sample size limits the confidence of this result, it confirms previous findings in paediatric cardiac surgery (Catchpole et al. 2006). Several team members suggested that operations were more frequently problematic with other surgeons. Consequently, we believe the data presented here are likely to provide a conservative estimate of the likely incidence of intra-operative failures in orthopaedic surgery across the UK.

The high incidence of distracters suggests that both the opportunity for and tolerance of external interference was high. Instances of reduced safety consciousness were also high, which was surprising considering the well-recognized and highly undesirable effect that nosocomial infection can have on the outcome of joint replacement surgery (Gao et al. 2000). Though equivocal evidence has been offered for the effectiveness of mask discipline for control of nosocomial infection (McLure et al. 1998, Mitchell and Hunt 1991), protocols should be applied consistently and particular attention should be paid to prosthetic implantation (Woodhead et al. 2002). Controlling the use of the telephone in theatre and reinforcing safety procedures are simple and direct solutions that could and should be applied. On a number of occasions senior team members attempted to maintain standards with little success, and in one instance an individual not involved with the operation entered the theatre during the procedure, initially without a mask, made a loud and argumentative phone call without the permission of anyone in the operating team, then left theatre, violating mask protocol on the way out. Failures to control distraction and safety are therefore symptomatic of the impact of culture on surgical quality (Baird et al. 2005), and rather than blaming individuals, the aetiology of this problem should be considered at all levels, from hospital management, through professional societies and associations, to national policy.

Unlike other types of surgery, which may be reliant on the scalpel-and-suture skills of the surgeon, TKR and TKR revision operations are reliant on the appropriate use of procedure-specific instruments. Achieving the correct equipment configuration is a key technical skill for this type of surgery. Though the instruments are usually reliable, the wide range of equipment required in a short space of time placed pressure on the operating team. For example, the ten-minute period from the first incision to completion of the femoral cuts for one make of implant requires the use of five specialist instruments (intra-medullary rod, femoral locating device, distal femoral cutting block, femoral sizing guide and anterior/posterior chamfer cutting block), as well as a range of other incidental equipment such as drills, saws, retractors, pins, hammers, scalpels, swabs, diathermy and suction. A surgeon cannot perform the operation without the scrub nurse to provide the appropriate instruments, and a scrub nurse cannot support the surgeon effectively if they are overloaded, distracted or unable to keep up with and anticipate the surgical tasks. Given the skill required for both roles, the mutual trust required and the authority gradient between them, this relationship is brittle. It was encouraging that in the present study the interaction between surgeons and scrub nurses was mutually supportive almost without exception, and remained solution-focused when things did not go according to plan.

In the TKR revision operations, which were always more demanding, the active participation of the prosthetic manufacturer sales representative helped the theatre and surgical staff to appropriately manipulate the even more complex and less familiar instrumentation, as well as providing an additional resource for aiding coordination and error capture. However, while this can have exceptional safety benefits, it can also have negative effects on the rest of the team, and often caused distraction, accounting for the high level of organizational/cultural threats in high risk operations. This also suggests a deficiency in the design of the instruments, which seemed too complex for surgical teams to use without a considerable amount of additional, manufacturer-specific training. It also raises ethical concerns. Overall, though patient-related difficulties were frequent, the difficulty of the operation was more dependent upon the design and management of the equipment, the coordination of the team, and the more frequent but generally less serious cultural threats.

This study provides further evidence of the value of expert observers in identifying threats to patient safety, and suggests several structured interventions to improve surgical quality. Since equipment management failures were closely associated with the effectiveness of the team, attention to non-technical skills could be immediately beneficial (Fletcher et al. 2002, Healy et al. 2004). Non-technical skills which are neither formally taught nor included in competency assessments can also be useful in avoiding or capturing problems before they can accumulate (Carthey et al. 2003, de Leval et al 2000, Helmreich 2000). Indeed the provision of pre-operative briefings, post-operative debriefings and non-technical skills development may provide a highly effective and long-term practitioner-driven safety and learning mechanism through which a broad range of inter-operative problems might be addressed. Further assessment of team-based non-technical skills was made during these operations, and has been independently reported (Catchpole et al. 2008). Attempts to improve the design and usability of equipment, and to reduce the number and range of specialist instruments (Nizard 2002, Nizard et al. 2004), should also be encouraged, provided appropriate human factors (Malhotra et al. 2005) and safety considerations (Lieberman and Wenger 2004) are present early in the design process. The observations of the computer-assisted system suggest that while equipment management issues are being partially addressed in new technologies, this can re-locate failures, making currently reliable and easy-to-configure instrumentation less reliable and more difficult to use in the future. Indeed, it is the opinion of the author after observing nearly 200 operations in at least six treatment centres that the systems for procuring, maintaining, and training for operating theatre equipment are either poorly managed or barely extant, compromising the safety of existing technologies, even before the increased risks associated with new technology are considered.

Conclusions

The most frequent failures may not always demonstrate the greatest threat to operative success or system function, but they can provide the environment in which major failures and adverse events are more likely. Examination of the fundamental properties of the system that these minor failure types display allows the identification of a small number of error reduction strategies that address the problem at the source. This is more advantageous than providing defences to a large number of unique deficiencies, since safety systems themselves can become brittle, ineffective and add to the problems in the system if too many defences are implemented (Cook and Woods 1994). The failure source model provides a diagnosis of the likely source of threats and errors in this operating theatre and in this type of surgery. An estimate based on current failure rates (Feinglass et al. 2004, Vincent et al. 2001) and projected surgical volume (Dixon et al. 2004) suggests that in 2010 between 2000 and 9000 patients in the UK will experience some form of adverse event following a TKR. By taking a prospective approach to the observation of system failures and human error in orthopaedic surgery, this chapter has identified problems with the organization and culture of safety, problems associated with the design and organization of the equipment in theatre which become amplified in more difficult operations, and the potential for improved non-technical performance in the operating team. Attention to these deficiencies in operating theatres would result in improvements in patient safety, surgical quality and system efficiency.

Acknowledgements

This project was funded by the Department of Health Patient Safety Research Programme. Thanks to Mr Tony Giddings and Prof Marc de Leval for their comments on earlier versions of this text, to Dr Paul Godden for his assistance in the data collection, and to Trevor Dale, Guy Hirst, Peter McCulloch and Michael Wilkinson for their assistance in various aspects of these studies. The preparation of this chapter was kindly supported through a Leverhulme Trust Early Career Fellowship.

References

Baird, C., Nunn, T., and Gregori, A. (2005) Inadequate standards of hygiene in an operating theatre changing room. *Journal of Hospital Infection* 59, 268–9.
Berlin, L. (2000) Hindsight bias. *American Journal of Roentgenology* 175, 597–601.
Bland, J.M. and Altman, D.G. (1986) Statistical methods for assessing agreement between two methods of clinical measurement. *Lancet* 1, 307–10.
Carthey, J., de Leval, M.R. and Reason, J.T. (2001) The human factor in cardiac surgery: Errors and near misses in a high technology medical domain. *Annals of Thoracic Surgery* 72, 300–305.
Carthey, J., de Leval, M.R ., Wright, D.J., Farewell, V.J., and Reason, J.T. (2003) Behavioural markers of surgical excellence. *Safety Science* 41, 409–25.
Catchpole, K., Godden, P.J., Giddings, A.E.B., Hirst, G., Dale, T., Utley, M. et al. (2005) *Identifying and Reducing Errors in the Operating Theatre* (Rep. No.

PS012). Patient Safety Research Programme. Available at <http://www.pcpoh. bham.ac.uk/publichealth/psrp/documents/PS012_Final_Report_DeLeval. pdf> [last accessed March 2009].

Catchpole, K.R., Giddings, A.E., de Leval, M.R., Peek, G.J., Godden, P.J., Utley, M. et al. (2006) Identification of systems failures in successful paediatric cardiac surgery. *Ergonomics* 49, 567–88.

Catchpole, K.R., Giddings, A.E., Hirst, G., Dale, T., Peek, G.J., and de Leval, M.R. (2008) A method for measuring threats and errors in surgery. *Cognition, Technology and Work* 10, 295–304.

Cook, R.I. and Woods, D. (1994) Operating at the sharp end: The complexity of human error. In M.S. Bogner (ed.), *Human Error in Medicine* (pp. 255–310). Hillsdale, NJ: Lawrence Erlbaum Associates Inc.

Cook, R.I. and Woods, D.D. (1996) Adapting to new technology in the operating room. *Human Factors* 38, 593–613.

de Leval, M.R., Carthey, J., Wright, D.J., Farewell, V.T. and Reason, J.T. (2000a) Human factors and cardiac surgery: A multicenter study. *Journal of Thoracic Cardiovascular Surgery* 119, 661–72.

Dixon, T., Shaw, M., Ebrahim, S. and Dieppe, P. (2004) Trends in hip and knee joint replacement: Socioeconomic inequalities and projections of need. *Annals of the Rheumatic Diseases* 63, 825–30.

Feinglass, J., Amir, H., Taylor, P., Lurie, I., Manheim, L. M. and Chang, R.W. (2004) How safe is primary knee replacement surgery? Perioperative complication rates in Northern Illinois, 1993–1999. *Arthritis Rheumetism* 51, 110–16.

Fennell, D. (1998) *Investigation into the King's Cross Underground Fire* (Rep. No. Cm 499). London: HMSO.

Fischhoff, B. (1975) Hindsight does not equal foresight: The effect of outcome knowledge on judgement under uncertainty. *Journal of Experimental Psychology: Human Perception and Performance* 1, 288–99.

Fletcher, G.C.L., McGeorge, P., Flin, R.H., Glavin, R.J., and Maran, N.J. (2002) The role of non-technical skills in anaesthesia: A review of current literature. *British Journal of Anaesthesia* 88, 418–29.

Gaba, D.M. (1989) Human error in anesthetic mishaps. *International Anesthesiology Clinics* 27, 137–47.

Gao, T., Lu, H., Zhou, D. and Guan, Z. (2000) Risk factors for nosocomial infections after total knee replacement. *Zhonghua Wai Ke.Za Zhi.* 38, 256–8.

Healey, A.N., Undre, S. and Vincent, C. (2004) Developing observational measures of performance in surgical teams. *Quality and Safety in Health Care* 13, i33–i40.

Helmreich, R.L. (1994) Anatomy of a system accident: The crash of Avianca Flight 052. *International Journal of Aviation Psychology* 4, 265–84.

Helmreich, R.L. (2000) On error management: Lessons from aviation. *British Medical Journal* 320, 781–5.

Kaplan, H.S., Battles, J.B., van der Schaaf, T.W., Shea, C.E. and Mercer, S.Q. (1998) Identification and classification of the causes of events in transfusion medicine. *Transfusion* 38, 1071–81.

Kennedy, I. (2001) *Learning from Bristol: The Report of the Public Inquiry into Children's Heart Surgery at the Bristol Royal Infirmary 1984–1995.* (Rep. No. Command Paper: CM 5207). London: HMSO.

Kirklin, J.W., Blackstone, E.H., Tchervenkov, C.I. and Castaneda, A.R. (1992) Clinical outcomes after the arterial switch operation for transposition: Patient, support, procedural, and institutional risk factors. *Circulation* 86, 1501–15.

Lawton, R. and Ward, N.J. (2005) A systems analysis of the Ladbroke Grove rail crash. *Accident Analysis and Prevention* 37, 235–44.

Lieberman, J.R. and Wenger, N. (2004) New technology and the orthopaedic surgeon: Are you protecting your patients? *Clinical Orthopaedics and Related Research,* 338–41.

Malhotra, S., Laxmisan, A., Keselman, A., Zhang, J. and Patel, V.L. (2005) Designing the design phase of critical care devices: A cognitive approach. *Journal of Biomedical Informatics* 38, 34–50.

McLure, H.A., Talboys, C.A., Yentis, S.M., and Azadian, B.S. (1998) Surgical face masks and downward dispersal of bacteria. *Anaesthesia* 53, 624–6.

Mitchell, N.J. and Hunt, S. (1991) Surgical face masks in modern operating rooms – a costly and unnecessary ritual? *Journal of Hospital Infection* 18, 242.

Nizard, R. (2002) Computer assisted surgery for total knee arthroplasty. *Acta Orthop.Belg.* 68, 215–30.

Nizard, R.S., Porcher, R., Ravaud, P., Vangaver, E., Hannouche, D., Bizot, P. et al. (2004) Use of the Cusum technique for evaluation of a CT-based navigation system for total knee replacement. *Clinical and Orthopaedic Related Research* 425, 180–8.

Vincent, C., Taylor-Adams, S. and Stanhope, N. (1998) Framework for analysing risk and safety in clinical medicine. *British Medical Journal* 316, 1154–7.

Vincent, C., Neale, G. and Woloshynowych, M. (2001) Adverse events in British hospitals: Preliminary retrospective record review. *British Medical Journal* 322, 517–19.

Vincent, C., Moorthy, K., Sarker, S.K., Chang, A. and Darzi, A.W. (2004) Systems approaches to surgical quality and safety: From concept to measurement. *Annals of Surgery* 239, 475–82.

Woodhead, K., Taylor, E. W., Bannister, G., Chesworth, T., Hoffman, P. and Humphreys, H. (2002) Behaviours and rituals in the operating theatre: A report from the Hospital Infection Society Working Group on Infection Control in the Operating Theatres. *Journal of Hospital Infection* 51, 241–55

Woods, D. and Cook, R.I. (1999) Hindsight biases and local rationality. In F.T. Durso, R.S. Nickerson, R.W. Schvaneveldt, S.T. Dumais, D.S. Lindsay, and M.T.H. Chi (eds), *Handbook of Applied Cognition* (pp. 141–71). New York: John Wiley and Sons Ltd.

Chapter 20

Remembering To Do Things Later and Resuming Interrupted Tasks: Prospective Memory and Patient Safety

Peter Dieckmann, Marlene Dyrløv Madsen, Silke Reddersen,
Marcus Rall and Theo Wehner

Introduction

In this chapter we take a closer look at tasks requiring some form of prospective memory (PM) which allows people to remember to do something in the future or to resume interrupted tasks.

Examples of Prospective Memory from the Operating Room

Example 1 – Treatment in Time

A patient is scheduled for surgery, requiring peri-operative antibiotics to prevent infection. It is absolutely critical that the antibiotics are applied some time before the surgeon cuts the skin. It is believed that allergic reactions are more frequent if antibiotics are given to conscious patients. So, when the patient arrives with the antibiotic taped to his chart, the anaesthesia team first induces anaesthesia and then has to remember to give the antibiotic, whilst preoccupied with many other tasks before the surgery starts.

Example 2 – Recurrent Measurements

A patient with insulin-dependent diabetes has to undergo major surgery, lasting several hours. After taking an initial blood glucose level measurement before anaesthesia, the anaesthetist must then repeatedly measure the blood glucose of the anaesthetized patient. Severe brain damage may result in the case of prolonged low blood glucose. There will be several occasions during the surgical procedure where the 'countdown timer' will beep, but the anaesthetist will not be able to respond, because of other ongoing critical tasks (e.g., blood transfusion, hemodynamic management). It will be a repeated challenge not to forget the checking of the blood glucose, which might be postponed for a while but must not be forgotten for too long.

Example 3 – Dynamic Change of Plans

A patient with a history of several laparotomies due to a renal disability in his childhood is admitted to the clinic with an *acute abdomen*. In the CT scan nothing specific can be found, so the patient is scheduled for an explorative laparoscopy and it is decided to perform an appendectomy, as 'no one would like to have to operate on this patient's abdomen again'. The operation is rather difficult due to multiple adhesions. There is a danger of abdominal injury, so the surgeon really has to concentrate on his task. Sometime during the operation he has to remember to also perform the appendectomy.

We will concentrate our discussion mainly on PM and its failures in the operating room (OR). We will explain the concept of prospective memory in some detail and explain how it is relevant for medical care and patient safety. We will use the PM theoretical framework (Brandimonte et al. 1996) to analyse the examples above and use data from a questionnaire and a simulator study to illustrate the relevance of PM for acute medical care. Finally, we will discuss implications for PM-related research and medical practice and patient safety. The longer-term goal of an improved understanding of this error form is to identify how best to deal with this challenge: removing error prone situations systematically, implementing protective measures and training people to optimize performance in PM situations. So far, we have only begun to investigate PM and its failures in acute care settings and it is too early to give sound advice on effective protection and countermeasures.

Relevance in the Operating Room (OR) and Other Acute Care Settings

The examples above emphasize the relevance and face value of prospective memory (PM) for medical practice. With rationalization, cost and time pressure, healthcare professionals are responsible for more than one and, sometimes several patients. Interruptions and delays are frequent in the different healthcare settings (Manser et al. 2003, Healey et al. 2006, Chisholm et al. 2000, Dieckmann et al. 2006, Dyrløv Madsen and Schou 2008). Interruptions in medical care have been found to be related to a preference for direct (synchronous) communication modes in medicine, for example face-to-face communications. Whilst using synchronous channels might help to decrease memory burden (e.g., by delegating tasks), it also increases the potential for interruptions when compared to asynchronous communication channels, like email or voice mails (Parker and Coiera 2000).

Delays and interruptions in the OR stem from task inherent difficulties (complications) and, the social, technical and organizational environment (Healey et al. 2006). For example, tasks are begun and finished, usually in a desynchronized fashion, by the separate *crews* (Gaba et al. 2001) involved in the treatment in the OR (e.g., anaesthesia crew, surgical crew, cleaning crew, etc.). While an individual starts a certain task (e.g., the anaesthetist places a nerve block before surgery to improve post-surgery care and comfort), the surgical crew might simply wait or fill the waiting time by beginning other tasks or taking a break – potentially outside the OR. The coordination of the interdependent tasks is at times imprecise (e.g., only rough or understated estimations of how long a task will take), leading to prolonged delays. While the above anaesthetist might underestimate the task duration ('I will be finished in five minutes' – where the task might actually take 15 minutes), the surgical crew might underestimate the duration of the task they do in between ('Anaesthesia will never finish in five minutes, so let's start our task – that might take 20 minutes'). After finishing placing the nerve block and waiting for the surgical crew to finish, the anaesthetic crew might then begin their next task to fill the waiting time, and so on. To exit this vicious circle, the interdisciplinary team would have to be very well coordinated, accept unproductive waiting time for some team members, or have to interrupt or speed up a task.

So far there are few data that directly link prospective memory and its failures to the quality and safety of care, but there is some implicit evidence, also from other disciplines, especially aviation, where PM failures were found to be important (Dismukes and Nowinski 2006). Some evidence within medicine stems from incident reporting systems. The MedMARx incident reporting system (<www.usp.org/medmarx>) collects information on medication errors. In a report, 6224 cases were analysed for underlying causes and contributing factors (US Pharmacopeia 2000). Interruptions of actions were found as contributing factors in 14 percent of the cases with negative consequences. Also, safety culture (Dyrløv Madsen et al. 2007, Itoh et al. 2007) seems to have an impact on interruptions. In an investigation with 2000 participants, a Danish safety culture questionnaire study showed that 69 percent of the participating healthcare professionals agree or highly agree that interruptions are reasons or contributing factors for adverse events (Dyrløv Madsen and Schou 2008). Finally, there is much anecdotal evidence from healthcare professionals who often respond enthusiastically to the concept of PM, claiming that it describes very common experiences of daily practice.

Interruptions as Situations with High PM Burdens

Many different situations place a high burden on PM: interruptions, distractions, parallel tasks, delays, etc. In the following section we focus on interruptions to narrow the scope of the discussion, allowing for more thorough analysis.

Interruptions and distractions are known to have a negative impact on performance, as they influence and minimize the professionals' ability to stay focused on a specific task (intention) (Beyea 2007). By analysing PM errors in interruption situations, it will also be possible to take a work analytical stance. Investigating PM errors in interruptions will help in understanding the personal redefinition of tasks. What do professionals see as an interruption (from the outside, e.g., by colleagues, alarms, telephone), a distraction (from the inside, e.g., sudden thoughts or ideas, difficulties in concentrating, inner resistances) and a task-inherent challenge (e.g., difficulties during intubation or finding the correct differential diagnosis)? This perspective is especially important in the multiple-crew, interdependent task context of most acute medical care settings. What does one crew accept as a legitimate task of the other crew? What do they see as a necessary interruption? What is accepted and what is not? These factors might influence the crew and team climate, the willingness to cooperate and thus, also patient safety.

Analysing PM errors in the interruption context will allow for supplementing the cognitive perspective with social aspects. Most professionals both expect and accept interruptions as part of their normal work day (Beyea 2007, Parker and Coiera 2000). From the cognitive perspective, those interruptions might be helpful to decrease one's own memory load interrupting a colleague and delegating the task frees one's own cognitive resources however, this interruption may increase that colleague's cognitive load. From the social perspective, interruptions might be related to reciprocal acceptance: accepting being disrupted and asked for help might, in turn, legitimize oneself interrupting others later. Interruptions are likely to be related to hierarchy as well: they could be seen as a status symbol ('I am important and needed – people interrupt me and I can help solve their problems') but also as an integral part of a certain position (by definition and job description, a consultant is a centre in a complex network of information flow with many 'inputs' and 'outputs' and thus interruptions) (Groopman 2007, Jauhar 2007). A recent observational study of nurses and doctors in an oncological ambulatory unit in a Danish hospital revealed many disturbances and interruptions in the daily workflow (Dyrløv Madsen and Schou 2008). Their study documented a large number of interruptions, especially for nurses, which often resulted in staff forgetting to finish tasks. Nevertheless, during post-observation interviews about the observed events, the professionals, on the whole, found them appropriate, legitimate and were able to justify their frequency. The interviewees claimed the interruptions were appropriate for the task at hand and/or to improve teamwork. On further reflection and discussion with the interviewer the professionals, however, recognized that many of the interruptions were a problem for patient safety and that they probably could be minimized or avoided if everyone was dedicated to do so. Therefore, how interruptions are perceived seems to be inherent to the professional culture.

Finally, interruptions are relevant for PM research as it might be easier to identify the underlying intention, as compared to other situations like delays in having the opportunity to execute a certain intention. We will discuss this aspect in more detail below. In summary, by studying interruptions in relation to PM in acute medical care, we hope to advance the knowledge about this error type.

Definition of Prospective Memory and its Failures

Prospective memory is defined as a psychological processes which enable humans to execute previously formed intentions during an appropriate but delayed 'window of opportunity' (Harris and Wilkins 1982) without being explicitly reminded to do so (Dieckmann et al. 2006; for an overview see Brandimonte et al. 1996). Not resuming the interrupted task, resuming the interrupted task at the wrong spot (missing a step or wrongly performing a step more than once) or not executing an intended task might be related to errors of PM. However, in order to make this 'error diagnosis', differential diagnoses need to be considered. Not resuming or executing a task might be related to a conscious decision (which might in itself be right or wrong), it might be because the window of opportunity was not recognized, or that other cognitive and emotional processes prevented the execution (e.g., unconscious resistances). Weimer (1925) suggested that one needs to distinguish between error forms (here: missing the execution of an intention, failing to resume a task or resuming it at the wrong spot) from the underlying error types, i.e., the underlying psychological processes (e.g., forgetting, denying, deciding against it). What might look like the same error from the 'outside' (error form: an intended task is not executed), might be very different from the 'inside'. Focusing on PM in interruptions as a situation type/error form helps in narrowing the search space for underlying error types.

In general, one can distinguish between different classes of PM tasks, depending on how the window of opportunity is to be described: activity-based PM tasks (i.e., do X after you are finished with M, see Example 3, 'Dynamic change of plans', above), event-based PM tasks (i.e., do X when Y occurs, see Example 1, 'Treatment in time') and time-based PM tasks (i.e., do X at time Z, see Example 2, 'Recurrent measurements').

Within the PM framework, five phases are distinguished that belong to a full PM cycle (Ellis 1996):

1. In the beginning, the *intention is formed and encoded*, containing three components: *that*, *what* and *when*. The *that component* can be seen as energizing the inner system, preparing the person to act at all (Goschke and Kuhl 1993, Lewin 1926). The *what component* specifies what needs to be done in more detail. The *when component* helps in anticipating the window of opportunity in a temporal and conditional sense.

2. During the *retention phase* the intention is kept in memory, more or less consciously, while the duration of the interval does not seem to have a large impact on the retention of the intention and its execution (Kvavilashvili and Ellis 1996). Short interruptions might be enough to hinder the execution of intentions.

3. The *window of opportunity* begins and the intention could be executed. It is a question of whether the person intending to act recognizes the beginning of the window of opportunity and is also able to retrieve the intention. For

it to be labelled a PM situation, there would not be an additional reminder about the intention.

4. The *execution action*, putting the intention into practice, is considered a separate phase in the model. It can contain specific errors, e.g., related to the ability to perform the intended task or meta-cognitive abilities to monitor the success of the intention implementation.

5. Finally, the acting person must *note whether or not the intention was fulfilled* and, if yes, also to what extent. On occasion, intentions are only partially fulfilled but seem to the acting person as though the task has already been completed.

6. Depending on the phase of the cycle in which this disturbance occurs, different error types would be responsible for the failed execution of the intention as error form. Future research should aim to better understand the error types. We will use the framework introduced here to more closely analyse the examples presented at the start of the chapter. This will necessarily involve some assumptions and even speculations – as PM failures are related to intentions, which can not be observed directly.

Analysis of the Clinical Examples within the PM Framework

Example 1 – Treatment in Time

The situation where the anaesthesia team must remember the antibiotic can be classified as an event-based PM task. This case is particularly difficult because the intention should be fulfilled before another event (skin cut) takes place. Therefore, the anaesthesia crew would need to create some kind of cue that could help them remember to provide the antibiotic before the skin cut. The *skin cut* is not an appropriate cue to trigger the action, as it occurs too late. The newly created cue could be 'internal': the crew could try to anticipate in detail the moment in which they want to remember to administer the drug. They could thus make their internal intention stronger, so that they would be more alert about the beginning of the window of opportunity (Gollwitzer and Schaal 1998, Schweiger Gallo and Gollwitzer 2007). Another strategy which is more 'external' and is already partially implemented according to the task description. The team can create some kind of external reminder (here the bottle that is taped to the chart). They could also use a combination of internal and external strategies when trying to remember to execute the intention: they could anticipate the moment in which they take the bottle off the chart and try to use this act as a cue to perform the intention of administering the drug as well. Potentially, it might be easy to forget to actually administer the drug if the bottle is taken away from the chart but not used immediately. Just handling the bottle carries the risk of psychologically 'finishing' the task (pars-pro-toto error type).

Example 2 – Recurrent Measurements

As opposed to the first example, the intention in this example (anaesthetist checking blood glucose) needs to be remembered by a single person, not a team. This has advantages and disadvantages. Research shows that asking other people to help remember might, at times, not be effective. One underlying mechanism might be the shared responsibility for forming and retaining the intention leads to lowered cognitive energy for all involved (Shaefer and Laing 2000). This example further involves a recurring time-based intention: the blood glucose needs to be checked at regular intervals. The anaesthetist relies on the alarm clock which acts as an external reminder. However, the effectiveness of this reminder might be compromised by the concurrent tasks during the operation – which might be even more obviously demanding (the negative effects of low blood glucose are not immediately obvious in anaesthetized patients). So, when the timer clock goes off and the anaesthetist is just performing another task, a new PM challenge is posed – the intended action is again interrupted or cannot even be started. The reminder does not have a memory for the execution of the task in the sense of the PM Phase 5, described above. Using such external reminders might have the drawback that their potential to help might not be usable in a specific moment and, in addition, using them requires resources in itself, thus adding to the complexity of the situation.

Example 3 – Dynamic Change of Plans

Unlike the first two examples, Example 3 (remembering to perform an appendectomy) involves changes of plans during the actions – a common situation in medicine as a dynamic field. During the demanding operation, the decision is made dynamically to extend the treatment by including an additional treatment after the originally planned steps are fulfilled. This situation requires either modification of the original intention or the formation of a new intention – a differentiation that might be difficult to make in practice but could be relevant for the strengths of the intention and thus the likelihood of the execution of this activity-based intention. In either case, due to the demanding operation, the forming of the intention might be weak and with little energy, increasing the likelihood of 'forgetting' it. In addition, this situation is error prone because of its 'pars-pro-toto' character (cf. (Dieckmann et al. 2006). When the originally planned part of the operation is finished, the fifth phase of the PM cycle becomes very relevant: the evaluation of the results. As the original intention is fulfilled completely, it might be easy to mistakenly see the whole, now enlarged intention as fulfilled, thus missing the newly formed part. Fulfilling a part of the intentions might feel as if they were being fulfilled completely.

Results from a Pilot Study

After the theoretical considerations during the analyses of the examples, we report empirical data from a pilot study about PM in acute care settings; it was meant as a first approximation to PM in acute medical care – a so far neglected connection (Dieckmann et al. 2006).

Simulator Study

In one study we used a patient simulator to investigate situations prone to PM failures and the effects of the missed execution of intentions (Dieckmann et al. 2006). In summary, we created ten different simulation scenarios for acute care settings. Each scenario contained between one and three PM situations, which differed in how closely they were related to the context of the scenario. The match to the context was the first independent variable. Participants were medical students who were close to or within their final year, and worked through the scenarios in pairs. The dependent variable was whether the team (i.e., one or both members) executed the intentions during the scenario. After each scenario, each student rated the importance of the intention and several other elements of the scenario. We used this rating as a second independent variable. We analysed the number and percentage of executed tasks in dependency of type and importance. No significant differences were found with regard to either factor. Subjectively, important tasks tended to be executed more often than unimportant tasks and the closer the task matched the overall goal of the situation (learning), the more often it tended to be executed. Despite the lack of significant results, since it was possible to trigger PM errors in these scenarios, we believe that the simulator is an appropriate research setting for studies on prospective memory.

Questionnaire Study

In another part of the study, we assessed the attitudes and experiences of elements of prospective memory in anaesthetists and intensive care physicians from diverse healthcare institutions in Germany. Based on the results of a workshop with eight anaesthetists of different experience levels, we developed a questionnaire, which described 24 PM-prone situations. The questionnaire briefly explained the concept of PM. Respondents rated the relevance of PM for their practice and estimated how often they had encountered each situation during the preceding month (see Table 20.1, mean count) and how often they failed to execute the specified intention. We computed percentages from these counts for every participant and averaged these percentages across situations (Table 20.1, mean percentage). Questionnaires were sent to 680 anaesthesiologists and intensive care physicians in German healthcare institutions of different sizes and types (university hospitals, community hospitals, private practice) from all 16 federal states in Germany. We sent every institution a letter that described the study, accompanied by the appropriate number of blank questionnaires and stamped return envelopes for the relevant staff.

There were 112 questionnaires returned (16.4 percent response rate). The mean duration of job experience of the respondents was 10 ± 8 years. A total of 69 percent of respondents rated the influence of PM failures on the development of critical incidents as 'very big', 'big' or 'somewhat big' (mean and standard deviation: 4.03 ± 1.01; n=107), while 59 percent estimated the threat of such failures to patient safety as 'somewhat big' or greater (3.78 ± .98; n=107). 'No impact at all' was not checked by any of the respondents. Table 20.1 shows the experiences of situations prone to failure of PM and the respondents' estimate of how often they are connected with missed executions of the intention.

Table 20.1   **Selected estimations of frequency of prospective memory based situations in medicine (mean count), error proneness of situations (mean %), and valid number of estimations for each situation (n)**

Situation	Mean count ± SD experienced	Mean % ± SD forgotten	Number of valid estimations (n)
A medical intervention is interrupted by a more important task and you want to correctly resume the interrupted treatment	36.3 ± 41.7	11.3 ± 9.0	98
You need to check whether another person executed the intention	28.9 ± 43.8	16.0 ± 17.0	61
You are disturbed by another person while you are about to execute an intention	25.7 ± 58.8	18.8 ± 19.5	83
You are disturbed by an alarm while you are about to execute an intention	24.7 ± 66.9	11.6 ± 14.6	78
You are not certain whether you already executed the intention or not	15.1 ± 36.6	15.5 ± 20.4	100
The intention concerns an action that is unimportant for you	10.5 ± 15.4	40.9 ± 29.7	82
You need to postpone a routine action and perform it later	10.2 ± 14.5	16.4 ± 19.4	81
You executed a very similar but not the intended action	9.3 ± 18.2	15.4 ± 20.0	86

Table 20.1   *Concluded*

Situation	Mean count ± SD experienced	Mean % ± SD forgotten	Number of valid estimations (n)
You know that you wanted to do something but cannot remember what it was	8.8 ± 11.4	36.2 ± 31.7	88
The intention concerns an action that is unpleasant for you	7.7 ± 9.0	8.1 ± 16.7	82
Problems using a device cause delays in executing an intention	6.9 ± 12.1	18.4 ± 20.8	91
You need to postpone an exceptional task and do it later	7.2 ± 11.6	16.0 ± 19.9	82

Because of the low response rate and an unrepresentative sampling, generalizations need to be drawn carefully from this questionnaire. Nevertheless, we think the results can generate hypotheses and emphasize the need for more research in this regard. One of the formed hypotheses is that interruptions appear to impact PM in different ways. Interruptions by persons are estimated to be more disruptive than those by alarms. This difference might be due to the fact that interruptions by other people tend to be stronger than those by alarms. Where it is possible to take a short time to finish a thought, task or part of a task when the alarm goes off, this is often more difficult with interruptions by other persons. Observations in the intensive care setting support this assumption: interruptions by other persons were followed by immediate reactions by those who were interrupted. These results fit also with the tendency for face-to-face communication in medical settings, described above. It is a question of further research to discover the underlying error types for this phenomenon.

Discussion of Research Related to Prospective Memory and its Failures in Acute Care Settings

There is a large body of basic psychological research on prospective memory, relying to a large extent on highly controlled studies in laboratories. While this type of research allows for looking more closely at the different error types underlying the missed execution of intentions, it seems difficult at times to use the results from those studies to improve patient care because it is difficult to directly apply the results from artificial research situations. The discussions showed that the theoretical PM framework is helpful to have a closer look at PM and how it relates to patient safety. However, there are challenges when trying to strictly apply the definitions within the PM framework to the dynamic settings of field research in the acute care settings. Intentions, as inner processes, are not directly observable but need to be inferred. In addition, they are not always conscious in all parts. It seems necessary to also conduct more applied studies under more ecologically valid conditions and to progress the knowledge by looking at prospective memory from both the applied and the basic science perspective.

As with all studies of errors, it is also a challenge in PM research, to define the 'unit of analysis', i.e., what is to be considered an error and what is correct performance (Wehner et al. forthcoming). In most PM studies, ours included, the investigation relies on the assumption that participants form an intention from instructions. If the instruction is never transformed into an intention, it would be wrong to assume an error, if no related task is executed. For this reason, we think it is beneficial to have a closer look at interruptions. It seems reasonable that tasks which are not yet completed are related to the intention of resuming and finishing it. In some cases there might also be the conscious decision not to pursue the intention any more, so that supplementary interviews and other data would still be helpful. In this regard, we acknowledge the smart methodological aspects of the first group studying PM-related issues in the 1920s around Kurt Lewin (Birenbaum 1930, Ovsiankina 1928, Lewin 1926, Zeigarnik 1927), who investigated, using interviews, how easily participants could remember intentions that were fulfilled as opposed to those that were not fulfilled.

Another challenge for research in PM and its failures stem from the fact that, in many cases, the window of opportunity is artificially strictly defined under study conditions, possibly decreasing the ecological validity of the results. In many clinical situations, the borders of the window of opportunity are not defined sharply, but more in terms of transitions (see Example 2 above). In many (certainly not all) cases it is not of significance whether a certain task is fulfilled in a specific time frame. The sequence of events might be more important in many cases (e.g., Example 1) than the absolute time and in some cases there might be discussions about the existence of a window of opportunity in the first place (i.e., in those cases where it is difficult to define the gold standard of medical practice).

There is much debate about the memory component of PM. As discussed above, the phenomenon of executing or not executing a certain intention involves many different processes during the phases of a PM cycle. In order to understand the underlying error mechanisms (error types), we would need a very fine-grained analysis – which is often not possible in applied studies. In this regard it might be better to (a) talk about intentions and their execution instead of PM in applied settings and (b) to integrate basic, laboratory-based research with more applied studies, with the aim of validating the findings.

Implications for Clinical Practice

For dealing with each threat to patient safety, it is important to work through at least three steps. The first step involves the removal of the threat from the system, reducing the number of PM-prone situations. One could analyse and optimize communication and interaction patterns, potentially decreasing the number of interruptions and the amount of time spent waiting for team members. This would be a question of work system design. In a second step, which should only be taken if the first step is not possible, one could try to build in safety measurements, to prevent errors in PM-prone situations. This can be external reminder systems, checklists and other (technical) devices that might help in optimizing PM performance. Thirdly, and this step should only be taken if the first two steps have failed, one could train people to handle the remaining PM situations better. The priority should be to systematically design weak points out of the system instead of training people to handle them. Such training could involve strategies that can help remembering and also showing the sometimes counter-intuitive effects of some of those strategies (e.g., asking someone to help remember, which might decrease the likelihood of executing the intention as discussed above). Here we do need deeper analyses, trying to understand how people redefine tasks into primary, secondary, etc. and decide what is the disturbance and what is the disturbed element.

Work system design can tailor the interplay of humans, technology and organization in a PM friendly and PM *error friendly* way (Wehner 1992, von Weizsäcker and von Weizsäcker 1984). Depending on the perspective of this interplay and the underlying error types, we need different ways for improvement. Those ways would necessarily involve cognitive, but also social and organizational, elements.

References

Beyea, S.C. (2007) Distractions, interruptions, and patient safety. *Aorn J* 86, 109–12.

Birenbaum, G. (1930) Das Vergessen einer Vornahme [The forgetting of an intention]. *Psychologische Forschung* 13, 218–84.

Brandimonte, M., Einstein, G.O. and Mcdaniel, M. (eds) (1996) *Prospective Memory: Theory and Applications*. Mahwah, NJ: Erlbaum.

Chisholm, C.D., Collison, E.K., Nelson, D.R. and Cordell, W.H. (2000) Emergency department workplace interruptions: Are emergency physicians 'interrupt-driven' and 'multitasking'? *Academic Emergency Medicine* 7, 1239–43.

Dieckmann, P., Reddersen, S., Wehner, T. and Rall, M. (2006) Prospective memory failures as an unexplored threat to patient safety: Results from a pilot study using patient simulators to investigate the missed execution of intentions. *Ergonomics* 49, 526–43.

Dismukes, K. and Nowinski, J. (2006) Prospective memory, concurrent task management, and pilot error. In A. Kramer and D. Wiegmann (eds) *Attention: From Theory to Practice*. New York: Oxford.

Dyrløv Madsen, M. and Schou, B. (2008) Forstyrrelser, afbrud og travlhed: Resultater af en pilotundersøgelse i et onkologisk ambulatorium [Interruptions, disruptions, and workload: Results of a pilot project in an oncological ambulatory department]. Unpublished internal work report, Danish Institute for Medical Simulation, Herlev Hospital, Herlev Denmark.

Dyrløv Madsen, M., Boje Andersen, H. and Itoh, K. (2007) Assessing safety culture and climate in health care. In P. Carayon (ed.) *Handbook of Human Factors and Ergonomics in Health Care and Patient Safety.* Mahwah, NJ: Erlbaum.

Ellis, J. (1996) Prospective memory or the realization of delayed intentions: A conceptual framework for research. In M. Brandimonte, G.O. Einstein and M. Mcdaniel (eds) *Prospective Memory: Theory and Applications.* Mahwah, NJ: Erlbaum.

Gaba, D.M., Howard, S.K., Fish, K.J., Smith, B.E. and Sowb, Y.A. (2001) Simulation based training in anesthesia crisis resource management (ACRM): A decade of experience. *Simulation and Gaming* 32, 175–93.

Gollwitzer, P.M. and Schaal, B. (1998) Metacognition in action: The importance of implementation intentions. *Pers Soc Psychol Rev* 2, 124–36.

Goschke, T. and Kuhl, J. (1993) Representation of intentions: Persisting activation in memory. *Journal of Experimental Psychology: Learning, Memory and Cognition* 19, 1221–6.

Groopman, J. (2007) *How Doctors Think.* Boston: Houghton Mifflin.

Harris, J.E. and Wilkins, A.J. (1982) Remembering to do things: A theoretical framework and an illustrative experiment. *Human Learning* 1, 123–6.

Healey, A.N., Sevdalis, N. and Vincent, C.A. (2006) Measuring intra-operative interference from distraction and interruption observed in the operating theatre. *Ergonomics* 49, 589–604.

Itoh, K., Boje Andersen, H. and Dyrløv Madsen, M. (2007) Safety culture in health care. In P. Carayon (ed.) *Handbook of Human Factors and Ergonomics in Health Care and Patient Safety.* Mahwah, NJ: Erlbaum.

Jauhar, S. (2007) *Intern. A Doctor's Initiation.* New York: Farrar, Straus and Giroux.

Kvavilashvili, L. and Ellis, J. (1996) Varieties of intention: Some distinctions and classifiactions. In M. Brandimonte, G.O. Einstein and M. Mcdaniel (eds) *Prospective Memory: Theory and Applications.* Mahwah, NJ: Erlbaum.

Lewin, K. (1926) Vorsatz, Wille und Bedürfnis [Intention, will, and need]. *Psychologische Forschung* 7, 330–85.

Manser, T., Thiele, K. and Wehner, T. (2003) Soziotechnische Systemanalyse im Krankenhaus – Eine Arbeispsychologische Fallstudie in der Anästhesiologie [Sociotechnical system analysis in the hospital – a work psychological case study in anaesthesiology]. In E. Ulich (ed.) *Arbeitspsychologie in Krankenhaus und Arztpraxis. Arbeitsbedingungen, Belastungen, Ressourcen.* Bern: Huber.

Ovsiankina, M. (1928) Die Wiederaufnahme unterbrochener Handlungen [The resumption of interrupted tasks]. *Psychologische Forschung* 11, 302–79.

Parker, J. and Coiera, E. (2000) Improving clinical communication: A view from psychology. *J Am Med Inform Assoc* 7, 453–61.

Schaefer, E.G. and Laing, M.L. (2000) 'Please Remind Me …': The role of others in prospective remembering. *Applied Cognitive Psychology* 14, S99–S114.

Schweiger Gallo, I. and Gollwitzer, P.M. (2007) Implementation intentions: A look back at fifteen years of progress. *Psicothema* 19, 37–42.

US Pharmacopeia (2000) *Summary of the 1999 Information Submitted to MedMARx - A National Database for Hospital Medication Error Reporting.* Available at: <http://www.usp.org/reporting/medmarx/1999/final.pdf>. Rockville: US Pharmacopeia.

Von Weizsäcker, C. and Von Weizsäcker, U. (1984) Fehlerfreundlichkeit [error friendliness]. In K. Kornwachs (ed.) *Offenheit – Zeitlichkeit – Komplexität: Zur Theorie der offenen Systeme [Openness – Timeliness – Complexity: On the Theory of Open Systems].* Frankfurt: Campus.

Wehner, T. (1992) *Sicherheit als Fehlerfreundlichkeit. Arbeits- und Sozialpsychologische Befunde für eine kritische Technikbewertung [Safety as Error Friendliness. Work- and Social Psychological Findings for a Critical Assessment of Technology].* Opladen: Westdeutscher Verlag.

Wehner, T., Mehl, K. and Dieckmann, P. (forthcoming) Fehlhandlungen und Prävention [errors and prevention]. In U. Kleinbeck (ed.) *Enzyklopädie der Psychologie. Band Ingenieurpsychologie.*

Zeigarnik, B. (1927) Über das Behalten von erledigten und unerledigten Handlungen [on the retention of executed and not executed tasks]. *Psychologische Forschung,* 9, 1–85.

Weimer, H. (1925) *Psychologie der Fehler* [Psychology of the errors]. Leipzig: Klinkhardt.

Chapter 21

Surgical Decision-Making: A Multimodal Approach

Nick Sevdalis, Rosamond Jacklin and Charles Vincent

Introduction

Surgeons, in conjunction with their patients and colleagues, have to make risky and irreversible choices. The ability to make clinical decisions, both within and outside the operating theatre, is a key feature of surgical expertise, which has been highlighted in attempts to define the essential competencies of a surgeon. For example, the CanMEDS model of clinical competency (Frank and Langer 2003), asserts that 'the role of *medical expert/clinical decision-maker* is central' (Frank et al. 1996, p. 4), and includes elements such as diagnostic reasoning, clinical judgement and clinical decision-making (Frank 2005). The CanMEDS model was influential in the development of the Intercollegiate Surgical Curriculum Project, which forms the framework for the postgraduate training of surgeons in the UK (Canter and Kelly 2007).

This chapter discusses surgical decision-making in both a clinical and research context and introduces a multimodal approach to measuring and assessing surgical decision-making. In what follows, we begin by outlining the role of decision-making within the 'systems approach' to surgical safety. Next, we describe some important features of surgical decision-making in its clinical context. Thirdly, we provide a brief overview of some of the methods available for studying surgical decision-making. Fourthly, we introduce the multimodal approach that we have taken to investigate, measure and train surgical decision-making in our research group and the results we have achieved so far. We conclude with a discussion of different research approaches, including limitations and implications for research in and assessment of surgical decision-making.

(i) The 'Systems Approach' to Surgical Safety

In recent years, there have been shifts in the understanding of surgical performance and surgical outcomes. Traditionally, surgical performance and outcomes were understood as a function of the patient's risk factors (i.e., the severity of the disease and existing co-morbidities). In the past ten years or so, with the surge in the use of surgical simulators and the associated development of the evidence base on surgical training and technical performance, the technical skill of the surgeon (i.e., surgeons' motor skill) has been recognized as a factor that mediates the relationship between patient risk factors and patient outcomes (e.g., Aggarwal et al. 2004, Dankelman and DiLorenzo 2005, Fried and Feldman 2008).

In the past five years, it has been proposed that this relationship should be qualified further. A number of other skills and factors have been suggested as potential determinants of performance and outcomes, alongside motor skills. These include cognitive and behavioural skills and also other factors, such as the operating theatre environment and procedures. Because of its multi-factorial perspective on surgical performance, error and outcome, this approach has been termed the 'systems approach' (Calland et al. 2002, Healey and Vincent 2007, Vincent et al. 2004).

The systems approach to surgical performance is novel, and thus the existing conceptual and empirical work that stems from it is still somewhat limited. Interpersonal and cognitive skills are required for many occupations; specific subsets of such skills have been identified in the relevant literature as being essential for surgeons (Healey et al. 2006a, Yule et al. 2006). On the one hand, there are skills that are related to the way the operating surgeon interacts with other members of the operating theatre team – including assistant surgeon(s) and members of the anaesthetic and nursing sub-teams. On the other hand, there are the skills that reflect surgeons' cognitive competence, such as decision-making. These skills are complementary to the manual dexterity of the surgeons and they have been termed, collectively, 'non-technical skills'. The working hypothesis for non-technical skills is that they contribute to surgical patient safety. The focus of this chapter is on one of these non-technical skills, namely decision-making.

Decision-making is becoming increasingly prominent in the surgical skills and training literature (e.g., Flin et al. 2007, Sevdalis and McCulloch 2006). Decision-making is a cognitive skill, involving a number of inter-related steps (which may occur in very rapid, often unconscious sequence):

1. recognition that choice between different courses of action is available;
2. perception of different courses of action;
3. evaluation of each course of action in relation to its potential risks and benefits;
4. actual choice;
5. monitoring of the patient's progress in relation to the decision taken (with review and change of plan if appropriate).

As in other high-risk environments, in surgery there are a number of different decision-making 'modes' (Flin et al. 2007, Sevdalis and McCulloch 2006). These modes of thinking span a continuum, ranging from implicit/cognitively untaxing modes, characterized by intuition and simply 'knowing what to do', (recognition-primed decisions; Klein 1998) to explicit/cognitively taxing (analytical decisions, in which the various options available are weighed up consciously and carefully). Typically, a surgeon applies different decision strategies to different problems, depending on a variety of factors including the type of problem, whether it is familiar or not, time pressure, the potential consequences, the surgeon's level of expertise, and other factors (Flin et al. 2007, Sevdalis and McCulloch 2006). For instance, the decision whether to offer surgery to a patient presenting with symptoms suggestive of gallstone disease may be intuitive (if the patient is significantly symptomatic from gallstones and fit for an operation, making the decision clear cut), or nearer the analytical end of the continuum if the patient is elderly and frail and the balance of risks and benefits is less clear cut. In contrast, the decision when a patient can eat and drink post-operatively appears to be a rule-based decision (with rules that differ somewhat between surgeons; Jacklin et al. 2008a).

(ii) Surgical Decision-Making in Context

Surgeons are faced with important choices at all stages of patient care and their decisions may be made in very different ways. At the pre-operative stage, deciding whether or not to operate can be a delicate balance of risks and benefits, made at leisure and collaboratively with the patient in the context of elective surgery. In the emergency situation, the same decision is likely to be made under time pressure. Intra-operatively, a sequence of operative steps is carried out, but decision-making continues – for example, deciding whether the anatomy has been clearly identified and whether the operation can proceed as anticipated, or the steps require re-evaluating. For instance, if a strangulated hernia is operated on, a decision must be made as to whether the bowel that was contained within it remains viable (and can be returned to the abdomen safely) or is beyond salvage (and must be resected), with attendant risks of leak from the anastomosis and longer post-operative recovery.

As in other high-risk environments, decision-making in surgery has some distinctive characteristics. Firstly, many surgical decisions carry high stakes. For the patient, the potential consequences of an operation (in addition to the desired ones) may include disability or death. Operating without causing some harm is impossible, so in every decision to operate there is a trade-off between the likely benefit and the inevitable anatomical (as well as physiological and psychological) damage caused to the patient as a primary consequence of the surgery itself.

Secondly, surgery is associated with complications and their consequences, which may be difficult to predict for any individual patient, but tend to have a relatively predictable incidence overall. In other words, surgical decisions are associated with uncertainty about their outcomes at the level of the individual patient. For example, elective open repair of abdominal aortic aneurysms has a mortality of up to 7 percent in some institutions (Hertzer 2006)

A third special feature of surgical decisions is their potential irreversibility. Once a laparotomy has been performed or tissue has been excised, this cannot be undone. Reversibility of surgical decisions is relative, as some aspects of an operation may be reversible. For example, where a stoma has been created and the gut left in discontinuity, the continuity may subsequently be restored at a further operation.

Finally, unlike many other medical decisions, intra-operative decision-making usually cannot be shared with the patient. Although operative details and likely findings can be discussed with patients pre-operatively, significant procedures take place under general anaesthetic or with spinal/local block often in combination with sedation. Patients are either unconscious or have impaired consciousness, with responsibility for operative aspects of decision-making resting with the primary or senior surgeon and their team.

(iii) Methods for Studying Surgical Decision-Making

There is a substantial established body of theory and experimental research into the psychology of decision-making and the related field of problem solving, and the cognitive processes that they involve. For a comprehensive summary of the field, see Koehler and Harvey's handbook (2004). In addition, there is a related literature on the nature of expert performance. Research into these areas has been published for the most part in a number of dedicated journals, such as the *Journal of Behavioral Decision Making, Organizational Behavior and Human Decision Processes*, the *Journal of Risk and Uncertainty, Group Decision and Negotiation* and *Medical Decision Making*.

Although the methods used by decision researchers are unfamiliar to many surgical researchers, many have been adapted for use in the healthcare setting. A number of theoretical approaches and empirical applications are described in Chapman and Sonnenberg's *Decision Making in Health Care* edited volume (2003). The book incorporates various decision research approaches to medical decision-making (including decision modelling, health economics and cognitive approaches) and covers a number of applications of this line of work (including decision support and assessment of patients' preferences). From a methodological viewpoint, Harries and Kostopoulou (2005) provide a thorough review of empirical approaches to the study of medical decision-making. Building on these reviews, in what follows we provide a brief overview of selected methodological approaches for empirical research into how surgeons actually make decisions in practice.

(iii-i) Self-report

Self-report, typically elicited in interviews, offers the opportunity for detailed exploration of particular decision-making issues. Interviewing surgeons about how they arrive(d) at a decision complements other methodological approaches by providing detailed information about the relevant cues to a decision, or identifying important contextual factors. Retrospective investigation of specific, recent, real-life decisions using detailed interviews forms the basis of the critical incident approach. This is used extensively within a research paradigm known as Naturalistic Decision-Making (NDM; Klein et al. 1993, Lipshitz et al. 2001). NDM approaches focus on how experts actually make decisions in naturally occurring working environments (e.g., in the operating theatre). In surgery, interviews have been used successfully to capture surgeons' subjective experience of stressors and impediments to their performance (Arora et al. 2009, Wetzel et al. 2006) and they can be useful additions to direct observation in the development of tools that capture expert knowledge in an accessible form and facilitate teaching/training of novice professionals, such as Hierarchical Task Analysis (e.g., Sarker et al. 2008). In the empirical section of this chapter, we describe an interview-based knowledge elicitation approach, in which interviews were used to capture expert knowledge on a given topic.

(iii-ii) Structural Approaches and Decision Modelling

Structural approaches are a group of methodologies that have in common their statistical approach to modelling relationships between inputs to a judgement or decision (i.e., decision cues) and their outputs. Judgement Analysis (Cooksey 1996a, 1996b) is one such structural approach. This methodology is based on presentation of a series of multiple-cue case profiles. The impact of different factors may be assessed by varying the values of the selected cues in differing combinations. Using linear regression it is then possible to determine the influence of different variables/factors on participants' judgements. The analysis yields multiple regression-derived beta weights for individual risk factors, and model fit. Data are typically analysed separately for each participant, but can also be aggregated to allow subgroup comparisons (e.g., novice vs. expert participants; Sevdalis and Jacklin 2008). Within surgery, this approach has been used to model surgeons' prioritization decision-making for cardiac surgery (Kee et al. 1998) and general surgery (MacCormick and Parry 2006), and treatment of prostate cancer (Clarke et al. 2007) – and there are other clinical applications, including management of typical non-end-stage renal disease (Pfister et al. 1999) and dental surgery (Koele and Hoogstraten 1999). One study described below used this approach to investigate how surgeons generate risk estimates on the basis of combinations of pre-operative risk factors.

(iii-iii) Observational and Process Approaches

Interpreted broadly, these approaches seek to characterize the decision-making process as it unfolds over time. Observation of real-life clinical work may focus on explicit information search, communication with colleagues and the patient during the decision-making process, the use of artefacts, or non-verbal interactions. In such approaches, researchers typically seek to capture clinicians' thinking and/or behaviours reliably and robustly as these unfold over the time it takes to complete the task under investigation (e.g., arrive at a diagnosis or treatment decision, or carry out a procedure). Such thinking or behavioural 'protocols' (verbal or non-verbal) have been reported in the medical literature – with 'think aloud' protocols being perhaps the most well known (Ericsson and Simon 1984). In such protocols, study participants report the content of working memory during a decision-making task (Denig and Haaijer-Ruskamp 1994). Non-verbal approaches, such as eye-tracking of gaze patterns, can give information about information search patterns, and can also be used to test the veracity of subjective accounts (e.g., Leong et al. 2007). Alternatively, researchers may choose to develop an observation protocol (usually after some pilot observations and testing), which is then used to collect data in real time. Such observational tools focus more on observable behaviours and less on underlying cognitive processes (as the former are easier to observe directly than the latter). Studies of medical and surgical working environments have used this approach successfully (e.g., Coiera and Tombs 1998, Healey et al. 2006b). The third set of empirical studies that we report below uses a simulated clinical setting (simulated operating theatre) to provide a safe and standardized setting to assess surgical decision-making (among other skills) via real time observation of key behaviours between team members.

(iv) A Multimodal Approach to Surgical Decision-making

To date, our research group has investigated surgical decision-making using the following three approaches:

1. knowledge elicitation from expert surgeons, used to model a care pathway from the decision-making perspective (Jacklin et al. 2008a);
2. experimental approaches to the modelling of surgical risk estimation (Jacklin et al. 2008b, Sevdalis and Jacklin 2008);
3. simulation-based assessment of decision-making, in which decision-making is assessed alongside other skills (Undre et al. 2007, Koutantji et al. 2008).

In what follows, we present the methodology and key findings of these studies (readers are referred to original publications for more detail). We discuss the findings and their implications in the concluding section of the chapter.

(iv-i) Knowledge elicitation

One of the distinguishing features of expertise is that when expert and novice professionals are presented with a situation that requires action or a problem that needs addressing, their perception of it (including their prioritization for actions to be taken and when) is markedly different. Training junior colleagues, therefore, involves an expert conveying how they grasp a situation – for instance, how they use just the relevant information and discard irrelevant 'noise'. In the context of surgery, however, such training is rather hard, as only rarely are surgical decisions of experts explicitly deconstructed into their constituent parts and explained to trainee surgeons. We conducted an interview study with the aim to provide such a method of deconstructing a series of interrelated surgical decisions (Jacklin et al. 2008a).

Methods Semi-structured interviews were conducted with ten expert surgeons (three senior specialist registrars and seven consultants), focusing on the care pathway of patients with symptomatic gallstone disease. First of all, participants were instructed to think of a patient attending an outpatient clinic with chronic symptoms of gallstone disease. Secondly, participants were asked to think of a patient presenting acutely at an emergency department, again with symptoms suggestive of a complication of gallstones. Participants were prompted to think about the decisions that they would be required to make throughout the patient's care (consultation, admission, surgery, recovery and discharge). They identified the decisions made in each setting, along with the relevant cues for each decision, and any strategies or rules of thumb.

A coding frame was developed to identify decisions and associated cues and rules from the text. Participants' responses were coded for content by a surgeon (RJ) and a psychologist (NS) and the relevant decisions identified. Decisions were defined as any nodal choice in the pathway of care.

Results The surgeon and the psychologist coders identified similar numbers of decisions per interview ($M_{Surgeon}$ = 16; $M_{Psychologist}$ = 15). A positive correlation between numbers of decisions per interview identified by each coder suggested reliable coding between raters (Spearman's $\rho = 0.61, N = 10, p < 0.06$). Interestingly, whereas the surgeon coder considered 'identification of anatomy' as a key intra-operative decision, the psychologist coder did not – perhaps due to differences in their training and ensuing focus.

Eighteen decisions that were identified in six or more of the interviews were extracted to form a decision 'hot list'. A sample of these decisions across the care pathways is given below:

- *Pre-operative*: are the symptoms due to gallstones or not? Should the patient be offered surgery or not?
- *Intra-operative*: open port insertion or Veress needle? Is an intra-operative cholangiogram needed or not?
- *Post-operative*: when to take drains out? When to discharge?

In addition, two distinct strategies for making these decisions were identified based on the surgeons' self-reports taken from the coded transcripts. The first was an intuitive strategy, described by participants as 'experience based', which was applied to decisions involving the assessment of a risk (e.g., decision whether the symptoms were due to gallstones or not; decision whether to operate or not). Such decisions were characterized by multiple features taken into account to balance risks and benefits, though how these were integrated into a decision could not be precisely articulated. Formal risk calculation tools were not used. The second, more rule-based strategy was associated with explicit criteria. For example, for the decision when to remove a drain post-operatively, surgeons often specified the absence of bile in the drain along with a volume criterion, the detail of which varied between individuals. Some technical aspects of the procedure (e.g., open port insertion or use of a Veress needle to create the pneumoperitoneum) were also subject to personal rules, again subject to individual variation.

(iv-ii) Experimental/modelling approach

A key limitation of self-report methodologies, such as knowledge elicitation as described above, is that participants may be unaware of some aspects of their own decision-making process (Nisbett and Wilson 1977). Thus, in addition to direct elicitation from experts, we also attempted in another study to model decision-making quantitatively, without resorting to the participants' own perceptions of their decision-making process.

We used Judgment Analysis (JA) to model surgeons' estimation of the risk of converting a laparoscopic (key-hole) cholecystectomy to open (Jacklin et al. 2008b, Sevdalis and Jacklin 2008).

Methods   Thirty junior surgeons (minimum six months' experience as trainee in general surgery after full registration as a doctor, or completion of the Royal College of Surgeons examination) participated in the study.

Participants were presented with 84 case vignettes – 64 design cases and 20 repeat cases to assess reliability. The clinical factors that were manipulated across vignettes were patient's biliary history, age/co-morbidity, previous surgery, obesity, sex and race (see Figure 21.1). In order to eliminate effects of the participants' position on the learning curve with respect to operative expertise, participants were instructed that the procedure would be carried out by Mr J, an experienced laparoscopic surgeon. Participants were asked to indicate the likelihood (0–100 percent) that, given the case presentation, the procedure would have to be converted from laparoscopic to open. One key feature of this study was the incorporation of an outcome-based 'gold standard' model against which each case could be scored. This provided an evidence-based estimate of the likelihood of conversion for each of the cases in the study, against which to assess participants' risk judgements.

We analysed the use of the available information (cues) across participants. We also analysed participants' reliability, accuracy and their use of the cues (i.e., cue beta weights in the regression models) with the gold standard model. Within the gold standard model, the biliary history, the patients' sex and previous abdominal surgery were the only variables that influenced the likelihood of conversion to open.

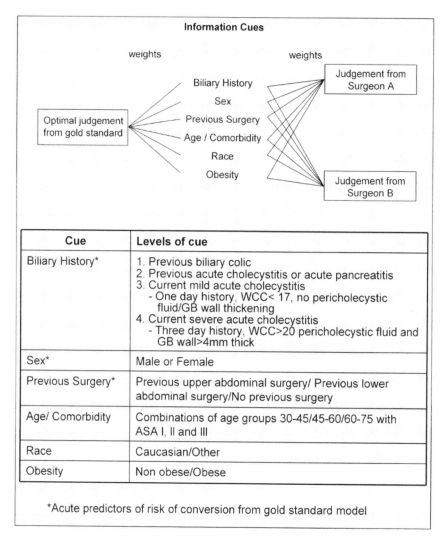

Figure 21.1   A model for the study, with the cues that were available to participating surgeons

Results   We observed significant variation across participants regarding the correlation of their estimates with the gold standard: we obtained a range of Pearson *r* correlation coefficients between 0.08 and 0.72 – with lower coefficients indicating lower agreement with the gold standard (i.e., lower accuracy). The average observed *r* was 0.48 (SD = 0.14). Similar variation was observed in the cue utilization across participants (see Figure 21.2).

Variability was obtained in model fit across individual participants as well. Obtained model fit ranged between $R^2_{adjusted}$ = 0.12 (poor fit) to $R^2_{adjusted}$ = 0.76

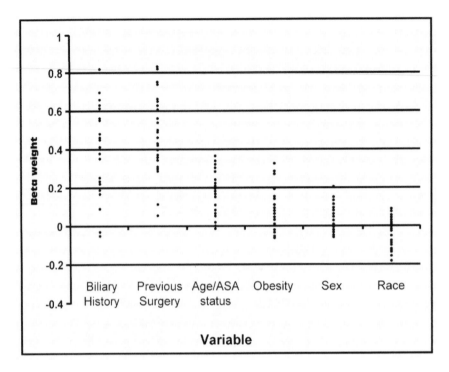

Figure 21.2   Cue utilization across individual surgeons

(very good fit), with mean $R^2_{adjusted}$ = 0.53. The data shows that judgement analysis methodology can be used to model of surgeons' risk judgements quantitatively, as well as to compare them with a gold standard model based on epidemiological data. Some participants were more consistent in their use of the cues, and, thereby, their responses were more amenable to modelling. The large variation in accuracy between individual surgeons was somewhat concerning clinically; for junior surgeons to be able to undertake tasks such as obtaining informed consent, from patients for procedures, there is a need for their understanding and estimation of surgical risks to improve.

(iv-iii) Simulation

In the past few years, simulation-based training has been used extensively for the honing of technical skill of surgical trainees (Aggarwal et al. 2004, Dankelman and DiLorenzo 2005, Fried and Feldman 2008). In commercial aviation (and other high risk industries), similar training modules have been developed for training pilots' non-technical and crisis-management skills (Helmreich et al. 1999, Klampfer et al. 2001).

We carried out two series of simulations, aiming to assess surgical teams' crisis management in a simulated operating theatre (Undre et al. 2007,

Koutantji et al. 2008). The simulated theatre is a fully equipped functional operating theatre separated from a control room by a one-way mirror and containing a standard operating table, operating lights, suction apparatus, anaesthetic machine and other equipment required for standard open or laparoscopic surgery, together with a moderate fidelity anaesthesia simulator mannequin (SimMan® Laerdal, UK). The mannequin is connected to a compressor and controlled by a computer from the control room, with software that enables the controller to create an anaesthesia crisis for training and feedback. We modified existing, standardized scales that assess non-technical skills in the context of commercial aviation, assessed their reliability, and used them to assess non-technical skills (including decision-making) in surgical crisis simulation.

Methods The first training series consisted of 20 half-day simulations, in which a full operating theatre team of trainees (surgeon, anaesthetist, scrub nurse and operating department practitioner (these practitioners are technicians trained to assist the anaesthetists performing tasks similar to those performed in some contexts by anaesthetic nurses)) completed a sapheno-femoral junction ligation procedure that involved a number of crises. For the surgeons, the crisis was bleeding halfway through the procedure, leading to cardiac arrest. The second series consisted of nine full-day simulations, very similarly formatted and carried out. The difference was a training module (on safety and crisis management) that the trainees underwent half way through the day – as a pilot intervention.

We used the NOn-TECHnical Skills (NOTECHS) observational tool. The NOTECHS was designed for use in the aviation industry to assess non-technical skills in cockpit crews – including decision-making, leadership skills, teamworking skills and situation awareness (Flin et al. 2003, van Avermaete and Kruijsen 1998). We revised the scale for use in surgical teams (Moorthy et al. 2005, Moorthy et al. 2006, Sevdalis et al. 2008). Here we focus on the assessment of surgical trainees' decision-making. The trainees were observed (via one-way mirror in the control room of the simulated operating theatre) and assessed in real time by expert trainers and at least one psychologist. Upon completion of the procedure, trainers and trainees completed a revised NOTECHS and received feedback on the training exercise.

Results Overall, the revised NOTECHS was found to be a reliable tool for the assessment of all non-technical skills in terms of internal consistency of the tool, and between participants and their trainers. Specifically for decision-making, we obtained a range of Cronbach α coefficients between 0.82 and 0.92.

Findings from the first series of simulations can be seen in Table 21.1. We did not observe significant differences between professional groups (surgeons, anaesthetists, scrub nurses and operating department practitioners) in relation to trainers' decision-making ratings. However, we did obtain significant differences across skills, with decision-making and leadership being rated significantly lower than the other skills ($F(4, 568) = 24.04$, $p < 0.001$). Finally, trainer surgeons'

Table 21.1   Non-technical skills in the first simulation series

Mean NOTECHS subscale rating (standard deviation)

	Communication	Vigilance	Teamworking	Leadership	Decision-making
Trainer	4.00 (0.97)	4.11 (1.17)	3.96 (1.15)	3.78 (1.01)	3.95 (1.10)
Trainee	3.69 (1.03)	3.67 (1.15)	3.76 (0.91)	3.73 (0.90)	3.74 (0.94)

ratings were not significantly different from trainee surgeons' self-ratings ($t(37) = 0.88, p > 0.05$), thus indicating agreement in the assessment of skill.

In the second series of simulations, decision-making was rated significantly lower than all other skills (all $ps < 0.05$). Moreover, there was a significant pre-post training improvement in the ratings of decision-making for the surgical trainees ($M_{Pre-training} = 2.51$ vs. $M_{Post-training} = 3.62$; $F(1, 15) = 6.59, p = 0.05$). Taken together, these studies suggest that simulation-based team training is feasible and has great potential as a training tool. From the decision-making perspective, simulations offer a unique environment, in which the skill can be observed and assessed 'in action' – in other words, in a dynamic, fluid, potentially stressful, but safe training environment.

(v) Concluding Remarks

Surgical decision-making is an important but under-researched field. The aim of the present chapter was to discuss the characteristics of surgical decision-making, highlight how some behavioural and naturalistic decision research approaches can be applied to surgery and, finally, present empirical work that has been carried out by our research team to date to assess decision-making processes and decision-making as a skill in surgery. We presented empirical applications of three different approaches to surgical decision-making – namely, knowledge elicitation from experts, experimentation and modelling using Judgement Analysis (JA), and, finally, simulation-based assessment of and training in decision-making (among other non-technical skills).

All approaches yielded promising findings. Knowledge elicitation resulted in the representation of the care pathway for patients presenting with symptomatic gallstone disease – both acute and non-acute. The approach was shown to be reliable. Its contribution is that it can be used to articulate key clinical decisions that need to be made in the process of care of such patients and, importantly, what are the cues (information or considerations) that feed into these decisions.

Experimentation and modelling using JA is a different approach, especially useful where cognitive processes that are not easy to articulate consciously are involved. In the presence of gold standard models of the type that we used in our study, JA can be used to assess surgeons' risk estimation and to provide individualized feedback regarding (in)appropriate cue utilization. Although accurate judgement of the likelihood of conversion of laparoscopic cholecystectomy to the open procedure is not a critical life-or-death issue, it is important in terms of informed consent. It may also be thought of as an 'exemplar judgement' – thus suggesting that findings from this study may be generalizable across other similar surgical risk judgements. Importantly, the technique does not rely on self-report.

Finally, simulation-based assessment allows the simultaneous assessment of decision-making and other skills, technical and non-technical. Simulation-based training that involves an entire operating theatre team recreates the working reality of the surgeon and can be used as a training environment for the whole surgical team. Existing observational tools, after appropriate revision, were shown to be reliable in the surgical context. Given the wide-spread use and face validity of surgical simulators, this approach can be used extensively both as a training tool, but also as a research environment. Currently, we are building on our initial experiences with each one of the three approaches presented here to expand the field of their application. We have used interviews to assess in detail surgeons' perceptions of the stressors that they face in the operating theatre (Arora et al. 2009, Wetzel et al. 2006). We found that technical issues (e.g., difficult anatomy; bleeding), malfunctioning/lack of availability of equipment, distractions/interruptions and poor teamwork/communication are the key stressors that surgeons have to cope with. We also found that surgeons recognize the impact of such stressors on their performance – including their intra-operative decision-making. Importantly, the interviews allowed us to capture a range of training needs that the surgeons articulated in relation to a stress management training module (Arora et al. 2009). We are now in the process of developing such a module, which will involve simulation-based team training. One of our key aims is to assess the impact of stress management training on intra-operative decision-making via observation (thus following up previous simulation-based assessment of decision-making and other non-technical skills).

We are also piloting the use of JA as a training tool. We recently used JA-derived feedback to improve accuracy and reliability of surgical risk estimation (Jacklin et al. 2009). Pre-feedback, we assessed accuracy and reliability of trainee surgeons' and medical students' estimates of operative mortality for major surgery using a number of patient vignettes with varying risk factors. Vignette construction was guided by a published risk model as a gold standard. Post-feedback, participants were retested on a second, equivalent case set. We found that feedback improved reliability of risk estimates in both groups and also accuracy in students' risk estimates: these estimates were significantly worse than those of the surgical group pre-feedback, but matched them in accuracy post-feedback. Accuracy of the surgeons' estimates did not improve (arguably, because of a ceiling effect). This is a novel application of JA, suggesting that the technique could be potentially useful for surgical training and assessment – at least in the field of risk estimation.

All approaches that we have used so far have limitations, both conceptual, but also practical. Over-reliance on self-report is an obvious limitation of knowledge elicitation/any interview-based technique. The usefulness of JA-type modelling will always be a function of the availability of robust epidemiological models to be used as gold standard comparisons, whilst the choice of modelling approach to be applied to the surgeons' judgements can be debated. Simulation is a rather expensive tool: it requires facilities and trained trainers. In addition, robust transfer of learning from simulated to real operating theatres remains to be empirically demonstrated.

These limitations, together with the variety of environments in which surgeons are required to make decisions and the range of potential applications of this line of research render a multimodal approach to surgical decision-making of paramount importance. First of all, surgical decision-making occurs in the operating theatre under time pressure and stress, but also in surgical wards and outpatient clinics, in which the surgeon has more opportunity to consider options and discuss them with the patient. Some of the decisions are grounded on highly technical knowledge and the required skill to execute them; others involve more reliance on patient's preferences; all of them require systematic use of the available evidence base. It is rather hard, if not impossible, to assume that all the approaches that we have described in this chapter are equally applicable to all decision situations.

Secondly, measuring surgeons' decision-making implies that it is feasible and conceptually sound to treat decision-making as an observable skill, in which surgeons can be trained. In turn, training involves demonstration of tangible improvement and also assessment (formative, summative, or both). Although some initial attempts can be found in the relevant literature (e.g., Sarker et al. 2009), these are still few and rather heavily knowledge-based – which suggests that their generalizability across decision-making situations remains to be demonstrated. Systematic, replicable empirical work across a variety of decision-making situations needs to be done in order to arrive at robust, valid tools to assess decision-making skill comprehensively. Such tools are not unlikely to consist of a range of different modules – thus representing the richness and variety of decisions that a modern surgeon is faced with. The multimodal approach that we propose here appears to be well suited to capture the various elements of real-life surgical decisions, thereby rendering surgical decision-making less of a 'black box' among other surgical skills.

Acknowledgements

The work that is reported in this chapter has been funded by a research fellowship of the Royal College of Surgeons of England (RJ), the Rosetrees Foundation (RJ), the Grand Lodge 250th Anniversary Fund (RJ), a research fellowship of the Economic and Social Research Council Centre for Economic Learning and Social Evolution (NS) and the British Academy (NS).

Authors' Note

Papers outlining methods of assessing surgical decision-making as described in this chapter were first presented at the 21st Society for Probability, Utility and Decision-Making (SPUDM) biennial research conference (Warsaw, 19–23 August, 2007) and at the 2nd Healthcare Systems, Ergonomics, and Patient Safety (HEPS) international conference (Strasbourg, 25–27 June, 2008). We would like to thank all our clinical and psychologist colleagues for their very useful feedback.

References

Aggarwal, R., Moorthy, K. and Darzi, A. (2004) Laparoscopic skills training and assessment. *British Journal of Surgery* 91, 1549–58.

Arora, S., Sevdalis, N., Nestel, D., Tierney, T., Woloshynowych, M. and Kneebone, R. (2009) Managing intra-operative stress: What do surgeons want from a crisis training programme? *American Journal of Surgery* 197, 537–43.

Calland J., Guerlain S., Adams R., et al. (2002) A systems approach to surgical safety. *Surgical Endoscopy* 16, 1005–14.

Canter, R. and Kelly, A. (2007) A new curriculum for surgical training within the United Kingdom: The first stages of implementation. *Journal of Surgical Education* 64, 20–6.

Chapman, G.B. and Sonnenberg, F.A. (2003) *Decision Making in Healthcare.* Cambridge: Cambridge University Press.

Clarke, M.G., Wilson, J.R.M., Kennedy, K.P. and MacDonald, R.P. (2007) Clinical judgment analysis of the parameters used by consultant urologists in the management of prostate cancer. *Journal of Urology* 178, 98–102.

Coiera, E. and Tombs, V. (1998) Communication behaviours in a hospital setting: An observational study. *British Medical Journal* 316, 673–6.

Cooksey, R.W. (1996a) *Judgment Analysis: Theory, Methods, and Applications.* San Diego, CA: Academic Press.

Cooksey, R.W. (1996b) The methodology of social judgement theory. *Thinking and Reasoning* 2, 141–73.

Dankelman, J. and Di Lorenzo, N. (2005) Surgical training and simulation. *Minimally Invasive Therapy and Allied Technologies* 14, 211–13.

Denig, P. and Haaijer-Ruskamp, F.M. (1994) 'Thinking aloud' as a method of analyzing the treatment decision of physicians. *European Journal of Public Health* 4, 55–9.

Ericsson, K.A. and Simon, H.A. (1984) *Protocol Analysis: Verbal Reports as Data.* Cambridge, MA: MIT Press.

Flin, R., Martin, L., Goeters, K.M., Hörmann, H.J., Amalberti, R., Valot, C., Nijhuis, H. (2003). Development of the NOTECHS (non-technical skills) system for assessing pilots' CRM skills. *Human Factors and Aerospace Safety* 3, 97–119.

Flin, R., Youngson, G. and Yule S. (2007) How do surgeons make intraoperative decisions? *Quality and Safety in Health Care* 16, 235–9.

Frank, J.R. (2005) *The CanMEDS 2005 Physician Competency Framework. Better Standards. Better Physicians. Better Care.* Ottawa: Royal College of Physicians and Surgeons of Canada.

Frank, J.R, Jabbour, M. and Tugwell P., et al. (1996) Skills for the new millennium: Report of the societal needs working group, CanMEDS 2000 Project. *Annals Royal College of Physicians and Surgeons of Canada* 29, 206–16.

Frank, J.R. and Langer, B. (2003) Collaboration, communication, management, and advocacy: Teaching surgeons new skills through the CanMEDS project. *World Journal of Surgery* 27, 972–8.

Fried, G.M. and Feldman, L.S. (2008) Objective assessment of technical performance. *World Journal of Surgery* 32, 156–60.

Harries, C. and Kostopoulou, O. (2005) Psychological approaches to measuring and modelling clinical decision-making. In A. Bowling and S. Ebrahim (eds) *Handbook of Health Research Methods: Investigation, Measurement and Analysis* (pp. 331–61). Maidenhead: Open University Press.

Healey, A.N. and Vincent, C.A. (2007) The systems of surgery. *Theoretical Issues in Ergonomic Science* 8, 429–43.

Healey, A.N., Sevdalis, N. and Vincent, C.A. (2006a) Measuring intra-operative interference from distraction and interruption observed in the operating theatre. *Ergonomics* 49, 589–604.

Healey, A.N., Undre, S. and Vincent, C.A. (2006b) Defining the technical skills of teamwork in surgery. *Quality and Safety in Health Care* 15, 231–4.

Helmreich, R.L., Merritt, A.C. and Wilhelm, J.A. (1999) The evolution of Crew Resource Management training in commercial aviation. *International Journal of Aviation Psychology, 9,* 19-32.

Hertzer, N.R. 2006. Current status of endovascular repair of infrarenal abdominal aortic aneurysms in the context of 50 years of conventional repair. *Ann N Y Acad Sci* 1085, 175–86.

Jacklin, R., Sevdalis, N., Darzi, A. and Vincent, C.A. (2008a) Mapping surgical practice decision making: An interview study to evaluate decisions in surgical care. *American Journal of Surgery* 195, 689–96.

Jacklin, R., Sevdalis, N., Harries, C., Darzi, A. and Vincent, C.A. (2008b) Judgment analysis: A method for quantitative evaluation of trainee surgeons' judgments of surgical risk. *American Journal of Surgery* 195, 193–8.

Jacklin, R., Sevdalis, N., Darzi, A. and Vincent, C.A. (2009) Efficacy of cognitive feedback in improving operative risk estimation. *American Journal of Surgery* 197, 76–81.

Kee, F., McDonald, P., Kirwan, .J.R. et al. (1998) Urgency and priority for cardiac surgery: A clinical judgment analysis. *British Medical Journal* 316, 925–9.

Klampfer, R., Flin, R., Helmreich, R.L., et al. (2001) *Enhancing Performance in High Risk Environments: Recommendations for the Use of Behavioural*

Markers. Report from the Behavioural Markers Workshop, Zurich, June. Berlin: Damler Benz Foundation.

Klein, G. (1998) *Sources of Power: How People Make Decisions*. London: MIT Press.

Klein, G., Orasanu, J., Calderwood, R. and Zsambok, C.E. (1993) *Decision Making in Action: Models and Methods*. Norwood, NJ: Ablex Publishing Corporation.

Koehler, D.J. and Harvey, N. (2004) *Blackwell Handbook of Judgment and Decision Making*. Oxford: Blackwell.

Koele, P. and Hoogstraten, J. (1999) Determinants of dentists' decisions to initiate dental implant treatment: A judgment analysis. *Journal of Prosthetic Dentistry* 81, 476–80.

Koutantji, M., McCulloch, P. and Undre, S., et al. (2008) Is team training in briefings for surgical teams feasible in simulation? *Cognition, Technology and Work* 10, 275–85

Leong, J.J., Nicolaou, M., Emery, R.J., Darzi, A. and Yang, G.Z. (2007) Visual search behaviour in skeletal radiographs: A cross-specialty study. *Clinical Radiology* 62, 1069–77.

Lipshitz, R., Klein, G., Orasanu, J. and Salas, E. (2001) Taking stock of naturalistic decision making. *Journal of Behavioral Decision Making* 14, 331–52.

MacCormick, A.D. and Parry, B.R. (2006) Judgment analysis of surgeons' prioritization of patients for elective general surgery. *Medical Decision Making* 26, 255–64.

Moorthy, K., Munz, Y. and Adams S. et al. (2005) A human factors analysis of technical and team skills among surgical trainees during procedural simulations in a Simulated Operating Theatre (SOT). *Annals of Surgery* 242, 631–9.

Moorthy, K., Munz, Y., Forrest, D., Pandey, V., Undre, S., Vincent, C. and Darzi, A. (2006) Surgical crisis management skills training and assessment. *Annals of Surgery* 244, 139–47.

Nisbett, R.E. and Wilson, T.D. (1997) Telling more than we can know: Verbal reports on mental processes. *Psychological Review* 84, 231–57.

Pfister, M., Jakob, S., Frey, F.J., Niederer, U., Schmidt, M. and Marti, H.P. (1999) Judgment analysis in clinical nephrology. *American Journal of Kidney Diseases* 34, 569–75.

Sarker, S., Chang, A., Albrani, T. and Vincent, C.A. (2008) Constructing hierarchical task analysis in surgery. *Surgical Endoscopy* 22, 107–11.

Sarker, S., Rehman, S., Ladwa, M., Chang, A. and Vincent, C.A. (2009) A decision-making learning and assessment tool in laparoscopic cholecystectomy. *Surgical Endoscopy* 23(1), 197–203.

Sevdalis, N. and McCulloch, P. (2006) Teaching evidence-based decision-making. *Surgical Clinics of North America* 86, 59–70.

Sevdalis, N. and Jacklin, R. (2008) Opening the 'black box' of surgeons' risk estimation: From intuition to quantitative modeling. *World Journal of Surgery* 32, 324–5.

Sevdalis, N., Davis, R,. Koutantji, M., Undre, S., Darzi, A. and Vincent, C.A. (2008) Reliability of a revised NOTECHS scale for use in surgical teams. *American Journal of Surgery* 196, 184–90.

Undre, S., Koutantji, M., Sevdalis, N., et al. (2007) Multi-disciplinary crisis simulations: The way forward for training surgical teams. *World Journal of Surgery* 31, 1843–53.

van Avermaete J.A.G. and Kruijsen E. (1998) *The Evaluation of Non-technical Skills of Multi-pilot Aircrew in Relation to the JAR-FCL Requirements* (project rep. CR-98443). Amsterdam: NLR, Amsterdam.

Vincent, C., Moorthy, K., Sarker, S.K., Chang, A. and Darzi, A. (2004) Systems approaches to surgical quality and safety: from concept to measurement. *Annals of Surgery* 239, 475–82.

Wetzel, C., Kneebone, R., Woloshynowych, M., Nestel, D., Moorthy, K., Kidd, K. and Darzi, A. (2006) The effects of stress on surgical performance. *American Journal of Surgery* 191, 5–10.

Yule, S., Flin, R., Paterson-Brown, S. and Maran, N. (2006) Non-technical skills for surgeons. A review of the literature. *Surgery* 139, 140–9.

Chapter 22

Simulator-Based Evaluation of Clinical Guidelines in Acute Medicine

Christoph Eich, Michael Müller, Andrea Nickut and Arnd Timmermann

Clinical Background

Guidelines in Acute Medicine

Guidelines and related algorithms play a major role in acute medicine, in particular for the handling of time critical and high-risk situations in anaesthesiology, emergency and critical care medicine. Well-known examples are the guidelines on cardiopulmonary resuscitation (ASA 2006, Biarent et al. 2005, 2006). Furthermore, numerous national and local guidelines exist on time-critical procedures and interventions, for example, on rapid-sequence induction (RSI) of anaesthesia in children (Schmidt et al. 2007). The new technique (RSI controlled) makes the potentially hazardous procedure of anaesthesia induction in a non-fasted infant less time critical. It is thought to produce less stress and fewer unsafe actions and critical incidents and hence may be safer for the child.

Characteristically, guidelines are based on a thoroughly performed consensus process on best scientific evidence, paired with expert knowledge and experience. Though guidelines aim to combine this with clinical feasibility, infrastructural conditions and educational aspects, evidence of their actual clinical superiority, and in particular of their whole entirety, is limited (Morley and Zaritsky 2005, Nolan 2005). A valid clinical evaluation frequently collides with ethical considerations, particularly when children are involved. Hence, a high proportion of guidelines in acute medicine may be evaluated by clinical observation, retrospective epidemiological analysis and expert appraisal only. The question is whether a high-fidelity simulator in an authentic clinical environment would be able to decrease this knowledge gap.

Stress and Safety

Stress is defined as a set of adaptive reactions of an individual undergoing aggression, stimulation, or effort. These stimuli provoke an increase in sympathetic activity that causes a raise of heart and respiratory rate, arterial blood pressure, and metabolic processes (Vrijkotte et al. 2000). Hence stress can generally be quantified by measuring cardiorespiratory and metabolic parameters.

Physical and mental stress in operating room team members are both thought to have negative impact on patient safety as high stress levels are likely to be related with unsafe actions and critical events (Lazarus et al. 1952, Gaba and Howard 2002, Howard et al. 2003, Moorthy et al. 2003, Metz 2007). As a consequence, clinical guidelines in acute medicine aim to reduce stress to increase patient safety. On the other hand, optimum stress levels which allow best individual performance are subject to interpersonal variations within a wide range (Metz 2007, Nater et al. 2007a). As there seems to be no direct or even linear correlation between stress levels and safety such as unsafe actions and critical incidents, stress measurement alone would have only limited analytical power for the evaluation of clinical guidelines. In order to get more valid answers, we combine objective stress measurement with observational criteria and self-assessment (perception).

The Model

High fidelity infant simulators have only been commercially available for a few years. There now exists a sizable body of experience with their use for training and assessment purposes (Gaba et al. 1998, Howard et al. 2003, Eppich et al. 2006, Eich et al. 2007b, Overly et al. 2007). In our view, and according to our experience, they should also be suitable for the evaluation of guidelines in acute medicine when placed in sufficiently realistic clinical environments.

Our research group at the medical simulation centres of Göttingen and Dresden aims to establish a model for simulator-based evaluation of clinical guidelines in order to decrease the evidence gap prior to their implementation. As a first pilot study of practical application, we compare a newly recommended controlled rapid-sequence-induction technique (RSI controlled) for non-fasted infants with the classic technique (RSI classic) using a high fidelity infant simulator (Eich et al. 2007a, Schmidt et al. 2007). Using an observational checklist we record critical events and unsafe actions. We simultaneously measure psycho-vegetative stress, based on ergospirometry (cardiorespiratory markers), saliva analyses (cortisol and alpha-amylase) and self-assessment (stress and safety perception).

The Infant Simulator and its Environment

For our current pilot study on RSI guidelines for infants, we work with a SimBaby™ infant simulator (Laerdal Medical), using software version 1.4 and its customary touch screen vital signs monitor. The baby mannequin is placed on an operating table in an authentic theatre environment within our simulation centre (see Figure 22.1).

SimBaby™ is a high fidelity integrated infant simulator which features all essential clinical and monitored vital signs. It is controlled via computer interface. It has no physiologic model implemented but scenarios and trends can be pre-programmed. For our RSI study, we programmed a standardized scenario on

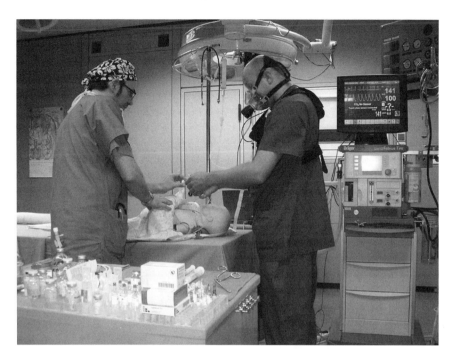

Figure 22.1   Study setting in theatres: infant simulator and anaesthesia work station, anaesthesia nurse (left) and candidate (right) with the mobile ergospirometry unit applied

anaesthesia induction in a four-week-old baby boy with pyloric stenosis. Initial respiratory rate, oxygen saturation, heart rate, blood pressure torso movement and vital signs monitor set-up were defined. Additionally we programmed three trends for respiratory rate, heart rate and oxygen saturation: 'RSI classic', 'RSI controlled' and 'recovery from hypoxemia' (oxygen desaturation). All trends are started manually on induction of anaesthesia or on appropriate ventilation respectively. The trends for oxygen saturation after breathing stops (apnoea) are based on oxygenation data derived from the Nottingham physiology simulator, as calculated for a one-month-old infant with no effective pre-oxygenation and open airway (Hardman and Wills 2006).

The Scenario

The techniques for RSI are standardized (see Figure 22.2).

The same anaesthesia nurse assists all procedures in an identical manner strictly following the protocol. The induction drugs are drawn up in the predetermined dose and are administered by the anesthesia nurse when prompted by the candidate. The nurse also provides exact timing to allow the first intubation attempt. In combination with programmed scenario and trends, this procedure ensures that all candidates are

Time [min]		
-10	1st saliva sample (pre-stress value)	
	Start of ergospirometry	
	5 min rest	
	Briefing of scenario	
0	Start of scenario	
	Pre-oxygenation	
	RSI classic	RSI controlled
+10	2nd saliva sample (first stress value)	
	3 min rest	
	End of ergospirometry	
+20	3rd saliva sample (second stress value)	
	4th saliva sample (post-stress value)	
+40	Questionnaire	
	End of trial	

Figure 22.2   Flow chart for simulated scenario and stress measurement

exposed to highly standardized conditions. However, if complications occur, the candidates are entitled to leave the algorithms for RSI classic and RSI controlled and act as they would do in clinical reality.

Observation of Unsafe Actions and Critical Events

The observation of unsafe actions and critical events is well established for human factor research using simulator environments (Gaba 1992, Gaba and Howard 2002, Howard et al. 2003, Overly et al. 2007). In this study we aim to evaluate a clinical guideline, applied to paediatric simulation; we are venturing into virtually unexplored territory. We record unsafe actions and critical events using a checklist.

These are defined as follows: oxygen saturation (SpO_2) < 90 percent, heart rate < 80 beats per min, forced mask ventilation with airway pressure (P_{AW}) > 20 cm H_2O, esophageal or endobronchial intubation, and more than one intubation attempt.

Stress Measurement

Our model comprises stress measurement by continuous ergospirometry, analyses of cortisol and alpha-amylase in saliva and a brief post-stress questionnaire.

Ergospirometry

We measure cardiorespiratory stress by ergospirometry, using a Cortex Metamax 3 B™ (Cortex Biophysik) (see Figures 22.3 and 22.4). This portable ergospirometry device with face mask comes combined with a Polar T 41™ (Polar Electro) heart rate meter. The following parameters are collected: respiratory rate (RR), minute volume (MV), oxygen consumption (VO2), carbon dioxide production (VCO2) and heart rate (HR). VO2 measurement is performed at STPD-conditions (Standard Temperature, Pressure, Dry).

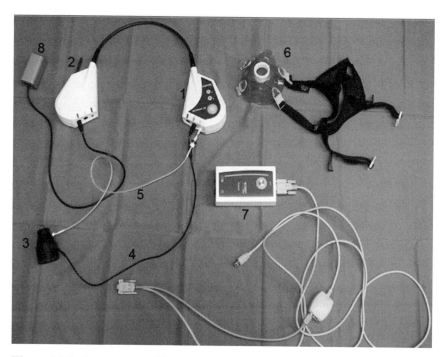

Figure 22.3   MetaMax 3B™

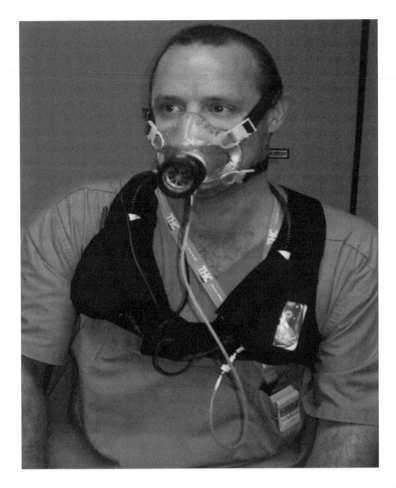

Figure 22.4 Candidate with mobile and wireless ergospirometry device attached

The portability of the ergospirometry device enables measurement of cardiorespiratory strain or stress under realistic working conditions with only minimal discomfort due to face mask, tubing and device. It allows virtually full range of motion for the candidate.

Cortex Metamax 3B™ uses a breath-by-breath technique. During ergospirometry, the candidate wears a breathing mask strapped to his face, breathing through a turbine-equipped volume sensor with a range of 0.05 to 20 l/sec, a sensitivity of 7 ml, and a precision of 2 percent. The oxygen analyser contains an electrochemical cell, allowing a measurement range from 0 to 35 percent. The infrared carbon dioxide sensor measures values from 0 to 13 percent (accuracy 0.1 Vol. percent). Both sensors have a measurement kinetic of 100 ms.

Ergospirometry data are wirelessly transmitted via telemetry with a maximum range of 1000 m. All parameters are continuously visualized and recorded with Windows™-based software (MetaSoft 3.3™, Cortex Biophysik) which allows for processing of the ergospirometry data and which is also compatible with other data-processing software such as Windows Excel™.

Before each trial (scenario), one-point calibration is performed before the ergospirometry device is attached to the candidates. They are then asked to sit in a comfortable arm chair in a shaded room for five minutes to relax, to get used to the face mask and to reach their individual cardiorespiratory baseline values on rest. This procedure is repeated after the scenario. The candidates are further advised to talk as little as possible in order to minimize any potential impact on spirometry. This requirement is quite easy to meet as both RSI procedures are highly standardized.

After this tuning phase, the candidate is informed about the scenario and the anaesthesia induction technique to be performed (RSI classic or RSI controlled). Then the scenario starts. Finally ergospirometry and recording are discontinued after the five-minute rest after the scenario.

Analysis of Cortisol and Alpha-amylase in Saliva

The second column of stress measurement consists of analyses of cortisol and alpha-amylase in saliva. These have been proved to be valid and reliable markers of adrenergic stress response in previous studies (Nater et al. 2006, Müller 2007, Yamaguchi et al. 2006).

Cortisol   Physical and mental stress is a stimulus for increased cortisol secretion. Cortisol levels can be determined either in serum, plasma or saliva, the latter reflecting its biologically effective fraction (Kirschbaum and Hellhammer 1994). Highest concentrations in saliva are seen approximately 20 minutes after the beginning of exposure to stress (Kirschbaum et al. 1995b) (see Figure 22.5).

In addition, cortisol follows a circadian rhythm with highest concentrations in the morning and lowest in the afternoon (Table 22.1). Hence we execute all trials in the afternoon between 2 and 6 pm.

Gender also has an impact on cortisol levels. During the follicle phase of the female cycle, cortisol values become significantly lower (Kirschbaum et al. 1995a). To rule out any impact of the female cycle on cortisol levels, we restricted the study to male candidates only. Furthermore, chronic nicotine consumption (e.g., inhalation of cigarette smoke) increases basal cortisol levels but diminishes stress response values whereas age does not have an influence on cortisol secretion (Kirschbaum and Hellhammer 1994).

Alpha-amylase   Apart from olfactory and gustatory trigger vegetative (ß2-adrenergic) stimuli provide the main pathway of secretion of alpha-amylase during acute stress response (Chatterton et al. 1996, Nater et al. 2006). This

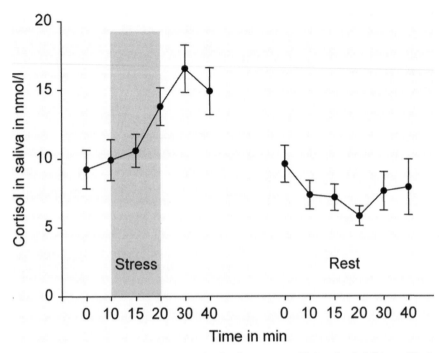

Figure 22.5 **Salivary cortisol levels during stress (Trier Social Stress Test, TSST) and rest conditions (Nater et al. 2006)**

Table 22.1 Reference intervals for plasma and salivary cortisol

	Reference intervals
Plasma	
a.m.	62- 195 µg/L (171- 536 nmol/L)
p.m.	23- 119 µg/L (64- 327 nmol/L)
Saliva	
a.m.	0,7- 6,9 µg/L (1,90- 19,1 nmol/L)
p.m.	0,7- 4,3 µg/L (2,05- 11,9 nmol/L)

Source: Methods Sheet Cortisol, version 10, Roche Diagnostics (2005)

relation has been validated with volunteers undergoing the Trier Social Stress Test (TSST). This study showed that stress induced increase of salivary alpha-amylase was related to heart rate, blood pressure and plasma-noradrenaline levels (Rohleder et al. 2004, Nater et al. 2006). Furthermore, van Stegeren et al. (2006) could demonstrate that secretion of salivary alpha-amylase is suppressed by non-selective beta-blocker propanolol. However, it remains unknown whether salivary alpha-amylase directly reflects noradrenaline release and would hence allow the replacement of the invasive measurement of plasma noradrenaline.

Peaks of salivary alpha-amylase are measured approximately 10 to 20 minutes after beginning of stress input and returns rapidly to baseline values (Nater and Rohleder 2005) (Figure 22.6).

Lowest salivary concentrations of alpha-amylase are found in the morning immediately after getting up and highest in the evening (Nater et al. 2007b). There are no well-defined reference intervals for salivary alpha-amylase but as we are interested in changes from baseline values only, this should not affect measurements and data interpretation. Salivary flow rate does not have an impact on alpha-amylase concentration in saliva and hence need not be calculated when cotton-wool Salivettes™ are used (Rohleder et al. 2006). In summary, salivary cortisol and alpha-amylase are valid and reliable parameters to determine adrenergic stress response. Saliva analyses are non-invasive and relatively easy to perform which make them popular for proband studies. However, their slow kinetics do not allow to measure rapid changes but rather peak levels of stress.

Saliva Sampling   The candidates are advised not to eat, drink or smoke two hours before beginning of the study. For each trial (simulated scenario), we obtain four saliva samples: –10, +10, +20 and +40 minutes from the beginning of the scenario,

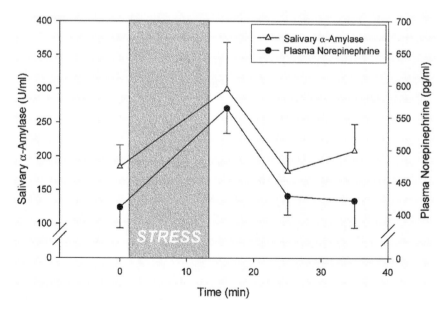

Figure 22.6   Salivary alpha-amylase and norepinephrine (noradrenaline) in response to stress (Trier Social Stress Test, TSST) (Rohleder et al. 2004)

representing pre-stress, stress (two samples), and post-stress conditions (Figure 22.2). As cortisol and alpha-amylase have slightly different peak times we obtain two samples at 10 and 20 minutes.

To gain saliva samples, the candidates have to rinse their mouth with water twice before they chew on a cotton roll (Salivette™, Sarstedt) for two minutes. The loaded Salivettes™ are centrifuged at 3000 rpm for five minutes and then immediately cooled to 5°C. All analyses are performed within 24 hours of collection at the Department for Clinical Chemistry at University Medical Centre Göttingen. According to previous studies, centrifuged salivary cortisol and alpha-amylase samples are stable at 5–8°C for up to five days (Kirschbaum and Hellhammer 1994, Nater forthcoming). Alpha-amylase in saliva is analysed with a Cobas Integra 800™ kit (Roche Diagnostics) which is based on an enzymatic extinction test. Salivary cortisol is determined with an immunoassay using a Cobas Modular Analytics E 170™ system (Roche Diagnostics).

Post-stress Questionnaire   Most simulator-based studies include some kind of self-assessment. Though much debated for its scientific validity, this methodology may help to identify individually perceived attitudes and behaviour (Gaba et al. 1998, Howard et al. 2003). In our study we compare perceived stress and safety levels with objectively measured values. After having obtained the fourth saliva sample, all candidates are asked to fill in a brief post-stress questionnaire which consists of two ratings and one open question: 'How was your perceived subjective stress level (scale 1–10)? How safe did you feel with the used RSI technique (1–10)? Which unsafe actions or critical events did you notice during the scenario?'

Statistical Analysis   All data from demography, observation, ergospirometry, saliva analyses and self-assessment are put into purpose-designed data templates (Excel™). All nine stress values obtained from ergospirometry, saliva analyses and self-assessment, such as respiratory rate, respiratory minute volume, oxygen consumption, carbon dioxide production, heart rate, salivary cortisol and alpha-amylase, stress and safety perception) are defined as dependent variables (DV). These DV will be tested for their dependence on method (RSI technique), professional experience (years in anaesthesiology) and interaction of both. We also aim to correlate stress (measurements and self-perception) with unsafe actions and critical incidents (observation) as well as the three methods of stress measurement (ergospirometry, salivary analyses and perception) with each other. Statistical analyses will be performed with SPSS Version 14. P-values lower than 0.05 will be regarded as significant.

Preliminary Results

At time of writing, our pilot study has just started. So far the key features of the model work reliably, including function of the infant simulator with its standardized scenario and trends, observation of unsafe actions and critical incidents, mobile ergospirometry, saliva analyses and self-assessment (questionnaire). Marked physical and mental stress has been induced hitherto in all candidates in the course of the scenarios, indicating an adequate level of suspension of disbelief. This is regarded to be an essential pre-requisite of simulator-based training, assessment and research. So far the scenarios have lasted about four to seven minutes. The main increase in respiratory rate, respiratory minute volume, oxygen consumption, carbon dioxide production and heart rate occur towards intubation of the infant mannequin. Salivary cortisol and alpha-amylase peaks are detected at 10 or 20 minutes and return towards baseline at 40 minutes after start of the scenario.

Summary

Our model of a simulator-based evaluation of clinical guidelines is methodologically feasible, using a combination of observation, stress measurement (ergospirometry and salivary cortisol and alpha-amylase) and self-assessment. Our preliminary data suggest that this evaluation method could endorse future developments of guidelines in acute medicine in order to produce less stress, less unsafe actions and critical incidents, and subsequently increase patient safety.

References

AHA (2006) American Heart Association guidelines for cardiopulmonary resuscitation (CPR) and emergency cardiovascular care (ECC) of pediatric and neonatal patients: Pediatric advanced life support. *Pediatrics* 117(5), e1005–28.

Biarent D., Bingham, R., Richmond, S., Maconochie, I. Wyllie, J., Simpson, S., Nunez, A.R. and Zideman, D. (2005) European Resuscitation Council guidelines for resuscitation. Section 6. Paediatric life support. *Resuscitation* 67, Suppl 1, S97–133.

Chatterton, R.T., Vogelsong, K.M., Lu, Y.C., Ellman, A.B. and Hudgens, G.A. (1996) Salivary alpha-amylase as a measure of endogenous adrenergic activity. *Clinical Physiology* 16(4), 433–48.

Eich, C., Timmermann, A., Russo, S.G., Wagner-Berger, H. (2007a) Simulator-based evaluation of clinical guidelines exemplary of a modified rapid-sequence-induction (RSI) technique for infants as compared to the classic technique. *Simulation in Healthcare* 2(3), 205.

Eich C., Timmermann A., Russo, S.G., Nickel E.A., McFadzean, J., Rowney, D. and Schwarz, S.K. (2007b) Simulator-based training in paediatric anaesthesia and emergency medicine – thrills, skills and attitudes. *British Journal of Anaesthesia* 98(4), 417–19.

Eppich, W.J., Adler, M.D., McGaghie, W.C. (2006) Emergency and critical care pediatrics: Use of medical simulation for training in acute pediatric emergencies. *Current Opinion in Pediatrics* 18(3), 266–71.

Gaba, D.M. (1992) Improving anesthesiologists' performance by simulating reality. *Anesthesiology* 76(4), 491–4.

Gaba, D. and Howard, S. (2002) Patient safety: Fatigue among clinicians and the safety of patients. *New England Journal of Medicine* 347(16), 1249–55.

Gaba, D. Howard, S., Flanagan, B., Smith, B.E., Fish, K.J. and Botney, R. (1998) Assessment of clinical performance during simulated crises using both technical and behavioral ratings. *Anesthesiology* 89(1), 8–18.

Hardman, J. and Wills, J. (2006) The development of hypoxaemia during apnoea in children: A computational modelling investigation. *British Journal of Anaesthesia* 97(4), 564–70.

Howard, S.K., Gaba, D.M., Smith, B.E., Weinger, M.B., Herndon, C., Keshavacharya, S. and Rosekind, M.R. (2003) Simulation study of rested versus sleep-deprived anesthesiologists. *Anesthesiology* 98(6), 1345–55, discussion 5A.

Kirschbaum, C. and Hellhammer, D. (1994) Salivary cortisol in psychoneuroendocrine research: Recent developments and applications. *Psychoneuroendocrinology* 19(4), 313–33.

Kirschbaum, C., Pirke, K.M., Hellhammer, D.H. (1995a) Preliminary evidence for reduced cortisol responsivity to psychological stress in women using oral contraceptive medication. *Psychoneuroendocrinology* 20(5), 509–14.

Kirschbaum, C., Prussner, J., Stone, A.A., Federenko, I., Gaab, J., Lintz, D., Schommer, N. and Hellhammer, D.H. (1995b) Persistent high cortisol responses to repeated psychological stress in a subpopulation of healthy men. *Psychosomatic Medicine* 57(5), 468–74.

Lazarus, R., Deese, J. and Osler, S.F. (1952) The effects of psychological stress upon performance. *Psychological Bulletin* 49, 293–317.

Metz, G.A. (2007) Stress as a modulator of motor system function and pathology. *Reviews in the Neurosciences* 18(3–4), 209–22.

Moorthy, K., Munz, Y., Dosis, A., Bann, S. and Darzi, A. (2003) The effect of stress-inducing conditions on the performance of a laparoscopic task. *Surgical Endoscopy* 17(9), 1481–4.

Morley, P. and Zaritsky, A. (2005) The evidence evaluation process for the 2005 International Consensus Conference on cardiopulmonary resuscitation and emergency cardiovascular care science with treatment recommendations. *Resuscitation* 67, 167–70.

Müller, M.P., Fichtner, A., Hardt, F., Hänsel, M., Weber, S., Kirschbaum, C., Eich, C. and Koch, T. (2008) Effects of simulator training on salivary amylase and cortisol levels in intensivists: A pilot study. *Simulation in Healthcare* 3, 86.

Nater, U.K. (forthcoming) Salivary Alpha-Amylase as a marker for stress. *Psychoneuroendocrinology Research Frontiers.*

Nater, U. and Rohleder, N. (2005) Human salivary alpha-amylase reactivity in a psychosocial stress paradigm. *International Journal of Psychophysiology* 55(3), 333–42.

Nater, U., La Marca, R., Florin, L., Moses, A., Langhans, W., Koller, M.M. and Ehlert, U. (2006) Stress-induced changes in human salivary alpha-amylase activity – associations with adrenergic activity. *Psychoneuroendocrinology* 31(1), 49–58.

Nater, U., Moor, C., Okere, U., Stallkamp, R., Martin, M., Ehlert, U. and Kliegel, M. (2007a) Performance on a declarative memory task is better in high than low cortisol responders to psychosocial stress. *Psychoneuroendocrinology* 32(6), 758–63.

Nater, U., Rohleder, N., Schlotz, W., Ehlert, U. and Kirschbaum, C. (2007b) Determinants of the diurnal course of salivary alpha-amylase. *Psychoneuroendocrinology* 32(4), 392–401.

Nolan, J. (2005) European Resuscitation Council guidelines for resuscitation 2005. Section 1. Introduction. *Resuscitation* 67 Suppl 1, S3–6.

Overly, F.L., Sudikoff, S.N. and Shapiro, M.J. (2007) High-fidelity medical simulation as an assessment tool for pediatric residents' airway management skills. *Pediatric Emergency Care* 23(1), 11–15.

Roche Diagnostics (2005) Cortisol. *Methodenblatt* V 10.

Rohleder, N., Nater, M., Wolf, J.M., Ehlert, U. and Kirschbaum, C. (2004) Psychosocial stress-induced activation of salivary alpha-amylase: An indicator of sympathetic activity? *Annals of the New York Academy of Sciences* 1032, 258–63.

Rohleder, N., Wolf, M., Maldonado, E.F. and Kirschbaum, C. (2006) The psychosocial stress-induced increase in salivary alpha-amylase is independent of saliva flow rate. *Psychophysiology* 43(6), 645–52.

Schmidt, J., Strauss, J.K.B, Giest, J. and Schmitz, B. (2007) Recommendation for rapid-sequence induction in children. *Anaesth Intensiv Med* 48, S88–93.

van Stegeren, A., Rohleder, N. et al. (2006) Salivary alpha amylase as marker for adrenergic activity during stress: Effect of betablockade. *Psychoneuroendocrinology* 31(1), 137–41.

Vrijkotte, T.G., van Doornen, L.J. and de Geus, E.J. (2000) Effects of work stress on ambulatory blood pressure heart rate and heart rate variability. *Hypertension* 35(4), 880–6.

Yamaguchi, M., Takeda, K., Onishi, M., Deguchi, M. and Higashi, T. (2006) Non-verbal communication method based on a biochemical marker for people with severe motor and intellectual disabilities. *Journal of International Medical Research* 34(1), 30–41.

Chapter 23

Measuring the Impact of Time Pressure on Team Task Performance

Colin F. Mackenzie, Shelly A. Jeffcott and Yan Xiao

Introduction and Background

Surgery often contains crisis-like moments, even for scheduled, elective procedures. Understanding team performance under time pressure provides a basis for developing counter-measures. However, prospective investigation to study team performance under stress is difficult, due to the unpredictable nature of crisis events. Time pressure is a hallmark of trauma care where breakdowns in coordination can result in errors which threaten the life of a patient and where decisions are frequently made with high levels of uncertainty (Xiao et al. 1998).

Trauma care thus provides a window for us to examine team performance under time stress. Under time pressure, problems with errors of commission and omission are particularly apparent when potentially life-saving decisions and actions must be carried out dynamically within a few critical minutes. For example, cognitive errors during emergency care were found to be a significant contributor to patient harm. Factors limiting the clinicians ability to make timely and correct diagnoses include multiple, concurrent tasks; uncertainty; changing plans; compressed work procedures; large workload and complexity (Xiao et al. 1996).

In comparison to teams in other domains, surgical teams are often ad hoc in nature for a number of reasons: in teaching hospitals, trainees rotate monthly through different services; trainee staff may even come from other institutions to gain experience; requirements for specialty services vary from patient to patient; nursing and anaesthesia care providers may have different staffing patterns than their surgical colleagues. Under time stress, teams may have to split to take care of multiple patients simultaneously. Such changing team composition adds to the challenge of providing optimal team performance under stress, because team members may have never worked together before. In addition, surgical teams usually do not have formal training in coordination.

Richer understanding of team performance under time pressure can benefit patient safety by assisting in team training development and can boost individual and team competencies in non-technical aspects of care, such as task prioritization, leadership and decision-making. The nature of anaesthesiology care for trauma patients makes it a rich test bed for team performance measurement since within the resuscitation and operating room environment, activities and decision-making must be coordinated between anaesthesia, surgery and nursing professionals, who all have their own group cultures and team dynamics.

Team performance depends on the ability to coordinate members' capabilities and efforts. Special skills are needed to synchronize individual members' activities especially when up to one third of the trauma centre deaths are reported as preventable and many can be attributed to non-optimal communication and coordination (Fitzgerald et al. 2006). Several strategies are available to coordinate teamwork, increase compliance with 'best practices' and improve patient outcomes including using established work procedures or standardized algorithmic approaches to assist decision-making and reduce errors. For instance, the protocol of airway, breathing and circulation (i.e., 'ABCs'), used in resuscitating cardiac-arrest patients, specifies goal and action priorities for resuscitation personnel (American College of Surgeons 1997, Mackenzie and Lippert 1999).

In emergency medical care (as in other medical settings) extensive on-the-job training and experience provide personnel with the ability to anticipate the needs of others and what they will do next without explicit (i.e., verbal or gestural) communication. Team members share the same workspace and event space (i.e., what is happening) and have continuous visual and auditory contact with one another. As a result, they can sense what others are doing or intend to do. A 'wait-and-see' strategy, for example, can be used in avoiding potential conflicts among several people who have access to the patient and equipment (Xiao et al. 1998); however, task complexity in emergency medical care can reduce the effectiveness of coordination strategies (Xiao et al. 1996).

This chapter examines the impact of time pressure on trauma resuscitation team performance, by using tracheal intubation as a model to contrast task performance at two levels of task urgency, emergency and elective interventions, depending on the clinical circumstances. The task of tracheal intubation is very relevant to understanding anaesthesia activities during surgery, as it is a task carried out after induction of anaesthesia in the operating room. Tracheal intubation includes rendering unconsciousness (using anaesthetic and paralysing drugs if the patient is awake or semi-conscious) to stop breathing efforts or patient resistance and allow placement of an endo-tracheal tube through the mouth and between the vocal cords. The 'airway management' achieved by tracheal intubation is a life-saving intervention when executed correctly in an emergency. However, it requires significant technical skill and has risks (vomiting and aspiration, detrimental changes in vital signs including cardiac arrest) that may even significantly outweigh the potential benefits of improved oxygenation and ventilation. The complications associated with task accomplishment may, themselves, become more life threatening than the problem that the intervention was intended to remedy. Several methods were considered to collect data to examine the impact of time pressure on tracheal intubation.

Methodological Consideration of Studying Team Performance under Time-Pressure

Direct observation is a valuable method for collecting information pertaining to team- and task-work performance when under time pressure. The structure and culture of healthcare organizations can act as a barrier to direct observation studies of task and team performance. However, provided free access, confidentiality and consent issues are resolved, observation can identify the individual, team and organizational precursors to breakdowns in team communication and coordination that might be expected when a task is carried out under time pressure (Carthey 2002). Understanding the relationships between the processes of care, including environmental and interpersonal interactions and outcomes, is thus essential to developing a complete understanding of how task accomplishment is influenced by time pressure. Research which adopts direct observation methods can be most useful, for example, for identifying recurrent and interrelated factors in communication during care delivery (Lingard et al. 2002, Shapiro et al. 2004).

To adequately synthesize and collect data by observation, the observer should understand the care providers and team psychological support and cultural norms. The observer must also have knowledge about what is uncertain about the shared plan of action and why certain tasks take preference or need completion expeditiously. Difficulty in understanding the situation in which trauma care specialists work is exacerbated by these intimate details that are often only gathered by being an experienced member of the team (Leonard et al. 2004).

Christian et al. (2006) used observation to identify major systems features influencing operating room team performance and carried out a quantitative analysis of factors linked to team performance and patient safety. Communication breakdowns, workload and competing tasks had a measurable negative impact on team performance. Observation of two different surgeries concluded that in both instances the results supported the concept that interventions designed to improve teamwork and communication may have beneficial effects on surgical technical performance and patient outcome (Catchpole et al. 2008).

Direct observation to measure aspects of surgical team performance has been carried out at a number of different levels of analysis. An example of a highly specific observation of an individual's team skills, excluding the performance of other team members is called Observational Teamwork Assessment for Surgery (OTAS) (Undre et al. 2007, Healey et al. 2005). Undre and colleagues developed OTAS to simultaneously assess specific tasks among environment, equipment, provisions and communications by one observer. A second observer rates clinical behaviours against five established components of teamwork: (1) cooperation; (2) leadership; (3) coordination; (4) awareness; and (5) communication among facets of the surgical process (Undre et al. 2007, see Undre et al. Chapter 6 in this volume).

An assessment which attempts to account for the whole team is called the Anaesthetists' Non-Technical Skills (ANTS) behavioural marker system (Fletcher et al. 2002, Fletcher et al. 2003b). ANTS comprises the following four skill categories: (1) task management; (2) teamworking; (3) situation awareness; and, (4) decision-making. It is the first tool for non-technical skills training in anaesthesia and supports the need for objective measures of teamwork to appropriately inform real and simulated training initiatives (Fletcher et al. 2003a, see Glavin and Patey, Chapter 11, and Graham et al., Chapter 12 in this volume, for examples). More recently non-technical performance measurement has been carried out in surgical and operating room teams. Using task analysis assessment to identify technical errors and non-technical team performance measures for surgery suggests that it may be possible to avoid errors associated with lack of surgeon situational awareness by intra-operative briefings and workload management (Mishra et al. 2008).

There is a role for both structured and unstructured observations to help capture and measure the complexity of team interactions. The rigour of these observations has been addressed by: employing strategies such as validating tools against best practice standards; using two independent observers to simultaneously collect data; and triangulating data using multiple data collection methods (Healey and Undre 2006). Additionally, further research is needed to ensure observation tools are robust and standardized, and, also importantly, remain consistent with current best practices (Undre et al. 2006).

Carthey points out that direct observation, especially of the structured variety, may not be suited to all healthcare environments. Those environments which are defined by emergent rather than elective procedures – where there is unpredictable diverse case mix, larger size and the greater movement of staff around a wider area while treating patients – can create difficulties for observers (Carthey 2002). It may be too great an attentional task to accurately record all teamwork communications due to the involvement of multiple actors and activities that can occur simultaneously (Wears 2000).

Alternatives to Observation to Determine Time Pressure Effects

Data collection is a major challenge, particularly in studies of emergency medical care because interesting care events are often unexpected. Real-time data collection is needed to counteract hindsight biases in retrospective construction of past events and to capture dynamically evolving emergency situations. Audio-video recording is an influential tool that may assist such data collection. Those analysing video data can repeatedly examine activities in emergency medical and trauma care settings and extract detailed qualitative and quantitative data (Mackenzie and Xiao 2003). Additionally, high risk medical providers can review their own care through audio-video records and provide comments on covert mental processes cued by audio-video records. Such a cognitive approach to examination of real emergency medical events is a powerful tool to uncover many facets of the nature of emergency care work, including time pressure, clinician performance, diagnosis, planning, and communications during stressful tasks and identification of patient and practitioner safety.

While observational studies illustrate types of errors and incidents in healthcare, they are not always effective at describing and analysing clinical conduct at the level of interactions within real complex clinical environments, such as detecting the influence of time pressure on task performance in trauma settings. Use of video is more appropriate than observation as it overcomes many of the disadvantages that direct observation has by enabling capture of fleeting events and communications and allowing repeated review and inter-rater reliability analyses of audio-video source material. Importantly video data allow the participant care providers to review and comment on the cognitive and uncertain aspects of the care that they provided, and the pressure they felt during task accomplishment. Video recordings can also be used in conjunction with direct observation to validate and supplement information collected by trained observers and other structured analysis.

When video is compared to direct observation, video data can help overcome difficulties in capturing subtle cues, fleeting errors, brief utterances or team interactions and communications. There is a great need to understand what occurs in uncertain emergency medicine workplaces, where risky but life-saving procedures such as tracheal intubation are carried out, often in non-optimal circumstances (Mackenzie et al. 2007, Mackenzie et al. 1996b). Video data may be helpful to identify what Reason has termed, unsafe acts, pre-cursor events (Reason 1980), accident opportunities, latent and systems failures that traditional observational data collection methodologies may fail to capture. Video based analyses in complex and high-risk medical settings offers advantages over direct observation since it allows for: (1) fine grained analysis; (2) repeated reviews by multiple experts; (3) the ability of multiple observers without compromising access to the patient; and, (4) playback for clinicians whose care is recorded.

Feedback to clinicians viewing their own care is potentially a most valuable advantage of video, providing systematic feedback and allowing team performance review. Such video review has the potential to advance the incorporation of non-technical skills training into healthcare and allow objective assessment of these skills (Moorthy et al. 2005). Also, in support of arguments elsewhere in this chapter, video records can identify problems and solutions to improve processes in emergency trauma care that are likely to be generalizable to other high risk medical domains (Mackenzie and Xiao 2003, Mackenzie et al. 1996b). Video data can also be used as input to root cause analyses or other quality improvement practices, and provide contextual detail, enable repeated raw data reviews by multiple reviewers and allow assessment of a critical event using measures developed subsequent to the video-recorded event. In this way, video analysis can be a powerful supplement to existing quality assurance methodologies for understanding the context and the proximal contributors to an adverse event.

Data Collection to Assess Time Pressure Effects during Tracheal Intubation Task

Audio-video recording was determined to be the optimal method to collect data on tracheal intubation. Before starting video data collection, non-structured interviews with subject matter experts (SME) among anaesthesiology faculty attending staff, were carried out to gain consensus about the task requirements and priorities. Interviews were conducted both at the trauma centre and a tertiary care hospital where mostly elective surgery was performed. From these interviews, some of which were audio-recorded and transcribed, the normative task model for tracheal intubation was derived and confirmed by SME's review. Capture of audio-video records from cameras and microphones installed on the ceilings of trauma resuscitation bays and operating rooms of a trauma centre provided data to identify details of the task performance. Patient vital signs including heart rate, blood pressure, blood oxygen saturation and exhaled carbon dioxide were continuously recorded.

Major components of video analysis included performance evaluation using the normative task analysis model as a performance template and completion of questionnaires based on this task model by SMEs during review of the video records. The questionnaires required completion of timing data for major task landmarks, subjective ratings of performance in tactic manoeuvres and decisions, and judgement of patient conditions. Aggregated results from the completed questionnaire produced the basis for further, often quantitative analysis.

Two types of task settings were emergency and elective, which reflect the urgency of decision-making and interventions. For tracheal intubation emergency was defined as within ten minutes of patient admission, identifying an urgent need to intervene rapidly to normalize oxygenation and ventilation. Semi-emergency intubation occurred 11–59 minutes after admission. Elective tracheal intubation included those newly admitted trauma patients who required airway management one hour or more later.

Findings Obtained from Video Analysis Illustrating Effects of Time Pressure

To measure different effects on performance of the tracheal intubation task under elective and emergency circumstances two experienced faculty anaesthesiologists were instrumented with ambulatory vital signs recording devices (automated blood pressure cuff [BP], electrocardiogram [ECG]). An example of the ECG tracings and BP results is shown in Figure 23.1 which shows the ambulatory electrocardiogram (ECG) and blood pressure (BP) of an anaesthesiologist during elective and emergency intubations. During the elective intubation (top panel) blood pressure and heart rate are normal. The same anaesthesiologist two hours later dealing with an emergency intubation has a greater than doubling of heart rate (lower panel) and clinically significant diastolic hypertension.

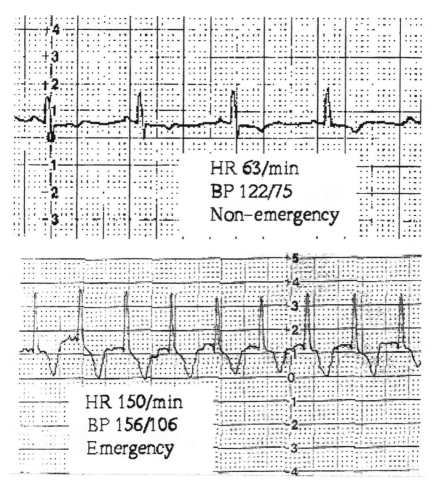

Figure 23.1   Ambulatory electrocardiograms (ECG) and blood pressure (BP) of an anaesthesiologist during elective (top panel) and emergency (lower panel) intubations

Figure 23.2 shows heart rate/minute (HR) and blood pressure (BP) of an experienced anaesthesiologist obtained by ambulatory monitors. Changes are recorded in BP and HR with increased physical exertion (d), during resting (c), and during elective intubation (a × 4) and emergency intubation (a/b) of a trauma patient. There are clinically significant increases in heart rate and systolic BP seen with emergency intubation (in comparison to elective intubation). These data show that the anaesthesiologist, despite being experienced, showed physiological signs of stress due to the time pressure of an emergency rather than elective tracheal intubation.

The results of the task analyses of tracheal intubation are shown in Table 23.1, decomposed into a sequence of steps, in preparation for, during and after task completion.

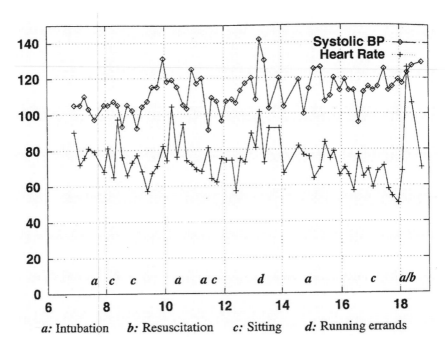

a: Intubation   *b:* Resuscitation   *c:* Sitting   *d:* Running errands

Figure 23.2   Heart rate (HR) and blood pressure (BP) of an experienced anaesthesiologist obtained by ambulatory monitors (Holler)

Among emergency tracheal intubations, there was associated increased workload (many tasks to do at once), time stress both due to the severity of the patient injury and on occasion due to the surgeon calling for induction of anaesthesia and tracheal intubation, so that other tasks in the resuscitation process could proceed more rapidly. Compared to elective tracheal intubation, there was also more uncertainty of information about patient status because more than half of the emergency intubations were required due to unconsciousness or patient-induced challenges such as combativeness or intoxication. Errors in emergency intubation could be attributed to knowledge-based shortcomings, for example, drug dosages were erroneous in three emergency intubations (Mackenzie et al. 1996a). Even though the majority of video recorded tracheal intubations (23/42) were performed by experienced personnel (>5 years in trauma centre), there were a greater number of tasks omitted from the task analysis model in emergency than elective tracheal intubation. Figure 23.3 shows the comparison of task omission (among those tasks shown in Table 23.1) during elective (EL), semi-emergency (SE) and emergency (E) airway management in 42 patients of whom 15 showed emergency, 13 semi-emergency and 14 elective airway management. Twelve SMEs prioritized the tasks that were checked during airway management. On video analysis a low weighting was given if a high priority task was omitted. Omission of a low priority task considered to be task shedding was given a high weighting that would have

Table 23.1   Task sequence tracheal intubation where X = cross, SpO$_2$ = O$_2$ saturation, BP = blood pressure, HR = heart rate, IV = intravenous, CO$_2$ = carbon dioxide

Preparatory tasks
Pre-oxygenation by facemask
Head positioning
Cricoid pressure applied correctly
In-line neck stabilization
Suction ready
SpO$_2$, BP, HR all monitored pre-induction of anaesthesia and muscle relaxation
IV running
Drugs drawn up
Stethoscope at hand
Assistance immediately available

During
Intubation equipment ready
Re-oxygenation after 3 attempts
Modification of technique between attempts
Re-oxygenation if SpO$_2$<95%
Cricoid pressure maintained until cuff sealed
Tube insertion distance checked
Auscultation of both sides of chest by intubator
Auscultation of upper abdomen

After
Listen to chest after ventilator connection
CO$_2$ monitored within 2 mins of intubation
Check neuromuscular blocker before non-depolarizer
Check ventilatory parameters

the effect of reducing the frequency of task omission. Despite weighting (grey background), there were still a greater number of tasks omitted in E than SE or EL airway management. Weighting decreased the percentage of tasks omitted in all three categories of airway management, indicating some task shedding occurred.

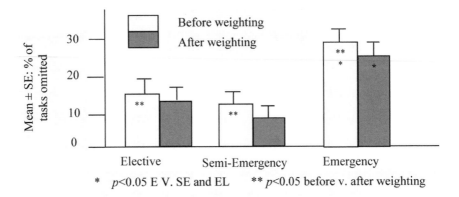

Figure 23.3 Comparison of task omission (among those tasks shown in Table 23.1)

Video analysis provided other evidence of increased time stress involved in emergency intubations and the additional shortcuts, task shedding and task deferral that can result, for example, fewer physiological monitors were used (p<0.05 unpaired t-test) during emergency and semi-emergency than during elective intubations, despite the same monitoring systems being present in all locations where video recording occurred (Table 23.2).

A major difference was in exhaled carbon dioxide monitoring. Time to achieve various landmarks in the task model for intubation showed that pre-oxygenation was shorter, duration between completion of tracheal tube insertion and monitoring of exhaled CO_2 was almost four times longer in emergency than elective intubation (Table 23.3).

Table 23.2   Monitors used: number of patients (%) of total n=48 at each level of airway management task urgency. Emergency = <10 mins after admission, semi-emergency < 10–60 mins after admission and elective = > 1 hour after admission

	Elective	Semi-emergency	Emergency*
SaO_2	12 (80%)	15 (100%)	15 (83%)
$ETCO_2$	7 (47%)	9 (60%)	4 (22%)
BP	13 (87%)	15 (100%)	14 (78%)
ECG	15 (100%)	15 (100%)	17 (94%)

* p<0.05 unpaired t-test, emergency v. elective, and semi-emergency

SaO_2 = oxygen saturation; $ETCO_2$ = end-tidal CO_2; BP = blood pressure; ECG = electocardiogram

Table 23.3   Task durations of intubation events. Mean and standard error of duration (in secs) of events in the intubation sequence among 11 elective and 12 emergency tracheal intubation

Event	Emergency intubation	Elective intubation
Preoxygenation before anaesthesia	234 ± 12.5*	92 ± 6.0
Preoxygenation before DL	310 ± 10.2*	145 ± 6.1
Duration of DL	31 ± 2.1	32 ± 2.4
Duration: DL to ventilate	41 ± 2.5	30 ± 1.3
Duration: Ventilation to listen to chest	10 ± 0.7	38 ± 5.9
Duration: Ventilation to ETCO$_2$ observe	52 ± 5.3*	205 ± 16.8

* significant at p <0.05

Commentary

Numerous studies show that under time pressure, people use less information in making decisions (Wallstein and Barton 1982, Rothstein 1986). Payne et al. (1988) describe the adaptive strategy that occurs under time stress where less complicated reasoning strategies occur in thinking and decision-making because extensive evaluation of multiple options are simply not feasible. Domain experts rely on their domain-specific expertise that enables them to identify the situation quickly and accurately and to use more intuitive decision processes in which actions are arranged with the appropriate action on the top (Klein 1989, Rasmussen 1987, Beach and Mitchell 1990). Training can explicitly address the speed/accuracy trade off issue to allow adaptation to changing time pressure (Means et al. 1993, Lipshitz 1993). In the tracheal intubation task analysis, time pressure was found to impair performance as judged against an idealized process model of the tracheal intubation task sequence. Overall, there was task shedding in emergencies, and this resulted in omission of low priority tasks, increasing the efficiency of achieving the end objective of rapid placement of a tracheal tube into the trachea. In emergency tracheal intubation, time pressure allowed the care providers to take care of patients whose condition was more critical with less available monitoring information. They accomplished the difficult task at a faster pace, but as a result there was a trade-off in speed and accuracy (Wickelgren 1977). Steps were omitted in the task analysis before, during and after tracheal tube placement. Under time pressure, tasks were omitted that were judged by subject matter experts to have high priority. The tasks that were shed, in some critical incidents, were life threatening and significantly impaired patient safety. In one patient, failure to check exhaled carbon dioxide after emergency tracheal intubation resulted in prolonged uncorrected oesophageal intubation. A task communication algorithm has been implemented to mitigate the problem of omitting high priority tasks and improving communication during tracheal intubation.

Video-record review, especially of emergency task accomplishment, provided fine-grained data analyses that identified errors of omission and non-optimal performance. Even the experienced team members who participated in the care that was video-recorded were not immune from these deficiencies and were unaware until receiving the feedback from the video record. Aggregate data from multiple task accomplishments compared at two levels of task urgency was a non-pejorative means of conveying the need for procedural change.

The importance of omission of a high priority task was confirmed by a critical incident that resulted in prolonged uncorrected misplacement of the tracheal tube in the oesophagus (Mackenzie et al. 1996b). In this incident, the anaesthesia care providers became fixated on lack of information about vital signs and oxygen levels. They failed to employ simpler but less technological contingency solutions to identifying patient status. As has been recognized in other critical incidents, there was a failure to utilize equipment that was at hand (end-tidal CO_2 monitoring) that could have definitively answered concerns about whether the tracheal tube was correctly placed (Mackenzie et al. 1996a, 1996b).

Several approaches are suggested to help teams cope with time pressure in emergency medical care. One approach is training in team coordination. Current training for patient resuscitation personnel is primarily oriented toward medical and technical aspects, not specifically toward the skills of performing in a time-critical team environment. For example, when novel approaches are adopted, verbalization can help the rest of the team orient and prepare themselves. Team training in resource management and attitude change has been advocated for highly skilled teams during crises (Foushee and Helmreich 1988, Howard et al. 1992) and for routine surgical operations. Although such training is important and necessary for teams in emergency care (Helmreich and Schaefer 1994), task complexity poses challenges that require more than changes in attitude and use of resources.

Training in explicit communication (Xiao et al. 1996, 1998) (e.g., statements such as 'stand clear' recommended for coordinating the activities of the resuscitation team before electric defibrillation) is needed for the purpose of team coordination to improve team performance in emergencies. Another approach to reducing the impact of time pressure and task complexity are work procedures, designed to reduce the ambiguity in terms of task distribution and increase the ability of team members to provide timely assistance in crisis situations (Boguslaw and Porter 1962). Part task training and variable priority training are techniques that have been used successfully to optimize human performance in adverse airway and respiratory events (Johnson et al. 2008) and have been implemented in a number of simulator-based training programmes resulting in an improved ability to multi-task (Gopher et al 1994).

Summary Messages in this Chapter

Collecting team performance measures in real clinical environments is a way to obtain data on time pressure and develop team training schemes

The clinic itself is the ultimate test bed for measurement of team performance. These measures enable assessment if and how team behaviours change with time pressure and after medical team training is carried out. The questions to answer with regard to team training effectiveness is what is the best way to train people in order that they will behave differently under time pressure – i.e., more efficiently, consistently and safely – within the real clinical environment and how would this be measured? Examination of real-world behaviour in the clinical domain can help us identify problem performance areas affected by time pressure that can be re-created in a simulated environment and help us learn more about the real world.

Better tools are needed to collect data and outcomes from time pressure effects on team performance

The available tools to collect data on time pressure effects on team performance are growing in number. However, all measures remain rather rudimentary and most are, as yet, unable to appropriately inform such team training schemes to minimize decrements in team performance because of time pressure due to lack of performance measurement reliability, validity and ability to generalize.

Video analysis provides many benefits over other measurement tools

Video allows fine-grained analysis, repeated reviews by multiple experts and playback for clinicians, whose care is recorded, thus providing systematic feedback and performance review allowing the details of when and how time pressure occurs and affects performance to be identified. Direct observation can not compete with such benefits, but is less intrusive and generally more accepted by clinicians.

To determine how time pressure affects clinical performance the many different contexts of care must be underpinned with the same conceptual model of team performance

Many of today's team performance measurement tools were designed with a particular context or specialist service in mind, for example, the operating room or neonatal care. As a result it is difficult to make comparisons between tools and establish what the effect of time pressure is on the generic processes and what supporting behaviours there are that minimize performance decrements due to time pressure. Consensus on a theoretical framework or model of team performance would provide researchers with the ability to describe the effects of time pressure on performance and test hypotheses concerning the interrelationships of various performance measures, as well as the interdependencies of the predictors and the outcome criteria from time-pressured performance decrements, across healthcare settings.

Ensuring competent teams that can perform optimally despite time pressure will help to boost patient safety efforts

Safety and quality in healthcare requires continuous training and competency assessment so that performance can be improved and maintained, even for experienced practitioners, under time pressure. Team dynamics such as responding to changing team composition, coordination and communication are fundamental skills to be incorporated into training curricula to counteract performance decrements due to time pressure, particularly through simulation involving interdisciplinary teams. There should also be an understanding that expertise at counteracting the effects of time pressure can occur independently of technical or clinical experience.

Team performance measurement must be evaluated against measures of team output

In the context of measuring team performance in trauma patient management, outcome measures are recorded at the point of discharge while the most intense, time pressured and crucial teamwork functions occur in the reception and resuscitation period (i.e., up to 30 minutes after admission). The intervening period, consists of a multitude of confounding variables making the process of linking initial management with outcome fraught with difficulty. However, process-based measures may be useful to measure the effects of time pressure, changes with training, and enable more effective correlation with team performance scores. These process measures might include time to execute key decisions, tasks or the number of repeated instructions to request task performance or requests to expedite interventions.

Research has identified many of the competencies necessary for effective teamwork but is not yet clear how best to measure and link these to outcomes, or how to continually assess competencies (Epstein and Hundert 2002). Training individuals in 'non-technical' skills to improve their team skills is a necessity since healthcare teams are typically temporary in their composition. Non-technical skills can be subdivided into: (i) cognitive or mental skills (e.g., decision-making, planning, situation awareness) and (ii) social and interpersonal skills (e.g., teamworking, communication, leadership) (Fletcher et al. 2002). Both team competency and non-technical skills sets are necessary for safe and effective performance across medical teams (Epstein and Hundert 2002).

Communication errors in teams are a major source of error and lead to failures within healthcare (Leonard et al. 2004). Specifically within anaesthesiology, communication problems contributed to 20 per cent of non-routine events reported by anaesthesia providers (Weinger et al. 2003). Similar to other high-risk medical settings, these problems can be linked to breakdowns in team coordination (Xiao et al. 1998). Varying levels of teamwork failures and the measurement of general attributes of medical teams are documented across different high risk settings, such as the operating room (Lingard et al. 2002), trauma (Morey et al. 2002), neonatal care (Thomas et al. 2004), critical care (Sherwood et al. 2002) and surgery (Undre et al. 2007). Research in these diverse domains, informed by human factors and high reliability organization theory, seeks to determine optimum teamwork within such complex and dynamic healthcare environments. In the complex environment in which anaesthetists are involved, communication remains problematic (Lingard et al. 2002, Healey and Undre 2006). Even when experienced clinicians are involved, communication of significant clinical decisions fails over 50 per cent of the time (McDermott et al. 2004). Linking computer-generated prompts via visual and auditory displays within trauma resuscitation bays may enhance clinicians' interaction and reduce errors of omission and miscommunication. Compliance with the prompts – rather than pre-learned algorithms – can then be undertaken using video-audit (Fitzgerald et al. 2006). Such an approach may allow an objective and streamlined means of audit, reducing the time consuming process associated with peer review. Video analyses of real medical care events are important in the development of the database necessary for simulation and to improve clinical practice and equipment in the future.

Teamwork training and measurement are necessary for advances in patient safety in emergencies

Measurement is a crucial aspect of understanding the effects of time pressure on medical team performance and the nature of interdisciplinary communication in teams. It can help asses the impact of time pressure and the effects of training to minimize decrements in performance by:

- creating a common language for defining team behaviours and performance;
- identifying possible areas of time-pressured decrements and implementing training;
- assessing how team input factors, such as new technology, affect time-critical teamwork;
- assessing how time pressure affects teamwork and patient outcomes and can be improved upon with training;
- developing team training to minimize the impact of time pressure and evaluation (in reality and simulation).

Teamwork has rightly been identified as a focus for safety and quality improvement initiatives. Systems-based patient safety interventions which target teamwork failures include mandatory audits and team checklists (Hales and Pronovost 2006, Ursprung et al. 2005). These may reduce some of the more conspicuous failures, but ultimately, research that identifies the most effective education and training strategies is needed to improve patient safety and outcomes (Musson and Helmreich 2004). This requires appropriate measurement in order to provide a foundation for evaluating emergency medical teams and team training; and, thus underpin attempts to improve teamwork in complex healthcare teams that perform in time critical settings.

References

American College of Surgeons Committee on Trauma (1997) *Advanced Trauma Life Support Courses.* Chicago: American College of Surgeons.

Beach, C.R. and Mitchell, J.R. (1990) Image theory: A behavioral theory of decisions in organizations. In B.M. Staw and L.L. Cummings (eds) *Research in Organizational Behavior*, Vol. 12. Greenwich, CT: JAI Press.

Boguslaw, R. and Porter, E.H. (1962) Team functions and training. In R.M. Gagne (ed.) *Psychological Principles in System Development* (pp. 387–416). New York: Holt, Rhinehart and Winston,.

Carthey, J. (2002) The role of structured observational research in health care. *Quality and Safety in Health Care 12* (Suppl II), i13–i16.

Catchpole, K., Mishra, A., Handa, A. and McCulloch, P. (2008) Teamwork and error in the operating room: Analysis of skills and roles. *Annals of Surgery* 274, 699–706.

Christian, C.K., Gustafson, M.L., Roth, E.M., Sheridan, T.B., Gandhi, T.K., Dwyer, K., Zinner, M.J. and Dierks, M.M. (2006) A prospective study of patient safety in the operating room. *Surgery* 139(2), 159–73.

Epstein, R.M. and Hundert, E.M. (2002) Defining and assessing professional competence. *Journal of the American Medical Association* 287(2), 226–35.

Fitzgerald, M.C., Gocentas, R., Dziukas, L., Cameron, P., Mackenzie, C.F. and Farrow, N. (2006) Using video audit to improve trauma resuscitation – time for a new approach. *Canadian Journal of Surgery* 49(3), 208–11.

Fletcher, G.C.L., McGeorge, P., Flin, R.H., Glavin, R.J. and Maran, N.J. (2002) The role of non-technical skills in anaesthesia: A review of current literature. *British Journal of Anaesthesia* 88(3), 418–29.

Fletcher, G., Flin, R. and McGeorge, P. (2003a) *Review of Human Factors Research in Anaesthesia Report.* Available at: <http//www.abdn.ac.uk/iprc/ants> [last accessed July 2008].

Fletcher, G., Flin, R., McGeorge, P., Galvin, R., Maran, N. and Patey, R. (2003b) Anaesthetists' Non-Technical Skills (ANTS): Evaluation of a behavioural marker system. *British Journal of Anaesthesia* 90(5), 580–8.

Foushee, H.C. and Helmreich, R.L. (1988) Group interaction and flight crew performance. In E.L. Wiener and D.C. Nagal (eds) *Human Factors in Aviation* (pp. 189–227). San Diego, CA: Academic Press.

Gopher, D., Weil, M. and Bareket, T. (1994) Transfer of skill from a computer game trainer to flight. *Human Factors* 36, 387–405.

Hales, H. and Pronovost, P. (2006) The checklist – a tool for error management and performance improvement. *Journal of Critical Care* 21(3), 231–5.

Healey, A.N. and Undre, S. (2006) The complexity of measuring interprofessional teamwork in the operating theatre. *Journal of Interprofessional Care* 20(5), 485–95.

Healey, A.N., Undre, S. and Vincent, C. (2005) Defining the technical skills of teamwork in surgery. *Quality and Safety in Health Care* 15, 231–4.

Helmreich, R.L. and Schaefer, H.G. (1994) Team performance in the operating room. In M.S. Bogner (ed.) *Human Error in Medicine* (pp. 225–53). Hillsdale, NJ: Erlbaum.

Howard, S.K., Gaba, D.M. Fish, K.J. Yang, G. and Sarnquist F.H. (1992) Anesthesia crisis resource management training: Teaching anesthesiologists to handle critical incidents. *Aviation Space and Environmental Medicine* 63, 763–70.

Johnson, K.B., Syroid, N.D., Drews, F.A., Ogden, L.L., Strayer, D.L., Pace, N.L., Tyler, D.L., White, J.L. and Westenskow, D.R. (2008) Part task and variable priority training in first-year anesthesia resident education. *Anesthesiology* 108, 831–40.

Klein, G.A. (1989) Recognition-primed decision. In W.B. Rouse (ed.) *Advances in Man-machine System Research*, Vol. 5. Greenwich, CT: JAI.

Leonard, M., Graham, S. and Bonacum, D. (2004) The human factor: The critical importance of effective teamwork and communication in providing safe care. *Quality and Safety in Health Care* 13 (suppl1), i85–90.

Lingard, L., Reznick, R., Espin, S., Regehr, G. and DeVito, I. (2002) Team communications in the operating room: Talk patterns, sites of tension, and implications for novices. *Academic Medicine* 77(3), 232–7.

Lipshitz, R. (1993) Conveying themes in the study of decision-making in realistic settings. In G.A. Klein, J. Orasanu, R. Calderwood and C.E. Zsambok (eds) *Decision Making in Action: Models and Methods* (pp. 103–37). Norwood NJ: Ablex.

Mackenzie, C.F. and Lippert, F.K. (1999) Emergency Department management of trauma. *Anesthesiology Clinics of North America* 17, 45–61.

Mackenzie, C. and Xiao, Y. (2003) Video techniques and data compared with observation in emergency trauma care. *Quality and Safety in Health Care* 12 (Suppl II), ii51–7.

Mackenzie, C.F., Jeffries, N.J., Hunter, W.A., Bernhard, W.N., Xiao, Y. and The Lotas Group (1996a) Comparison of self-reporting of deficiencies in airway management with video analyses of actual performance. *Human Factors* 38, 623–5.

Mackenzie, C.F., Martin, P. and Xiao, Y. (1996b) Video analysis of prolonged uncorrected esophageal intubation. *Anesthesiology* 84, 1494–503.

Mackenzie, C.F., Xiao, Y., Hu, F., Seagull, F. and Fitzgerald, M. (2007) Video as a tool for improving tracheal intubation tasks for emergency medical and trauma care. *Annals of Emergency Medicine* 50(4), 436–42.

McDermott, F.T., Rosenfeld, J.V., Laidlaw, J.D., Cordner, S.M., Tremayne, A.B. (2004) Evaluation of management of road trauma survivors with brain injury and neurologic disability in Victoria. *The Journal of Trauma* 56(1), 137–49.

Means, B., Salas, E., Crandall, B., Jacobs, T.O. (1993) Training decision-making for the real world. In G.A. Klein, J. Orasanu, R. Calderwood, C.E. Zsambok (eds), *Decision-Making in Action: Models and Methods* (pp. 306–26). Norwood, NJ: Ablex.

Mishra, A., Catchpole, K., Dale, T. and McCulloch, P. (2008) The influence of non-technical performance on technical outcomes in laparoscopic cholecystectomy. *Surgical Endoscopy* 22, 68–73

Moorthy, K., Munz, Y. and Adams, S. (2005) A human factors analysis of technical and team skills among surgical trainees during procedural simulations in a simulated operating theatre. *Annals of Surgery* 242(5), 631–9.

Morey, J.C., Simon, R. and Jay, G.D. (2002) Error reduction and performance improvement in the emergency department through formal teaching training: Evaluation results of the MedTeams project. *Health Services Research* 37, 1553–81.

Musson, D.M. and Helmreich, R.L. (2004) Team training and resource management in health care: Current issues and future directions. *Harvard Health Policy Review* 5(1), 25–35.

Payne, J.W., Bethman, J.R. and Johnson, E.J. (1988) Adaptive strategy reflection in decision-making. *Journal of Experimental Psychology, Learning, Memory and Cognition* 14, 534–52.

Rasmussen, J. (1987) Mental models and the control of actions in complex environments. In J.M. Tamber and D. Ackerman (eds) *Mental-models and Human-Computer Interactions* (pp. 41–69). Amsterdam: North Holland.

Reason, J. (1980) *Human Error*. New York: Cambridge University Press.

Rothstein, H.G. (1986) The effect of time pressure on judgment in multiple cue probability learning. *Organizational Behaviors and Human Decision-Making* 37, 83–92.

Shapiro, M.J., Morey, J.C., Small, S.D., Langford, V., Kaylor, C.J., Jagminas, L., Suner, S., Salisbury, M.L., Simon, R. and Jay, G.D. (2004) Simulation based teamwork training for emergency department staff: Does it improve clinical team performance when added to an existing didactic teamwork curriculum? *Quality and Safety in Health Care* 13(6), 417–21.

Sherwood, G., Thomas, E.J., Bennett, D.S. and Lewis, P. (2002) A teamwork model to promote patient safety in critical care. *Critical Care Nursing Clinics of North America* 14(4), 333–40.

Thomas, E.J., Sexton, J.B. and Helmreich, R.L. (2004) Translating teamwork behaviors from aviation to healthcare: Development of behavioural markers for neonatal resuscitation. *Quality and Safety in Health Care* 13 (Suppl 1), i57–i64.

Undre, S., Sevdalis, N. and Healey, A.N. (2006) Teamwork in the operating theatre: Cohesion or confusion? *Journal of Evaluation in Clinical Practice* 12, 182–9.

Undre, S., Sevdalis, N., Healey, A.N., Darzi, A. and Vincent, C.A. (2007) Observational teamwork assessment for surgery (OTAS): Refinement and application in urological surgery. *World Journal of Surgery* 31, 1373–81.

Ursprung, R., Gray, J.E., Edwards, W.H., Horbar, J.D., Nickerson, J., Plsek, P, Shiono, P.H., Suresh, G.K. and Goldmann, D.A. (2005) Real time patient safety audits: Improving safety every day. *Quality and Safety in Health Care* 14(4), 284–9.

Wallstein, T.S. and Barton, C. (1982) Processing probabilistic multidimensional information for decisions. *Journal of Experimental Psychology, Learning, Memory and Cognition* 8, 361–84.

Wears, R.L. (2000) Beyond error. *Academic Emergency Medicine* 7, 1175–6.

Weinger, M.B., Slagle, J., Jain, S. Ordonez, N. (2003) Retrospective data collection and analytical techniques for patient safety studies. *Journal of Biomedical Informatics* 36, 106–19.

Wickelgren, W.A. (1977) Speed-accuracy trade off and information processing dynamics. *Acta Psychologica* 41, 67–85.

Xiao, Y., Hunter, A., Jeffrey, N., Mackenzie and Lotas Group (1996) Task complexity in emergency medical care and its implication for team coordination. *Human Factors* 38, 636–45.

Xiao, Y., Mackenzie, C.F., Patey, R., Lotas Group (1998) *Team coordination and breakdowns in a real life stressful environment.* Proceedings of the Human Factors and Ergonomic Soc 42nd Annual Meeting, 186–90. Chicago, Human Factors Society, Santa Monica CA.

Chapter 24

Distractions and Interruptions in the Operating Room

Nick Sevdalis, Sonal Arora, Shabnam Undre and Charles Vincent

Introduction

In recent years, there have been significant attempts in the surgical literature to re-conceptualize the way surgical performance, errors and outcomes are understood. Key drivers behind such attempts are the recent focus on the safety and the quality of the care delivered to surgical patients (e.g., Greenberg et al. 2007, Gawande et al. 2003), the dramatic changes in surgical training – with reduced time to train and exposure to cases in the operating room (OR) (Royal College of Surgeons of England 2007), and recent technological as well as educational advances in surgical simulators (Aggarwal et al. 2004, 2008; Dankelman and DiLorenzo 2005, Issenberg et al. 2005).

One such promising re-conceptualization is the 'systems view' of surgical performance (Calland et al. 2002, Healey and Vincent 2007, Vincent et al. 2004). According to the systems view, surgical performance (and error/outcome) can be thought of as a composite function of:

- individual surgical skills (including technical and non-technical skills; Yule et al. 2006);
- teamworking in OR teams (Undre et al. 2006a, 2006b, 2007a);
- OR environment.

The systems view is currently a working hypothesis. As such, it has sparked interest amongst surgical researchers and a number of papers have started to emerge in the literature examining various skills, especially non-technical skills and teamworking in surgical teams, on the one hand, and their relationship with surgical performance, on the other. The OR environment, however, has been conspicuously absent from these developments. The empirical evidence on the role of the OR environment in the safety and the quality of surgical care (as proposed in the systems view) is almost non-existent. In addition to the lack of empirical evidence, conceptual thinking in relation to the OR environment and its contribution to the delivery of safe surgical care is rather in its infancy.

The present chapter is a first attempt at filling this lacuna. Specifically, we focus on distractions and interruptions to clinical work that occur in the OR.

We begin by reviewing relevant evidence from other (i.e., non-OR) clinical domains. We then review the available evidence on the incidence of distractions and interruptions in the OR and the evidence for a link between this aspect of the OR environment and deteriorated performance/increased stress in surgeons. We conclude with suggestions regarding future empirical research and potential relevant interventions in the OR.

Distractions/Interruptions to Surgical Work: Incidence and Severity

Empirical evidence on what the OR environment is like and what its potential impact is on surgical performance is scarce. To an outsider, the lack of research appears rather surprising. Psychological research has been investigating links and interactions between human environments and human actions, emotions and well-being over a number of years. An entire branch of psychology is focused on such interactions (environmental psychology). As a result of this research, there is now a large body of evidence that suggests that an environment might be more or less conducive to the success of human action (e.g., Saegert and Winkel 1990, Sundstrom et al. 1996).

Early studies of what the clinical environment is like in specialities outside surgery focused on interruptions of clinical work. The motivation behind these studies was anecdotal experience of clinicians that their work is more often than not interrupted (by their colleagues, phones or bleepers) and that continuous interruptions led to loss of concentration and thus increased likelihood of error. An early such study was reported by Coiera and Tombs (1998). The researchers observed medical and nursing staff in a British hospital during approximately 30 working hours and recorded communications between staff. They found that staff were generating twice as many calls/bleeps as they received (65 vs. 31, respectively) and concluded that, with their own behaviour, staff were contributing to a disruptive workplace, potentially conducive to error. Similar findings emerged from a study by Alvarez and Coiera (2005) conducted in an intensive care unit of a large teaching hospital in Sydney, Australia. The researchers observed nine participants (doctors and nurses) for 24 hours and recorded communications between them. In this study, distracting communications accounted for a significant 37 percent of total communication time between doctors (junior and senior) and nurses, with 14 'turn-taking interruptions' (i.e., someone talking before the other person had finished) recorded per hour of clinical work.

Other studies have examined distractions in the emergency department (ED). Brixey at al. (2008) carried out an observational study in a trauma centre in a tertiary teaching hospital in the United States. After observing five attending/consultant physicians for 29.5 hours and 9 nurses for 40 hours, the researchers devised a ten-level taxonomy of interruptions (e.g., 'intended recipient', 'unintended recipient', 'recipient blocked', etc.), which they used to code their observations. The researchers found that physicians and nurses received approximately 10 and 12 interruptions per hour of work, respectively. The vast majority of the interruptions for both professional groups were initiated by other people (i.e., their colleagues and patients). In another study, Chisholm et al. (2001) compared five non-teaching community hospital EDs with 22 primary care offices in five central cities of Indiana in the United States. Twenty-two physicians were sampled from each clinical setting and the observations were based on a task analysis. The researchers found that ED physicians spent an average 6.4 mins/hour multi-tasking (i.e., dealing with more than one task at the same time) and 9.7 mins/hour being interrupted. The figures for the primary care physicians were 11.4 mins/hour and 3.9 mins/hour, respectively. Taken together, these findings suggest that the working environment in the ED is as disruptive as those in the intensive care unit and in the wards.

In the light of these studies in non-surgical specialities, our research group carried out a number of systematic studies of the OR environment (Healey et al. 2006, 2007, Primus et al. 2007, Sevdalis et al. 2007, 2008). The focus of this work has been disruptions and distractions that occur during procedures. Distractions were defined as events that visibly diverted the surgeon's (and any other OR member's) attention from the task s/he was carrying out. We sought to determine the incidence of such events, as well as the level of disruption that they introduce. Most of the studies that we have carried out to date were observational, but we have also developed a self-report tool, appropriate for surveying OR staff.

In a first study (Healey et al. 2006), we observed 29 laparoscopic and 21 open general surgical procedures (lasting between 30 and 240 minutes each) in a large teaching hospital in London. A number of categories were derived a priori (through observation) to code the distracting events as they occurred; these included staff flow in/out of the OR, auditory distractions (e.g., irrelevant communications), visual distractions (e.g., movement around the laparoscopic monitor), and operational distractions (related to equipment and ergonomic issues). In addition, each distraction was rated on a 1–9 level behaviourally anchored scale:

- Levels 1–3 were allocated to relatively inconsequential distractions, dealt with by a 'floating' member of staff.
- Levels 4–6 were allocated to distractions that visibly affected one team member.
- Levels 7–9 were allocated to distractions that visibly affected the entire team.

The rating scale was reliable, as assessed by two observers rating distractions concurrently in the OR (Spearman ρ correlation between observers for level of first observed distraction per category = 0.61, $p < 0.0001$; ρ between observers for aggregated level of observed distractions = 0.89, $p < 0.0001$). We observed an average of 13 distracting events per procedure. Operational distractions (including equipment problems), case-irrelevant communications, movement around the laparoscopic monitor and staff flow in/out of the OR were the most commonly observed distractions. Case-irrelevant communications and operational distractions caused the most disruption to the team.

Focusing specifically on the irrelevant communications in the above data set, we found 3.5 events per procedure. Equipment/provisions-related communications were significantly more disruptive than patient-related communications, 'small talk' and teaching. Surgeons were the most likely initiators as well as recipients of these distracting communications (Sevdalis et al. 2007).

These findings were replicated in 30 urological procedures (Healey at al. 2007, Primus et al. 2007). In this study, we also sought to establish whether distractions add to the length of a procedure – as might be expected. During an average procedure duration of just over 50 minutes ($M = 52.35$ mins), the rate of visibly distracting events was 0.45/min – one distracting event every other minute of the procedure. Average staff flow through the OR was quite high: 1.08/min (i.e., someone walking in/out of the OR every minute). Importantly, these disruptions increased operative time by an average of 5.66 mins.

Other researchers have adopted a narrower focus. Verdaasdonk et al. (2007) observed 30 laparoscopic procedures focusing on equipment-related incidents – i.e., what we have defined above as equipment-related distractions. These researchers found 49 such incidents (i.e., 1.6 incidents per procedure), with one or more incident occurring in 87 percent of the observed cases. Of the 49 incidents, 55 percent related to equipment malfunctioning in some way and 45 percent related to equipment being absent or positioned erroneously. In a subsequent study, Verdaasdonk et al. (2008) showed that use of a simple checklist reduced the number of equipment-related distractions that they observed in a similar set of cases.

In addition to the distractions discussed so far, noise is a potential source of distraction in the OR. A number of older and more recent studies appear to be in agreement regarding the levels of noise in the OR, which usually exceed recommended guidelines (of about 45dB(A); Moorthy et al. 2004, Cabrera and Lee 2000). Early studies have recorded OR noise levels around 80–85dB(A) (Shapiro and Berland 1972, Hodge and Thompson 1990) – a level that matches noise at a motorway. In our studies (Healey et al. 2006, 2007), we observed average (mean) noise levels of 57.80dB(A) (general surgery) and 56.92dB(A) (urology), but maximum noise levels across cases averaged at 62.94dB(A) (general surgery) and 80.28dB(A) (urology). In both sets of cases, the absolute maximum level of noise observed was 94.40dB(A) (general surgery) and 92.60dB(A) (urology).

On the basis of these observational studies, we have devised a tool that captures distractions and disruptions in surgical work as self-reported by OR staff – the Disruptions in Surgery Index (DiSI; Sevdalis et al. 2008). DiSI covers the following categories of disruption:

- individuals' skills, performance, and personality;
- OR environment;
- communication;
- coordination and situation awareness;

- patient-related disruptions;
- team cohesion and organizational disruptions.

DiSI is a self-report survey tool. Each one of the above categories comprises two to six relevant items. For each item, participants are asked to rate how often they experience a disruption associated with it (percent), and to what extent the disruption obstructs them from accomplishing their goals and/or to what extent it contributed to error (0–9 scales). For example, one (of four) patient-related disruption items reads 'Unavailable pre-operative notes'. Participants are asked to estimate the frequency of this disruption and its contribution to error/goal obstruction. In a pilot study, we administered DiSI to 62 OR staff (surgeons, anaesthetists, nurses, Operating Department Practitioners) and asked them to make the above estimates and judgements for themselves and for their colleagues. We found that disruptions listed in DiSI occur in 25 percent (surgeons) to 42 percent (nurses) of procedures – a high level of occurrence by any standards. Interestingly, OR staff judged that coordination issues, patient-related disruptions and team cohesion/organizational disruptions occur equally to themselves and to their colleagues. In contrast, all professional groups reported that disruptions related to individuals' skill, the OR environment, and communication occur to others more than they occur to themselves – a paradoxical finding that perhaps mirrors preparedness to accept organizational-level issues that affect everyone equally, but reluctance to accept disruptions that somehow feel more personal.

Distractions/Interruptions, Stress and Surgical Performance

The studies that we have reviewed so far suggest that distractions do occur in the OR and that they are disruptive to surgical work (some of them more so than others). An important question, however, remains: is there a link between distractions/ interruptions and surgical performance, technical and/or non-technical?

Few studies have assessed the impact of distractions on technical performance and most of them have done so in simulated settings (e.g., Goodell et al. 2006, Hsu et al. 2008, Miskovic et al. 2008). Wiegmann et al. (2007), however, did carry out a study in real time in real cardiac procedures. The researchers observed operation flow disruptions and technical errors in 32 cardiac procedures in a United States hospital. Technical errors were agreed on among surgical members of the research team by consensus. Five categories of disruption were observed:

1. teamwork related;
2. extraneous interruptions;
3. equipment/technology related;
4. resource-based issues;
5. supervisory/training-related issues.

Wiegmann et al. (2008) observed five technical errors and 11 disruptive events per procedure. Importantly, teamwork-related disruptions correlated positively with technical errors: higher number of disruptive events was associated with higher number of errors per procedure. In addition to providing a link between distractions/disruptions and surgical performance, these findings are important because they corroborate the types of distractions that surgical teams are likely to be exposed to. The disruption categories that were obtained by Wiegmann et al. (2007) in cardiac procedures mirror those that we have found in general surgical (open and laparoscopic) and urological procedures in our observational studies of disruptions in the OR (Healey et al. 2006, 2007; Primus et al. 2007, Sevdalis et al. 2007) – thus suggesting an emerging empirical consensus.

Other studies have investigated the impact of distractions on technical performance using simulators – and have thus focused on laparoscopic surgery. Goodell et al. (2006) asked 13 medical students and surgical trainees to carry out six tasks on a laparoscopic virtual reality simulator with and without distraction. The distractions consisted of mental arithmetic problems. The researchers found that time to complete the laparoscopic tasks increased significantly with distractions, but overall performance score and economy of motion were not significantly affected (although they were worse in the distractions condition). Hsu et al. (2008) compared nine more experienced with 31 less experienced participants' performance at a laparoscopic task when distraction was added (consisting of mathematical addition questions). They found that whereas the less experienced participants' performance deteriorated with distraction, no such deterioration was observed in the performance of the more experienced participants and attributed the findings to the automaticity in task execution that the expert participants had developed.

Noise and music in the OR and their impact on performance have attracted some research attention, but the findings to date seem to be inconclusive. In an experimental study, Murthy et al. (1995) exposed anaesthetists to noise levels of 77.32dB(A) – the levels of noise that they had previously observed in a local OR. The researchers assessed the participants' performance on two standardized psychometric tests of mental efficiency and one such test of short-term memory and found that pre-exposure performance on all tests was significantly higher than post-exposure performance. In a survey regarding music in the OR and its impact on anaesthetic performance reported by Hawksworth et al. (1997), 72 percent of 144 surveyed anaesthetists reported that music is a regular feature of the ORs in which they work. Approximately 26 percent of the participants reported that music potentially reduces their vigilance and impairs communication with other OR staff, whereas 11.5 percent of them felt that music might distract them from alarms. However, a subsequent study by the same research group on 12 trainee anaesthetists using a computer-based psychomotor performance assessment failed to show any adverse effects of music or noise on performance (Hawksworth et al. 1998). Similar null findings emerged from a surgical study that investigated the effects of noise (80–85dB) and music on laparoscopic performance in 12 surgeons of various levels of expertise (Moorthy et al. 2004). The researchers failed to show any effects of noise or music on any performance parameter (time taken, path length, number of movement, and others). Miskovic et al. (2008), however, found that trainee surgeons reached top performance at a laparoscopic task without music. In addition, music that the subjects liked affected their performance less than music that they did not like. The authors concluded that trainee surgeons should switch off the radio that is often on in the OR to reduce the potential for error in real procedures.

Additional evidence on the impact of distractions on surgical performance comes from studies that have investigated acute intra-operative stress in surgeons. Two qualitative interview studies that have recently been carried out by our group provide links between distractions and key stressors in operative surgery (Wetzel et al. 2006, Arora et al. 2009). In both studies, distractions in the OR featured as a prominent source of stress. This is illustrated by a quote from a surgeon in the Arora et al. (2009) study: 'What annoys me is not being able to do what I can do. Too much interference, for example from managerial staff [whilst operating]. Also, nurses relating to you cost issues when you're dealing with life and death can be enough to drive you mad.'

The same participant went on to highlight that the resulting stress means 'the chances of getting things wrong are a lot higher ... and because we are dealing with lives, the stakes are that much higher still'. Additional examples of distractions mentioned by participants included being interrupted, noise, multiple demands, phone calls, bleeps and people walking in and out of the OR (i.e., all the distractions that our observational studies have furnished). Despite the lack of objective performance data in these two studies, surgeons felt that distractions impair their technical as well as non-technical skills (including judgement and decision-making, communication and teamwork), thus potentially jeopardizing patient safety.

Other studies have investigated the impact of distractions using useless chatter during the procedure (Hassan et al. 2006), introduced increased cognitive demands (e.g., being asked to do a mathematical task whilst simultaneously doing the procedure; Moorthy et al. 2003, Schuetz et al. 2007), increased noise in the OR (Moorthy et al. 2003, Schuetz et al. 2008), external visitors in the OR (Schuetz et al. 2008) and equipment problems (Undre et al. 2007b).

Of those, three studies investigated the effect of distractions on performance and showed that, overall, increased distractions correlated with poorer performance on laparoscopic tasks. Hassan et al. (2006) found that distractions in the form of useless chatter from the investigators led to a longer time to complete the task, increased number of errors and poorer economy of motion. The authors speculated that distractions are particularly 'counterproductive because the operator must concentrate on the task at hand' – and distractions are not conducive to attention focus. The studies by Moorthy et al. (2003) and by Schuetz et al. (2008) examined the effects of multiple stressors on performance. This is particularly relevant, because frequently surgeons are subject to a variety of distractions in the OR that can compound together to increase stress. Moorthy et al. (2003) found that certain distractions (noise, doing a mathematical task and time pressure) led to impaired dexterity of surgeons performing a laparoscopic transfer task compared to quiet conditions. The effect was even more pronounced when all distractions co-occurred. Schuetz et al. (2008) subjected their participants to multiple stressors in the form of sequential distractions (asked to do a mathematical task, time pressure, increased volume of pulse oximeter, presence of external visitor) whilst asking them to perform a laparoscopic cholecystectomy on a virtual reality simulator. The researchers found that surgeons who experienced stress but recovered demonstrated better manual skill than those who experienced stress but did not recover (an expected finding). This suggests that coping with stressful distractions could potentially be important for maintaining high performance.

Taken together, the above studies in the OR and on surgical simulators suggest that distractions are likely to lead or contribute to impaired surgical performance, both technical and non-technical, and increased stress in operating surgeons.

Current Evidence and Future Research

The OR is anecdotally characterized as a disruptive place to work, often conducive to loss of cognitive focus and attention and, thus, rendering OR staff potentially vulnerable to errors. In the present chapter, we reviewed existing evidence on the incidence and disruptiveness of distractions that occur in the OR. We also examined the impact that such distractions have on surgical performance.

Although the evidence for incidence and disruptiveness of distractions in the OR is slim, their occurrence appears to be a regular feature of the OR environments across continents (Europe, America, Australia) and specialities (general surgery, cardiac surgery, urology). Types of distractions are also consistent across studies, with equipment-related and other operational issues and staff/teamwork-related distractions being most disruptive. These patterns are not inconsistent with patterns obtained in non-surgical specialities, such as intensive care units and EDs – suggesting that distractions are not a feature peculiar to the OR but they affect all of healthcare. The evidence is equally inconclusive regarding the impact that such distractions have on surgical performance. Few studies have addressed this question and most of them have been carried out using surgical simulators. Although more research is necessary to elucidate the relationship between distractions/interruptions and surgical performance, it appears that distractions introduce potential for increased stress and subsequent performance impairment, especially in trainee surgeons.

Clearly more and more focused empirical research is needed for a better understanding of the OR environment as a performance-shaping factor, as hypothesized by the systems view of surgical performance. In what follows, we outline what we believe are the key research questions that should be tackled by future research on distractions and interruptions in the OR environment.

Question 1: What is the Incidence and Severity of Distractions/Interruptions in the OR?

This question addresses the size of the problem. In light of the existing empirical evidence, we propose that future studies assess a quasi-standardized set of distractors. As a minimum, the following should be assessed:

- *Equipment-related distractions* – these should cover lack of availability of necessary equipment and equipment failure.
- *Staff/teamwork-related distractions* – these should include irrelevant communications (e.g., external requests).
- *Managerial/training issues* – these should cover training in the OR and operating list issues.
- *Phones/bleeps.*
- *Noise levels.*

Standardizing to some extent the types of distractions that are assessed will allow better comparability across studies and, thus, a more robust evidence base.

Question 2: What is the Relationship between Distractions and Surgical Performance?

Two types of studies are likely to be informative. Firstly, studies using surgical simulators and the performance metrics that they provide (path length, time taken, economy of motion, and others) are useful in that they provide a micro-level analysis of the impact of distractions on performance. Secondly, observational studies in real ORs are needed, in which distractions should be assessed alongside performance. Both technical and non-technical aspects of surgeons' performance should be assessed. Technical performance can be assessed in real time by an expert observer, or via recording of a procedure and retrospective assessment outside the OR. Similarly, a number of tools are now available that assess teamworking in OR teams (e.g., Undre et al. 2007a) and surgeons' non-technical skills (e.g., Sevdalis et al. 2008, Yule et al. 2008). Concurrent administration of these tools will provide evidence of the impact of different distractors on performance and will also function as cross-validation studies for the tools involved.

At least three important considerations are likely to emerge from this stream of work. A first consideration is the role of expertise in managing distractions. Some of the studies that we reviewed suggest that expert surgeons are better equipped to cope with the disruptive working environment of the OR. If this finding is replicated and shown to be robust, it will carry obvious implications for how an OR should be managed when more junior surgeons are performing procedures (e.g., the radio should be switched off and phones/bleepers left outside). A second consideration is the role of individual differences in multi-tasking ability. Being disrupted from a task means that a surgeon is asked to multi-task – i.e., to shift attentional focus from the primary task to one or more secondary tasks. Psychological research suggests that such shifts come at a cost, as performance at the primary task deteriorates (e.g., Altmann and Trafton 2007, Monsell 2003, Trafton and Monk 2008) and that different people are affected to different degrees by such demands to multi-task (e.g., Ishizaka et al. 2001). This means that some surgeons will fare better than others in coping with distracting events in the OR – an individual difference that should be assessed systematically. A final consideration is the interaction of expertise and individual differences with the level of disruptiveness in the OR. Simply put, junior surgeons might be able to cope with an equipment failure when everything else is going smoothly in a procedure. However, if a technical problem appears jointly with an equipment failure in an OR team that does not communicate information very well, the same situation will become more stressful and the potential for impaired performance will increase. Multilayered disruptions to surgical work are likely to have an effect on performance significantly more pronounced than the effect of individual distracting events.

Question 3: Can the OR be Designed in Such a Way that Unnecessary Disruptions are Minimized?

The preliminary links between distractions, stress and performance are important from a patient safety perspective. Demirtas et al. (2004, p. 929) suggested that the 'aroused emotional state of surgeons during an operation make them more prone to make mistakes as a result of physical and mental fatigue and strain' and concluded that surgeons may have a legal responsibility to consider the negative impact of factors such as stressors, distractions and mental strain on their performance. Distractions can greatly add to stressors that are inherent in surgery and thus significantly increase stress by increasing demand upon the individual (see Figure 24.1). It follows that minimizing distractions in the OR environment wherever possible and/or by training surgeons in how best to cope with them when they occur is an important step towards safer surgery.

Some distractions, typically those associated with equipment, cannot be anticipated. Equipment might be checked in the beginning of the operating list and still fail unexpectedly. Adequate planning (part of efficient teamwork in the OR and potentially enhanced using simple interventions, such as an equipment checklist), however, should allow quick replacement and minimize disruption to the operative process. Other distractions are more amenable to control. Number of visitors in the OR can be reduced, phones/bleepers could be left outside the OR and answered by a floating member of staff, who can filter the information for urgency and decide whether the surgeon, or any other team member, should be interrupted. Vincent et al. (2006) and Bates (2000) have commented that most healthcare processes were not designed; instead, they evolved. Socio-technically complex, the OR is a workspace that could potentially benefit from evidence-base design, with user input (e.g., Reiling et al. 2004). Importantly, smaller- and larger-

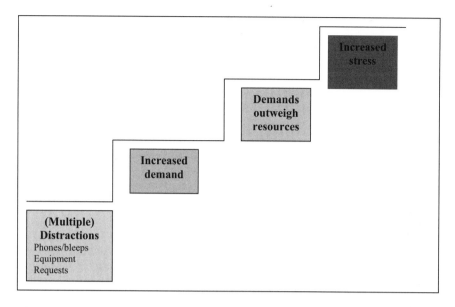

Figure 24.1   The distractions–stress ladder

scale design intervention should be evaluated for efficacy in reducing overall level of disruption and enhancing the flow of the surgical process (Campbell et al. 2000).

Acknowledgements

This chapter is based on an ongoing research programme on safety implications of the surgical environment that is being carried out by our research group. Dr Andrew N. Healey, former member of the group, played an instrumental role in the shaping and development of this work since its inception and over a number of years.

The authors would like to thank the Department of Health: Patient Safety Research Programme (CAV), the BUPA Foundation (CAV), the Smith and Nephew foundation (CAV), the Engineering and Physical Sciences Research Council (EPSRC) (CAV), and the Economic and Social Research Council (ESRC) Centre for Economic Learning and Social Evolution (NS) for providing funding for the work reported in this chapter.

References

Altmann, E.M. and Trafton, J.G. (2007) Timecourse of recovery from task interruption: Data and a model. *Psychonomic Bulletin and Review* 14, 1079–84.

Aggarwal, R., Moorthy, K. and Darzi, A. (2004) Laparoscopic skills training and assessment. *British Journal of Surgery* 91, 1549–58.

Aggarwal, R., Balasundaram, I. and Darzi, A. (2008) Training opportunities and the role of virtual reality simulation in acquisition of basic laparoscopic skills. *Journal of Surgical Research* 145, 80–6.

Alvarez, G. and Coiera, E. (2005) Interruptive communication patterns in the intensive care unit ward round. *International Journal of Medical Informatics* 74, 791–6.

Arora, S., Sevdalis, N., Nestel, D., Tierney, T., Woloshynowych, M. and Kneebone, R. (2009) Managing intra-operative stress: What do surgeons want from a crisis training program? *American Journal of Surgery*, 197, 537–543.

Bates, D.W. (2000) Using information technology to reduce rates of medication errors in hospitals. *British Medical Journal* 320, 788–91.

Brixey, J.J., Tang, Z., Robinson, D.J., Johnson, C.W., Johnson, T.R., Turley, J.P., Patel, V.L. and Zhang, J. (2008) Interruptions in one trauma center: A case study. *International Journal of Medical Informatics* 77, 235–41

Cabrera, I.N., and Lee, M.H. 2000. Reducing noise pollution in the hospital setting by establishing a department of sound: A survey of recent research on the effects of noise and music in health care. *Preventive Medicine* 30, 339–45.

Calland, J.F., Guerlain, S., Adams, R.B., Tribble, C.G., Foley, E. and Chekan, E.G. (2002) A systems approach to surgical safety. *Surgical Endoscopy* 16, 1005–14.

Campbell, M., Fitzpatrick, R., Haines, A., Kinmonth, A.L., Sandercock, P., Spiegelhalter, D. and Tyrer P. (2000) Framework for design and evaluation of complex interventions to improve health. *British Medical Journal* 321, 694–6.

Chisholm, C.D., Dornfeld, A.M., Nelson, D.R. and Cordell, W.H. (2001) Work interrupted: A comparison of workplace interruptions in emergency department and primary care offices. *Annals of Emergency Medicine* 38, 146–51.

Coiera, E. and Tombs, V. (1998) Communication behaviours in a hospital setting: An observational study. *British Medical Journal* 316, 673–7.

Dankelman, J. and Di Lorenzo, N. (2005) Surgical training and simulation. *Minimally Invasive Therapy and Allied Technologies* 14, 211–13.

Demirtas, Y., Tulmac, M., Yavuzer, R., Yalcin, R., Ayhan, S., Latifoglu, O. and Atabay, K. (2004) Plastic surgeon's life: Marvellous for mind, exhausting for body. *Plastic and Reconstructive Surgery* 114, 923–31.

Gawande, A.A., Zinner, M.J., Studdert, D.M. and Brennan, T.A. (2003) Analysis of errors reported by surgeons at three teaching hospitals. *Surgery* 133, 614–21.

Goodell, K.H., Cao, C.G.L. and Schwaitzberg, S.D. (2006) Effects of cognitive distraction on performance on laparoscopic tasks. *Journal of Laparoendoscopic and Advanced Surgical Techniques* 16, 94–8.

Greenberg, C.C., Regenbogen, S.E., Studdert, D.M., Lipsitz, S.R., Rogers, S.O., Zinner, M.J. and Gawande, A.A. (2007) Patterns of communication breakdowns resulting in injury to surgical patients. *Journal of the American College of Surgeons* 204, 533–40.

Hassan, I., Weyers, P., Maschuw, K., Dick, B., Gerdes, B., Rothmund, M. and Zielke, A. (2006) Negative stress-coping strategies among novices in surgery correlate with poor virtual laparoscopic performance. *British Journal of Surgery* 93, 1554–9.

Hawksworth, C.R., Asbury, A.J. and Millar, K. (1997) Music in theater: Not so harmonious. A survey of attitudes to music played in the operatic theater. *Anaethesia* 52, 79–83.

Hawksworth, C.R., Sivalingam, P. and Asbury, A.J. (1998) The effect of music on anaesthetists' psychomotor performance. *Anaethesia* 53, 195–7.

Healey, A.N. and Vincent, C. (2007) The systems of surgery. *Theoretical Issues in Ergonomic Science* 8, 429–43.

Healey, A.N., Sevdalis, N. and Vincent, C.A. (2006) Measuring intra-operative interference from distraction and interruption observed in the operating theatre. *Ergonomics* 49, 589–604.

Healey, A.N., Primus, C.P. and Koutantji M. (2007) Quantifying distraction and interruption in urological surgery. *Quality and Safety in Health Care* 16, 135–9.

Hodge, B. and Thompson, J.F. (1990) Noise pollution in the operating theatre. *Lancet* 335, 891–4.

Hsu, K.E., Man, F.Y., Gizicki, R.A., Feldman, L.S. and Fried, G.M. (2008) Experienced surgeons can do more than one thing at a time: Effect of distractions on performance of a simple laparoscopic and cognitive task by experienced and novice surgeons. *Surgical Endoscopy* 22, 196–201.

Ishizaka, K., Marshall, S.P. and Conte, J.M. (2001) Individual differences in attentional strategies in multitasking situations. *Human Performance* 14, 339–58.

Issenberg, S., Gordon, M.S., Gordon, D.L., Safford, R.E. and Hart, I.R. (2001) Simulation and new learning technologies. *Medical Teacher* 16, 16–23.

Miskovic, D., Rosenthal, R., Zingg, U., Oertli, D., Metzger, U. and Jancke, L. (2008) Randomised controlled trial investigating the effect of music on the virtual reality laparoscopic learning performance of novice surgeons. *Surgical Endoscopy* 22, 2416–20.

Monsell, S. (2003) Task switching. *Trends in Cognitive Science* 7, 134–40.

Moorthy, K., Munz, Y., Dosis, A., Bann, S. and Darzi, A. (2003) The effect of stress-inducing conditions on the performance of a laparoscopic task. *Surgical Endoscopy* 17, 1481–4.

Moorthy, K., Munz, Y., Undre, S. and Darzi, A. (2004) Objective evaluation of the effect of noise on the performance of a complex laparoscopic task. *Surgery* 136, 25–30.

Murthy, V.S.S.N., Mlhotra, S.K., Bala, I. and Raghunathan, M. (1995) Detrimental effects of noise on anaesthetists. *Canadian Journal of Anaesthesia* 42, 608–11.

Primus, C.P., Healey, A.N. and Undre, S. (2007) Distraction in the urology operating theatre. *BJU International* 99, 493–4.

Reiling, J.G., Knutzen, B.L., Wallen, T.K., McCullough, S., Miller, R. and Chernos, S. (2004) Enhancing the traditional hospital design process: A focus on patient safety. *Joint Commission Journal on Quality and Patient Safety* 3, 1–10.

Royal College of Surgeons of England (2007) Safe Shift Working for Surgeons in Training: Revised Policy Statement from the Working Time Directive Working Party. London: Royal College of Surgeons of England

Saegert, S. and Winkel, G.H. (1990) Environmental psychology. *Annual Review of Psychology* 41, 441–77.

Schuetz, M., Gockel, I., Beardi, J., Hakman, P., Dunschede, F., Moenk, S., Heinrichs, W. and Junginger, T. (2008) Three different types of surgeon-specific stress reactions identified by laparoscopic simulation in a virtual scenario. *Surgical Endoscopy* 22, 1263-7.

Shapiro, K.A. and Berland, T. (1972) Noise in the operating room. *New England Journal of Medicine* 287, 1236–8.

Sevdalis, N., Healey, A.N. and Vincent, C.A. (2007) Distracting communications in the operating theatre. *Journal of Evaluation in Clinical Practice* 13, 390–4.

Sevdalis, N., Forrest, D., Undre, S., Darzi, A. and Vincent, C.A. (2008) Annoyances, disruptions, and interruptions in surgery: The Disruptions in Surgery Index (Disi). *World Journal of Surgery* 32, 1643–50.

Sundstrom, E., Bell, P.A., Busby, P.L. and Asmus, C. (1996) Environmental psychology 1989–1994. *Annual Review of Psychology* 47, 485–512.

Trafton, J.G. and Monk, C.M. (2008) Task interruptions. In D.A. Boehm-Davis (ed.), *Reviews of Human Factors and Ergonomics, Volume 3* (pp. 111–26). Santa Monica, CA: Human Factors and Ergonomics Society.

Undre, S., Sevdalis, N., Healey, A.N., Darzi, A. and Vincent, C.A. (2006a) Teamwork in the operating theatre: Cohesion or confusion? *Journal of Evaluation in Clinical Practice* 12, 182–9.

Undre, S., Healey, A.N., Darzi, A. and Vincent C.A. (2006b) Observational assessment of surgical teamwork: A feasibility study. *World Journal of Surgery* 30, 1774–83.

Undre, S., Sevdalis, N., Healey, A.N., Darzi, A. and Vincent, C.A. (2007a) Observational teamwork assessment for surgery (OTAS): Refinement and application in urological surgery. *World Journal of Surgery* 31, 1373–81.

Undre, S., Koutantji, M., Sevdalis, N., Gautama, S., Selvapatt, N., Williams, S., Sains, P., McCulloch, P., Darzi, A. and Vincent, C.A. (2007b) Multidisciplinary crisis simulations: The way forward for training surgical teams. *World Journal of Surgery* 31, 1843–53.

Verdaasdonk, E.G.G., Stassen, L.P.S., van der Elst, M., Karsten, T.M. and Dankelman, J. (2007) Problems with equipment during laparoscopic surgery. *Surgical Endoscopy* 21, 275–9.

Verdaasdonk, E.G.G., Stassen, L.P.S., Hoffman, W.F., van der Elst, M. and Dankelman, J. (2008) Can a structured checklist prevent problems with laparoscopic equipment? *Surgical Endoscopy* 22, 2238–43.

Vincent, C., Moorthy, K., Sarker, S. K., Chang, A. and Darzi, A.W. (2004) Systems approaches to surgical quality and safety: From concept to measurement. *Ann. Surg.* 239(4), 475–82.

Vincent, C.A., Lee, A.C.H. and Hanna, G.B. (2006) Patient safety alerts: A balance between evidence and action. *Archives of Disease in Childhood Fetal and Neonatal Edition* 91, 314–15.

Wetzel, C.M., Kneebone, R.L., Woloshynowych, M., Nestel, D., Moorthy, K., Kidd, J. and Darzi, A. (2006) The effects of stress on surgical performance. *American Journal of Surgery* 191, 5–10.

Wiegmann, D.A., ElBardissi, A.W., Dearani, J.A., Daly, R.C., and Sundt, T.M. (2007). Disruptions in surgical flow and their relationship to surgical errors: An exploratory investigation. *Surgery* 142, 658–65.

Yule, S., Flin, R., Paterson-Brown, S. and Maran, N. (2006) Non-technical skills for surgeons. A review of the literature. *Surgery* 139, 140–9.

Yule, S., Flin, R., Maran, N., Rowley, D.R., Youngson, G.G. and Paterson-Brown, S. (2008) Surgeons' non-technical skills in the operating room: Reliability testing of the NOTSS behaviour rating system. *World Journal of Surgery* 32, 548–56.

Part IV
Discussions

Chapter 25

Putting Behavioural Markers to Work: Developing and Evaluating Safety Training in Healthcare Settings

David Musson

Introduction

Like others in this book, the impetus to write this chapter came from a meeting that was held in Edinburgh in 2007 that brought together some of us who were active or interested in research aimed at understanding and improving the performance of teams in the operating room (or the operating theatre, as my friends in the United Kingdom would say). As I sat listening to colleagues from Europe and North America describe their excellent work in defining and training non-technical skills, I was left with a nagging sense that we were missing something important.

Although I had started my career in medicine, I had spent many of the last 15 years immersed in aviation safety – first in the Canadian Air Force, and more recently at the University of Texas at Austin studying under, then working alongside, Bob Helmreich, with whose work some readers are likely familiar. Arriving in Austin in 1998, I had essentially parachuted into the world of CRM – crew resource management. Crew resource management is the term that has been given to training programmes developed within the aviation world to teach or train commercial and military pilots in human factors, leadership and crew management with the ultimate goal of improving flight safety. As a physician landing in one of the major CRM research groups in the world, it took some time to adjust to the differences in the ways my new colleagues looked at teamwork and the way I had been used to thinking of it in medicine. It would have been fair to say that I was not used to thinking about teamwork at all, but rather was comfortable looking at performance in terms of individual (or more specifically *my own*) competence in what I now realized were team settings. I do not think I was unique in that sense, and in fact my impression since that time has been that most physicians are worried about, first and foremost, their own competence. Indeed, one can argue that individual practitioner competence has long been perceived as the fundamental cornerstone of quality medical care. It is why medical schools are supposed to be difficult to get into, and why medical school curricula are typically challenging and the study load demanding. It is also why the training hours are long and arduous, and why current efforts to reduce those hours are sometimes met with resistance. Like many physicians, I had prided myself on believing I was competent (and I think I actually was competent…), and, again, like many physicians, I was not overly keen to delve into human error in medicine and team performance in healthcare. For many of us, that topic feels just a little too close to home, at least at first take. Rather, I focused most of my interest and efforts on our work in aviation safety. I learned about CRM training, which by that time had ceased to be a controversial topic in aviation and by then had become the standard of practice for any good airline.

Rather than defining CRM and developing training programmes for aviation, our lab's efforts at that time were focused on in-flight data collection – trying to understand what worked and what did not in the cockpit; on what practices the good pilots demonstrated, and what we thought the rest should try and emulate. These were the early days of LOSA – the Line Operations Safety Audit. The University of Texas LOSA programme involved sending observers from our lab group out onto aircraft flight decks to watch crews at work as they flew routine flights, recording crew behaviours and errors, and noting their responses to safety threats (Helmreich et al. 2002). Our experience was showing us that when LOSA audits went ahead without management support, then resources were scarce and the projects tended to stall. When senior management pushed for an audit, but the pilots were mired in labour disputes or felt they were being used as scapegoats for problems on the flight line, observers from our lab were greeted with suspicion in the cockpit and again, safety audits stalled. When everyone in the organization was on board, and when both senior management and pilot unions were enthusiastic supporters of the safety audit, the process was typically a major success, and the organizations would devour the findings produced by the audit. There was a sense that everything was moving forward as it should, and that we were all contributing to something valuable.

I was fortunate to be a part of those efforts. We all had the sense we were doing something worthwhile. Despite the difficulties associated with research and the challenges in producing empirical validation, few in our lab group or in commercial aviation for that matter seemed to doubt the effectiveness of CRM, or the value of trying to improve it. During this time, many of the first efforts in trying to bring CRM to healthcare were underway. David Gaba at Stanford had already started his Anesthesia Crisis Resource Management training programme (Gaba et al. 1992), which was receiving positive reviews in the safety community. Bob Helmreich had been working with Swiss collaborators to bring CRM to operating room teams in that country (Helmreich et al. 1994). MedTeams, a commercial training group out of Boston, had produced a consulting and training product and had brought their version of healthcare CRM to several sites in the United States (Morey et al. 2002). By the late 1990s, Rhona Flin and colleagues in Scotland had started work on the Anaesthesia Non-Technical Skills project, an empirically derived, non-technical skills rating system (Fletcher et al. 2003) that remains one of the stand-out efforts to date in our growing field (see also Chapter 12 in this volume). In the US, healthcare team training (or CRM, or non-technical skills programmes) is offered at a number of simulation centres, and such courses tend to be focused on the operating room, the intensive care unit or cardiac arrest management. Training is also offered through professional consulting organizations providing a range of related leadership training, organizational assessment, culture change, and team training services. Around 2003, Bob Helmreich and I wrote some of our impressions and thoughts in a paper entitled 'Team training and resource management in healthcare: current issues and future directions' (Musson and Helmreich 2004). Details of these early programmes are described in that paper, along with some worries about how things were proceeding. Our concern at that time was primarily that CRM was becoming a private consulting project in many quarters, and that the open, collaborative environment that fostered the growth and success of CRM in aviation was almost nowhere to be found. Thankfully, this is changing, as demonstrated by the behavioural markers researchers meeting in Edinburgh, 2007 that was organized by Rhona Flin and that spawned this book. However, there is still a nagging discomfort in the back of my mind that has been present since I first became aware of the potential promise of CRM to improve healthcare delivery. That discomfort stems from the sense that there are fundamental differences between healthcare and aviation, and that these differences stand to undermine the many efforts underway that are trying to improve how teams work in critical healthcare settings. This chapter, hopefully, articulates some of those concerns and helps shed light on how some of us should proceed on this important, though sometimes frustrating path.

CRM in Aviation

There is some value in briefly revisiting what CRM really is in aviation. In that industry, CRM has undergone a long evolution over the past 30 years – this has been described elsewhere, and I will not belabour the chronology of increments and evolutions in this chapter. As seen through the eyes of those in healthcare who have looked to aviation for system improvement, CRM has been interpreted as a set of skills that should be trained in order to improve teamwork and improve safety. In a sense this is true, though some key points seem to have been lost in transition. CRM is as much an organizational philosophy as it is a training programme. I was not around in the earliest days, but if I had to guess, I would imagine that this has not always been the case. CRM started as a means of training better cockpit leadership skills, but soon became integrated with human factors training in general – a more comprehensive training movement that dealt with the risks posed by the ways humans operate in complex settings. For example, good CRM courses include didactic teaching or small group workshops that focus on such things as the effects of fatigue on concentration, memory and decision-making; curricula include discussions on how family stressors can serve as distractions and how telling your crewmates of such stressors helps alert everyone to the potential impact of those stressors in the cockpit on that day. Such material serves not only to add to the base of knowledge essential for understanding how good CRM works, it also serves to shift attitudes among trainees from one of autonomous independence to one of team-centred interdependence. The concept of safety as an underlying fundamental (or super-ordinate) goal that serves to unify team members' motivations and behaviours is stressed as a fundamental principle of crew management.

Over time, as new pilots are indoctrinated into CRM and adopt its principles of crew management and as the majority of pilots in various airlines adopt a team-centred approach to daily operations, the principles expounded by CRM seem to have permeated the senior ranks of commercial aviation and the very culture of flight operations. This is not surprising, as senior pilots tend to fill both middle and upper management positions at most airlines. It is not uncommon to hear pilots describe management's actions and decisions in terms of 'good CRM' or 'bad CRM'.

All that is CRM, of course, has taken root in the pre-existing operating environments of aviation and over the pre-existing cultures of piloting. Cockpits are small, both in terms of space and in terms of crew numbers – always at least two in number (in commercial aircraft, at least), and seldom more than three. Everyone in the cockpit has essentially the same training, often very common backgrounds, and even similar personality types. Pilots did their jobs very well before CRM ever came along, and in that light, CRM can be thought of as the icing on the cake of high-level team performance. CRM provided a framework to help highly functioning teams become even better. The infrequent mishaps that had occurred in aviation in the years prior to the introduction of CRM, where miscommunication between or intimidation of crew members contributed to mishaps, became even less common thanks to improved awareness of human factors and to the skills introduced into crew training through CRM. It is important to remember that CRM was never brought in at the expense of existing good practices. What we used to call good 'airmanship' has been expanded to include the fundamental elements and principles of CRM, and the culture has undergone a re-conceptualization of piloting competency that integrates both technical proficiency and CRM as essential skill sets.

CRM in Medicine

As mentioned above, a number of individuals began looking at developing CRM, or non-technical skills training programs for healthcare in the 1990s. In 1999, the Institute of Medicine (IOM) released its report *To Err is Human: Building a Safer Health System* (Kohn et al. 2000). In it, aviation-based CRM was identified as a key strategy that held great promise for reducing error in the complex treatment teams that are ubiquitous in modern healthcare. This triggered immediate interest in CRM and the activities of our lab in Texas, and set in motion a growing interest in the subject that has only gotten stronger with time.

But, as I mentioned at the opening of this chapter, I have had a nagging feeling that CRM was not quite the answer that many thought. The parallels between the operating room and the cockpit seemed obvious to many and to me as well, but I thought that there seemed as many differences as similarities. Compared to the civilized two-person teams I had seen in cockpits, the operating room had always felt like a jungle to me. People came and went throughout each operation. As a medical student and intern, I never knew the identities of at least half of the masked people in the room, and I was never sure if anyone could actually name each person who came and went. Maybe the circulating nurse knew who they were, but I sure didn't. Sometimes, she would switch out mid-procedure when her shift ended, and a new person (whose identity was also unknown to me) would come into the room to take her place without a word being spoken. At times the atmosphere was casual and light-hearted, at other times it was tense and sometimes hostile. Instruments do get thrown – that is not an urban legend; I have seen it happen on more than one occasion. More often, insults were thrown, usually directed to residents or interns, though also at times they would be cast at entire groups (non-surgical specialties were a frequent target). Eyebrows were used to communicate disapproval and irritation, and could be used to do so quite effectively. The humour was at times bawdy, and as the lowly medical student you were not always quite sure when you should laugh and when you should remain quiet. It was always safer to just hold the retractor as instructed, though one could never go wrong nodding in silent agreement with whoever was most senior. Production pressure was paramount. Anything that delayed the completion of the case had the potential to upset the rest of the day's list and a number of people in the room. Everyone seemed to have their own job; there was seldom any sharing of tasks and there seemed little awareness about what others' jobs entailed. The ether screen, suspended between two poles on either side of the patient's head, served to separate the world of surgery from the world of anaesthesia. Sometimes it seemed higher than it needed to be. Maybe it was to protect against flying instruments, I wondered. As a doctor in training, I knew virtually nothing of the world of nurses, except that in the operating room they seemed efficient and key to everything that transpired, though they were typically silent. This was my impression of surgical operating teams, and to me, introducing CRM skills like briefing and cross-checking would not necessarily make things run all that much better. The idea that CRM would fix everything I had seen in training and later in practice seemed a tall order.

Undaunted by the challenge and motivated by a sincere desire to make healthcare safer, a number of parties have forged onward in their attempts to improve the performance of operating room teams, and of teams elsewhere in healthcare through the development and implementation of CRM-like training. At the time of writing this chapter, I have since moved on from Bob Helmreich's group (and he has retired) and I now oversee simulation and non-technical skills at McMaster University. As such, I find myself dealing with the front line issues of integrating CRM or non-technical skills into the postgraduate medical curriculum at our university, and with integrating simulation and patient safety into a number of undergraduate programmes. Indeed, simulation is by many accounts a valuable tool in our arsenal as we look for the best ways to improve healthcare team behaviour. There are many challenges, such as how we first introduce these concepts and at what level. Or, how we educate the practising provider population so that our trainees do not meet resistance to using their new-found skills as they move on from our educational programmes and into the day-to-day working environment of healthcare? I, like others, am grateful for the work of our Scottish colleagues who have developed the ANTS methodologies, and the more recent Non-Technical Skills for Surgeons (NOTSS) system that you will find described elsewhere in this book (see Chapter 2). I remain convinced that these programmes are on the right track and should be integrated into any efforts to improve operating room team performance.

There are a number of us struggling with these same challenges of how best to design, deliver and evaluate CRM or non-technical skills training for healthcare. Many efforts in this area have stalled, or have produced less radical change in the day-to-day behaviour of operating room teams than some had hoped. Anecdotally, it is common to hear frustrations from those who have attempted to implement such programmes. Beginning with early programmes, such as MedTeams, and progressing to the current day, trainers and course developers lament the difficulty of getting the simplest of interventions to be adopted, though often these frustrations are voiced in private since many of these efforts involve either commercial consulting groups or academic centres where project failure is not well regarded. Efforts to bring team skills training to healthcare are resource intensive and expensive. When clinical champions and institutional leaders have fought hard to bring in expensive training programmes into their local institutions, challenges are not usually discussed openly and outright failures are sometimes denied.

So, why does this training sometimes seem less successful than we would like? Why is there resistance among highly competent professionals to adopt practices that we think make perfect sense? Presumably these individuals are interested in delivering quality care, regardless of what other competing demands may be present. Aviation had its difficulties and challenges for sure, but either the challenges in healthcare are greater or the standard for success is higher. Possibly both are factors. The threshold for determining success in healthcare is frankly more rigorous than it ever was for aviation. Decision-makers want hard evidence of success before scant resources are directed towards CRM and team training courses. A poorly known (and seldom communicated) fact of aviation safety is that evidence for the success of CRM has actually been quite elusive. Eduardo Salas at the University of Central Florida has written extensively and thoroughly on issues related to the validation of CRM training, and in particular on the challenges of validating such training in the complex operational environments of healthcare and aviation (for detailed reviews of CRM evaluation, see Salas et al. 1999, 2006). In this chapter, however, we will assume that improving teamwork, sharing expectations associated with the task at hand, informing others of one's plans, improving communication in general, task redundancy, reducing needless variability and having team members monitor each other to improve reliability are all good things, and that programmes to encourage these behaviours should have at least some positive benefit on team performance in healthcare.

In this chapter, I want to examine what it is that seems to be standing in the way of many sincere and diligent efforts to improve team performance. Take the example of the 'surgical time out' or 'surgical pause' (WHO 2008). This is the practice of ensuring everyone is present at the start of a surgical case, where the identity of the patient is confirmed, along with the site of surgery and confirmation of the specific nature of the procedure. This was introduced to prevent wrong-site, wrong-patient surgical errors. It can also serve as a tool to communicate expectations between team members, brief potential contingencies and possible complications, and provide an opportunity to clarify everyone's mental model of what is about to transpire. This is what those of us in aviation safety would call 'basic CRM', and is an example of how we would get team members to 'share their mental model' amongst each other. It is current best practice for surgical care, and in North America is encouraged or required by agencies such as the Joint Commission, the Institute for Healthcare Improvement (IHI), and the Canadian Patient Safety Institute. To most of us in the error/CRM/non-technical skills world, the value of the surgical time out is obvious, and any downsides are almost impossible to identify. Yet, accounts of difficulties in implementing this simplest of practices abound. Some surgeons refuse to do it, others roll their eyes, while yet others are reported to ridicule the resident or nurse who reminds them that the practice be followed. In other centres, certainly, the practice is adopted and enthusiastically supported. The question remains, why the difference and why would anyone resist? It is a simple behaviour. The theoretical basis for it is strong. The amount of effort is minimal. Is it because it is being forced, and anti-authoritarian tendencies cause some to rebel? Is it seen as a loss of professional autonomy? Do they not believe that it makes any sense? Is there a perceived loss of efficiency in the operating room? Surely, if such a simple practice meets with resistance, more complex and less concrete practices are also doomed, at least in some settings.

Let's start with the basics. CRM, or non-technical skills programmes, involve the process of describing the behaviours of highly competent, safe individuals. A current approach in healthcare is to develop a comprehensive list of such behaviours and develop a training programme around that list. Surely ANTS and NOTSS are excellent examples. Those systems have been empirically derived, agreed upon by a consensus of experienced practitioners, and the face validity of their component elements is strong. Good training programmes may also involve a significant amount of supporting theory, didactically delivered and well founded in psychology and experience. Some programmes even involve significant coaching with ongoing reinforcement. Yet the desired behavioural changes in team members have not been consistently observed following training and even in well-designed programmes, resistance is not uncommon.

There are certainly examples of poorly run training programmes, some lasting only an afternoon, without opportunity to practise skills or provide feedback, and without a plan for reinforcement over time. Some programmes are simply copies of aviation programmes, with little domain specificity, and we would not expect such programmes to result in major changes in team behaviour. But, some courses seem extremely well designed, and much effort has gone into their delivery and implementation. Yet, still, many of these programmes have failed to produce the desired outcomes.

Are we right to be focusing on behaviours? The term in our field is *behavioural markers*, and it refers to the explicit, observable actions of team members. Our thinking to date has largely been to identify the optimal behaviour set employed by ideal practitioners, usually arrived at through consensus methods, and teach everyone to practise those same behaviours. Seems straightforward. But, what are human behaviours? Why do people behave the way they do? Why do good team players naturally share their plans with their team members, even without being told to do so? Why do some people resist changes even when they seem to make sense? If we think of behaviour as stemming from our cognition – action from thought, as some would say – then the question becomes: what are they thinking and why? If we are going to change the way people behave in the operating room, or elsewhere in healthcare for that matter, we need to be examining why they do what they do.

Behind the observable behaviours of an individual lie the various processes of human cognition. This includes all of the things that influence our moment-to-moment and day-to-day thinking, working away in our minds, often below the surface and out of sight: our values, attitudes, perceived responsibilities, memories, and even our own personality characteristic tendencies. Furthermore, we can ask what has led us to have those attitudes and beliefs. In our work settings, this may be the professional cultures into which we have been acculturated, or the many interactions we have had with others over our careers, or even the national and organizational cultures that surround us at home and work. All of these factors influence who we are and how we think. You can picture an iceberg, with the base being the social structures, cultural backgrounds and organizational milieu in which we live lying deeply below the surface of the water. Examples of these deep-seated influences may include pre-existing social attitudes about gender and roles, or more concrete factors like the lounge that allows surgeons, but not nurses, to relax and make telephone calls between cases and the messages that this gives us. These factors serve as the foundation for the middle layer, which lies just below the surface: our day-to-day thinking; the attitudes, values and cognitive processes. The top of the iceberg, rising above the surface, represents our observable behaviours; the only thing others can see from the outside. I have drawn this below in Figure 25.1.

This chapter is about behavioural markers, training and learning from aviation, so let's go back to aviation for a minute. CRM had its challenges, to be sure, but the healthcare experience, I believe, is proving more problematic and the road

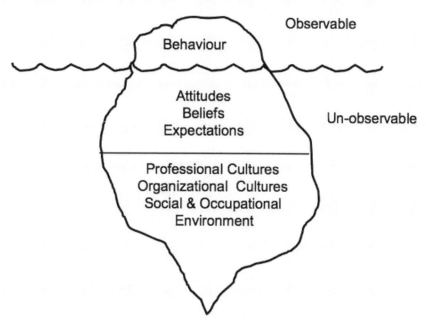

Figure 25.1   An iceberg model for observed behaviours

more uneven. Why did CRM seem to work more easily in aviation, or at least why is it more readily accepted now? If we examine the nature of aviation teams, what do we find? Captains and first officers, as I have mentioned, are similar – similar backgrounds (flight school), similar interests (airplanes), similar frustrations (Air Traffic Control), and even similar haircuts. They share their jobs – often alternating who is in command and who is monitoring on each successive flight. There is little confusion about the goal – a smooth flight and safe landing. The only major barriers to communication are usually hierarchy, experience and sometimes a tendency to work as an individual and not as a team. CRM was designed to address these barriers; hence, much of its focus is on overcoming hierarchical barriers to communication, sharing plans for the purpose of mutual understanding and the importance of coordinating tasks in cockpit crews.

An important question to ask is this: do surgical teams encounter the same challenges as those encountered by pilots? By this I am not referring to flap settings vs. intubation difficulties; obviously the technical challenges are different. But, are the barriers to the fluid flow of information due to the same issues of command hierarchy? Sometimes, perhaps, but is this always the case? Are there other barriers? Interprofessional friction, for example? Is there a perception that the job of the anaesthesiologist is separate from that of the surgeon? Do surgeons, anaesthesiologists and operating room nurses have similar personalities, similar experiences and identical goals? Professional subgroups, or occupational subcultures as some call them, are everywhere in healthcare. Doctors, nurses, medical sub-specialists, technicians and therapists – all see themselves as groups distinct from each other. They relax in different lounges, use language and jargon specific to their subgroups, and wear trappings and symbols of their group membership. There are hierarchical barriers within disciplines (residents/registrars and consultants) and between disciplines (who is in charge in the operating room: anaesthesia or surgery? Asking this can start a brawl...) and of course, between professions (doctors, nurses and others).

Each sub-group or discipline has its own perceived strengths and roles. Some see themselves as doing the primary job at hand (such as surgery), while others may see themselves as risk mitigators (such as anaesthesia). Each believes they are doing their job to the best of their ability; the surgeons are typically technically competent, the anaesthesiologists maintain stability of the patient, the nurses ensure order in the room, produce equipment for the surgeon as needed without delay and count sponges to make certain nothing is left behind. Friction between sub-groups and sub-cultures is common. Humour may be directed at one group or another, and disparaging generalizations about one profession or another, or about one specialty or another are not rare.

If we return to our iceberg diagram, we can picture a schism or a fault in the base – a rift between groups, or dysfunctional professional cultures. The problem may be specific to one team, or characteristic of a given culture in an entire hospital or teaching centre. It may be the doctors-only lounge that was mentioned earlier. This fault in the foundation of team structure leads to dysfunctional attitudes, biases and differing values within those teams, and eventually manifests as poor team behaviours – perhaps a tendency toward individualistic behaviour or a reluctance to help out with heavy workload. An example of such behaviour would be a reluctance to ask for help with a busy taskload, either because mutual support is not part of the culture, or because a practitioner could be self-conscious about appearing to not be able to cope with his or her workload. A particular work setting may well evolve its own fixes and informal countermeasures to deal with perceived risks to safety or deficiencies in team performance. These may take the shape of unofficial rules, or things nurses do without the physicians' awareness to try and ensure safety and quality. The visible behaviours resulting from deep-seated fractures within the team structure can be more egregious: insults, disrespect or open hostility.

Anecdotes of team dysfunction are rampant in healthcare, though systematic analysis is seldom found in the literature. These are stories shared in the nurses' or residents' lounges or over drinks with colleagues on a Friday night. Few of us would expect that CRM training or non-technical skills courses would likely eradicate these problems, and resistance to change can come from either a perception that the new skills offered will undermine existing practices, or because the underlying team structure is so dysfunctional that no brief training programme is likely to repair the existing degree of damage.

So, back to aviation. Is there anything that the aviation industry can teach us about how to implement changes in team behaviour? Our experience with LOSA, as you might remember from earlier in this chapter, was that without both senior management and workforce buy-in, our efforts often proved futile. In healthcare, this would mean getting senior administrative personnel to support team improvement efforts (specifically, the chief executive officer, the chief of medical staff and the chief nursing officer, at a minimum), and in the case of the operating room, the heads of surgery, anaesthesia and nursing. Why is this important? Without the support of the senior executive of an organization, resources will not be adequate and those trying to implement change will find institutional resistance acting as a major barrier to their efforts. It strikes me that I have not defined 'support'. By support, I mean money (which is rare), not a letter of support (which is more common). These projects require resources. They may require operating rooms to close for training, which means loss of revenue. Senior management in one institution may choose to pay staff to attend training, while in other institutions they may be expected to attend on their own time. Without buy-in from key physicians and nurses, medical and nursing staff are unlikely to role model and encourage the proposed changes, and desired behaviours and practices will likely disappear after training, despite best intentions.

Our experiences in healthcare CRM, however, suggest that top-level and practitioner support alone is not likely to be enough. Many of us in this field often say that healthcare is more complex than aviation, but what does that mean? This belief really relates to the nature of our work groups more than it does to the actual work itself. Teams in healthcare are unstable; their members come and go through the course of the week, the day and even the procedure. Multiple professions and disciplines, as discussed above, must work together, and often must deal with unusual stresses and sources of friction. It is no secret that in many institutions, bad behaviour on the part of some senior staff is tolerated. The growing numbers of formal codes of conduct currently appearing in our hospitals attest to this fact, as institutions try to find administrative tools to deal with the problem of disrespectful and offensive behaviour. Such issues must be dealt with if any attempt to improve team performance is going to succeed. Our experience in aviation was that disruptive and abusive pilots were strong resistors of CRM and actively tried to subvert those programmes when they first appeared.

Will CRM or Non-Technical Skills Training Work in Healthcare?

There is probably little doubt that in well-functioning operating rooms teams (and for teams elsewhere in healthcare), CRM and non-technical skills training can raise reliability and safety to a higher level. The important question is how do we go about implementing this, or what else needs be done? Paul Uhlig, another participant at the Edinburgh meeting in 2007 and contributor to this book (see Chapter 26), has written and spoken extensively about the need to reform healthcare. He has suggested that the future of healthcare is to reform the working relationships that exist throughout our systems, and he probably has the right idea. Without addressing the underlying dysfunction of the work environment in this industry, without addressing interprofessional friction, and without addressing organizational issues in how we encourage (or fail to encourage) optimal team performance, it is difficult to see how behavioural marker-based, CRM-oriented team training programmes will take hold and be able to deliver their potential in improving the quality of care that is delivered in our current systems.

So, looking back, what was it that made me worry that adapting CRM and similar practices from aviation would fail to produce the benefits that many had expected? It was the suspicion that CRM alone was too easy a solution to the complex problems that surround medical error and team dysfunction. Physician, surgeon, and nursing cultures have evolved to function within the systems in which they operate, and indeed have created key elements of the very system itself. Well-designed CRM programmes may address some of the issues that arise in those teams, and may provide a safety net that traps potential errors before they occur. But will a training programme, once delivered, continue to influence behaviour in any one setting or surgical unit? Possibly, but our experience from aviation and our early experience from healthcare suggests the impact of training may quickly decay. If the programme itself suffers from a perceived lack of relevance, then its decay will be almost immediate.

So, how do we ensure that trained safety behaviours persist? How do we make training relevant to front-line personnel? To be relevant, programmes must be well designed conceptually and must address practical issues in the environment in which they are introduced. Basing such training programmes on front-line safety and error data was responsible for major improvements in the effectiveness of CRM in aviation. Often now called threat and error management (or TEM), this most recent variant of CRM is more proactive, more relevant and likely more effective than earlier generations of training. Does this mean that behavioural markers are no longer pertinent? Certainly not; they still form the foundation of CRM and TEM. Markers represent the behavioural tools that good crews and good practitioners continue to use to manage and perform in effective teams, but behavioural markers alone do not a training programme make. Continually incorporated front-line data allow course designers and trainers to shape programmes and produce training products that are not only more effective, but also more likely to be perceived as effective by front-line personnel. In a sense, data tell one where and when to apply CRM, and tells the organization where to restructure operations to improve safety.

In healthcare, we often lack the data for any given organization that tells us where vulnerabilities lie. We also often lack the understanding of what the underlying cultural issues are at work below the surface that leads to the problems in team performance we see all too frequently. This book describes some of the best research currently being done in the area of behavioural markers in surgical and other healthcare settings. For those of us who now seem to be spending more time on the training and education side of the equation, the question becomes what do we do with the outcomes of this impressive body of research? Somewhere between fixing the underlying dysfunctional cultural of healthcare and finding a way of measuring what goes wrong on the front lines of healthcare delivery, training programmes to improve teamwork represent the future of improved healthcare quality. Behavioural markers will be the key to those programmes, and improved team culture will be the fertile ground on which they will take root.

References

Fletcher, G., Flin, R., McGeorge, P., Glavin, R., Maran, N. and Patey, R. (2003) Anaesthetists' Non-Technical Skills (ANTS): Evaluation of a behavioural marker system. *British Journal of Anesthesia* 90, 580–8.

Gaba, D.M., Howard, S.K., Fish, K.J., Yang, G. and Sarnquist, F. (1992) Anesthesia crisis resource management training: Teaching anesthesiologists to handle critical incidents. *Aviation Space and Environmental Medicine* 63, 763–70.

Helmreich, R.L., Schaefer, H.G. and Bogner, M.S. (1994) Team performance in the operating room. *Human Error in Medicine.* Hillsdale, NJ: Lawrence Erlbaum Associates.

Helmreich, R.L., Klinect, J.R., Wilhelm, J., Tesmer, B., Gunther, D., Thomas, R., Romeo, C., Sumwalt, R. and Maurino, D. (2002) *Line Operations Safety Audit (LOSA).* Montreal. Available at: <http://homepage.psy.utexas.edu/homepage/group/HelmreichLAB/Aviation/LOSA/LOSA.html> [last accessed June 2009].

Kohn, L.T., Corrigan, J. and Donaldson, M.S. (2000) *To Err is Human: Building a Safer Health System.* Washington, DC: National Academies Press.

Morey, J., Simon, R., Jay, G., Wears, R., Salisbury, M., Dukes, K. and Berns, S. (2002) Error reduction and performance improvement in the emergency department through formal teamwork training: Evaluation results of the MedTeams Project. *Health Services Research* 37, 1553–81.

Musson, D. M. and Helmreich, R.L. (2004) Team training and resource management in healthcare: Current issues and future directions. *Harvard Health Policy Review* 5, 25–35.

Salas, E., Burke, C.S., Bowers, C.A. and Wilson, K.A. (1999) Team training in the skies: Does crew resource management (CRM) training work? *Human Factors* 43, 641–74.

Salas, E., Wilson, K.A., Burke, C.S. and Wightman, D.C. (2006) Does crew resource management training work? An update, an extension, and some critical needs. *Human Factors* 48, 392–412.

WHO (2008) *World Alliance for Patient Safety. WHO Guidelines for Safe Surgery.* Geneva: World Health Organization.

Chapter 26

Commentary and Clinical Perspective

Paul Uhlig

Introduction

Eight years ago the cardiac surgery team that I led at Concord Hospital, Concord, New Hampshire, began a remarkable association with an expert in aviation safety and human factors science.

I remember the first day that Jeff Brown accompanied our care team as we made rounds in the ICU and on the post-operative floor. During the course of the morning Jeff made many notes on a yellow legal pad as he watched and listened attentively. I was very curious about what he was observing and writing.

Later a small group of us sat down with Jeff to review his observations. It became quickly apparent that Jeff was interpreting the work of our team from a conceptual framework we had never heard of before. It was humbling and surprising to learn from Jeff about safety science, high reliability organization theory and what is known about optimum teamwork in high risk settings. We literally had no idea.

Over time our care team undertook the challenge of translating these concepts of safety and high reliability into our daily interactions and work processes. We began having weekly team meetings. We started making rounds together each day using a consistent method of information sharing and action planning that we called the 'collaborative communications cycle'. We took steps to lower the hierarchy of our team to actively protect and seek out the insights of the quietest voices on our team. We built in ways of reflecting together about our work so we could identify problems together and correct them at a system level. We involved patients and family members in ways we had never considered before.

As we adopted these new ways of working together many things changed. Our outcomes became measurably better in multiple dimensions – safety, efficiency, patient satisfaction and professional satisfaction. Our thinking changed, from an individual emphasis to a system focus. Other things changed as well: how we felt about each other and about our work, and even what we considered important.

Our patients told us they had never experienced anything like this before, and never wanted us to go back to the old ways. Our team received the Eisenberg Patient Safety Award, the highest award in patient safety given by the Joint Commission on Accreditation of Healthcare Organizations and the National Quality Forum (The Joint Commission 2008). It is fair to say that my life as a surgeon has never been the same since.

Pioneering Work

I am reminded of these experiences as I reflect about the research studies reported in this book. The time is exactly right for the kind of pioneering scholarship presented here. The authors of these studies are scholars who, like Jeff Brown, are working at the frontiers of their disciplines, translating safety science into the day-to-day interactions of healthcare teams.

Healthcare is at a crucial juncture – time-honoured ways of working are insufficient to meet evolving needs of patients and society, yet new ways of working have not been invented yet. It is increasingly clear that challenges of safety, quality, cost, access and other important concerns in healthcare will be solved only from new perspectives leading to transformation of care processes. It is not sufficient to trade one goal against another. New approaches are needed that achieve all of these goals at the same time: improved safety, higher quality, lower cost, greater access and better experiences of care for patients, families and practitioners alike.

These goals will not be achieved by asking healthcare practitioners to work harder. People in healthcare are already working as hard as they can. Rather, these goals will be achieved by finding ways to work and relate *differently*. It is important to realize that 'modern scientific medical practice' is over one hundred years old. Organizational structures and practice models that were breakthroughs years ago no longer serve us well. Healthcare needs truly fresh ideas and methods. Healthcare needs innovation.

Two things are certain about innovation: it is hard work, and it is always surprising. Of course, that is the nature of innovation: by definition innovation means doing things in ways that have not been done before. Creating innovation in healthcare is exciting, hopeful, meaningful work but it is certainly not easy. If better ways of working were known and proven, clinicians would be using them already.

Many Questions

This book is about a particular kind of innovation that is needed in healthcare, the transformation from healthcare as the work of individuals, to healthcare as the work of teams. Healthcare has grown beyond the capabilities of any one individual, yet is still organized, taught and practised from deep cultures of autonomous individual effort.

Pioneering practitioners working to create teamwork in healthcare, and pioneering researchers working to understand and measure teamwork, learn quickly that there are many unanswered questions: What will optimum teamwork look like in healthcare? How should it be measured? How can it be achieved? How can it be sustained?

Understanding Teamwork

One way of understanding what optimum teamwork will look like in healthcare is to ask what happens already on our 'great days'. In any of the settings where I work, great days for me happen when I have the good fortune of working with others that I know and trust. Even when an operation is difficult or a patient very sick, everything is easier on great days. Things flow more smoothly, people intuitively understand and anticipate each other's needs, tensions are lower and there is a lot of mutual support.

There is a personal dimension as well on great days: it is satisfying to be part of a team like that, feeling that your contributions are part of something greater than yourself, with meaning and purpose. In my experience, great teamwork feels very 'alive'. By 'alive' I mean a satisfying kind of mutual engagement and intrinsic energy that feels different than 'just working'. Great teamwork should look and feel like great days, every day.

Measuring Teamwork

Based on the 'great days' approach, teamwork should be measured by variables that reflect the following characteristics: knowledge of one another, trust, flow, intuitive understanding, anticipation, lowered tension, mutual support, satisfaction, mutual engagement, meaning and purpose. If we could somehow measure 'aliveness' I would add that, too.

It is interesting that present measures of teamwork are frequently based on observations of individual behaviour. Measuring teamwork by observing individual behaviour, and focusing on individual behaviour for teamwork training and professional evaluation, may miss the essential point of teamwork which is that teamwork is about the team, not the individual. In the same way that practitioners may have difficulty moving beyond deep cultures of individual accountability in which they are trained to think and work effectively in teams, researchers trained in observing and analysing the behaviour of individuals may be challenged to break free of their training to approach the study of teamwork at the level of the team as a whole using analytical models.

Most of the papers in this book are about operating room (OR) teamwork. As a cardiac surgeon, the OR is an important part of my professional life. But I also care for patients in the intensive care unit (ICU), on the post-operative floor, and before and after their hospitalization. Each of these settings presents different challenges regarding teamwork.

In the OR, a small group of people work together in close physical proximity with a high level of intensity and focus for the duration of a several-hour operation. In the ICU, a critical-care nurse is consistently present with the patient and a respiratory therapist is close by, but other members of the care team usually do not work in consistent physical proximity except during times of crisis. Care in the

ICU requires a different kind of teamwork than the OR – coordinating information and care activities across roles and disciplines, across space and time, and among different individuals as shifts, schedules and assignments change. On the post-operative floor and in outpatient settings the challenge of coordinating care across roles, disciplines, people, space and time is different still. In each case the needs for teamwork are different, and the resources available for achieving teamwork are different.

These realities point to the need for new research approaches that consider teams inclusively with their contexts. I believe that socio-technical research approaches based on concepts of distributed cognition, situated learning and activity theory will become increasingly important for understanding healthcare teamwork and implementing teamwork across various clinical environments.

It is also possible that present methods of observing and analysing teamwork by observers trained in a particular discipline such as human factors science may give way to new methods and new insights that are likely to be achieved through the interactions of an interdisciplinary research approach. Innovation almost always arises at the edges and intersections of disciplines, rarely within the core of a discipline.

I was part of an interdisciplinary research team that analysed clinical teamwork from the intersecting perspectives of the assembled team members: a cognitive engineer, organizational psychologist, human factors scientist, anthropologist, computer scientist, communications analyst, knowledge management expert, patient advocate and surgeon. It was an extraordinary experience, as thought provoking and transformational for the research team as collaborative practice was for the clinical teams we studied.

A communications teacher once told me that, to be effective, the structure of a change message must match the desired final result. In other words, if the desired final result is teamwork, then the structure of the change message (the research that we do) must demonstrate teamwork as well. I believe that we are only just beginning to understand healthcare teamwork, and how to research it. Advances in teamwork research will proceed hand-in-hand with advances in healthcare teamwork itself.

Implementing Teamwork

If the 'great days' approach is right, teamwork in healthcare means 'working with others that I know and trust'. If so, teamwork is achieved by actions that help teams develop mutual knowledge and trust.

I am increasingly convinced that care teams develop mutual knowledge and trust more reliably through social interventions at the level of the team as a whole than by cognitive or behavioural interventions directed at individual team members. Exceptional teamwork arises when organizational structures and activities exist or are created in the local team environment that provide opportunities for mutual reflection and dialogue among team members. In my experience teams achieve exceptional teamwork by creating structures that promote interactions and establishing activities that improve relationships.

The key insight for implementing teamwork is that mutual knowledge and trust – which I believe are foundational for teamwork – are team-level resources that arise and are continually renewed over time through interactions, conversations and other relationally based experiences among team members. These and other team-level resources such as team-level ability to change and adapt are more or less likely to arise depending upon the presence or absence of supportive structural and social preconditions in the local environment. From this perspective, teamwork is socially constructed and always changing.

When we first developed our collaborative care model and received the Eisenberg Award, a number of other teams contacted us to learn from us and replicate our methods. At that time we believed our teamwork success was due to specific things we did during our collaborative rounds process based on crew resource management principles. When other teams replicated these methods they often did not achieve our results. Over time we realized that our success was the result of many small changes we had made in our team structures and routines, especially the weekly team meetings, that helped us get to know one another, understand each other's roles, motivations and contributions, and develop trust. Specific behaviours were much less important than structural changes that led to better relationships.

Sustaining Teamwork

One of the most interesting unsolved challenges regarding healthcare teamwork is how it can be sustained. This is a question of culture and how cultures change. It is important for clinicians and researchers to consider teamwork and safety with respectful awareness of the complex and powerful forces that surround clinical healthcare education and practice. Aviation reached a tipping point and successfully achieved a sustainable culture of safety, but that is a 40-year story still in evolution.

I have watched with excitement then sadness as healthcare teams train together in simulations or successfully implement teamwork in their own clinical environments, then slip inexorably back to their previous status quo in the face of overwhelming cultural and contextual forces. Most of the clinical teams I have helped or observed have been successful at first at achieving degrees of teamwork, but then gradually or suddenly lost ground later. That is the heartbreak of this otherwise joyous work.

I do not yet know how to sustain teamwork. I understand what great teamwork is like and have experienced it first hand. I know teamwork when I see it, and believe measurement is increasingly possible. I am learning how to implement teamwork and can do that reliably. But I do not know yet how to sustain teamwork. This is the state of our art: we can bring teams to life, but they do not live long.

I think the key to sustainability has to do with the nature of the connections between the local team environment and its larger organizational context. Whereas implementing teamwork depends on structures and social preconditions at the local team level, sustaining teamwork depends on the nature of the context in which the local environment exists and how it connects to the larger organization.

In my experience, creating exceptional teamwork more often than not induces an 'organizational immune response' against the transformed local team environment, as the local unit begins to function and relate within the larger organization in unfamiliar ways. The local unit is perceived as overly autonomous and out of control. High reliability teamwork may not appear to be reliable at all from a traditional hierarchical management viewpoint. In fact, it can be downright irritating.

Creating exceptional front-line teamwork disturbs the connections between the local unit and the larger organization. It affects management methods and organizational functions throughout the entire organization, far removed from the front-line team environment. It is important to recognize that teamwork threatens traditional methods of organizational operation and management. Understanding, measuring, implementing and sustaining teamwork require research and insights at all these levels.

Looking Forward

In a few years it will be clear which of the ideas and approaches described in this book will have withstood tests of time and usefulness. A direction that I believe will not withstand the test of time is a tendency to approach diagnosis and treatment as a commodity and healthcare as a transaction. I believe something very important is lost by this approach. Teamwork and safety science can be used to support a commodity approach to healthcare, but I hope they will not be used that way. One of the most powerful ways to avoid this mistake is to include the patient in our conceptualization of the team.

The most important lesson I have learned caring for patients and studying teamwork in healthcare is that healthcare comes first from the human spirit. We need to understand, measure and implement this aspect of teamwork, which I believe is the relational dimension. If we do this, I am convinced that what we achieve will stand the test of time. Think about how a single smile can brighten your day, and a single bad interaction can close the world down around you. Healthcare and teamwork are built from these moments of human connection. The essential nature of healthcare – and teamwork – is relational.

It was a pleasure being present in Edinburgh to hear these presentations first hand. It is a privilege being asked to contribute to this book. A learning community is being established through these activities, and I am excited to be part of it. A growing network of practitioners and researchers is making contributions that will change how healthcare is thought about and practised for years to come.

I am reminded of one of our former surgery residents, Prakash Pendali, at the University of Cincinnati. Something Prakash said frequently may be an appropriate final comment for this chapter. Whenever anyone asked Prakash how he was doing he always gave the same answer. He would smile and say:

Living the dream, sir!

References

The Joint Commission (2008) *John M Eisenberg award for Patient Safety*. Available at <http://www.jointcommission.org/PatientSafety/EisenbergAward/> [last accessed November 2008].

Chapter 27

Behaviour in the Operating Theatre: A Clinical Perspective

Nikki Maran and Simon Paterson-Brown

As clinicians, we have spent many thousands of hours working in operating theatres over the last 20 years. As a senior anaesthetist and surgeon, we recognize that we have a great deal of influence on the atmosphere created in the operating theatre and that our behaviour influences those around us. However, as trainees we experienced many different 'regimes' in a variety of theatres in which we were trained. There has always been a steep hierarchy within any surgical team and there was no question but that the senior surgeon was the leader. The only time this might ever have been in doubt was where there was an equally formidable theatre sister or anaesthetist in post. Voices were raised, instruments thrown, brows mopped and tears shed. These were not environments in which one questioned decision-making or challenged leadership if one wished to set foot in the operating theatre again! We tended to work in small clinical teams or 'firms' with little turnover of staff so everyone knew each other fairly well and teams became well oiled in 'routine practice'. Although few protocols as we recognize them today existed, deviation from the team routine was seldom tolerated.

Patients died, usually because they had co-existing medical disease and occasionally, due to some technical failure during surgery, at least these were the only things we measured. Occasional emergency situations arose which resulted in a patient's death and these 'unfortunate' events were often regarded as 'unavoidable' complications of surgery. Occasionally a culprit was identified and usually publically vilified in departmental mortality meetings.

As junior doctors, we provided continuity of care by working over 100 hours per week and specialist training lasted eight to ten years. The major focus of training was in the development of good technical skills and these were honed to a high level through an apprenticeship style of training by 'practising' on patients. Examinations measured knowledge and everyone knew the trainees who were 'good with their hands'. The system had massive training redundancy which gave us all plenty of time to 'absorb' the implicit skills which were not part of the curriculum – those of picking up cues in the clinical environment – Situation Awareness (SA), developing good clinical judgement – decision-making and developing our own teamwork and leadership skills by modelling our behaviours on those demonstrated to us by our seniors. Many of those who did not develop good SA or decision-making would fail to reach the senior registrar grade, however, leadership behaviours, styles of communication and modes of teamworking were more subjective. The development of non-technical skills (NTS) has therefore been an implicit, though recognized, part of the medical curriculum for generations.

Although the focus of scrutiny in health care is often on failures and adverse events, we are well aware that, in clinical practice, many potential adverse events are avoided when individuals within the team pick up and act on early warning signs. This phenomenon is recorded in studies (de Leval et al. 2000, Catchpole et al. 2007) which demonstrate that high performing teams show greater ability to recover from minor errors.

Over the last 20 years, the health service has changed enormously. Medicine and surgery have become more complex, we are able to keep frail patients alive for much longer and so our patient population is becoming older and sicker. This is well summed up by a quote from Chantler who said that where 'Medicine used to be simple, ineffective and relatively safe, now it is complex, effective and potentially dangerous' (Chantler 1999, p. 1181). We have learned from other high reliability domains and are now aware that human factors are implicated in many of the things which go wrong in hospitals and indeed in the operating theatre. Indeed, the underlying causes of adverse events in healthcare are more likely to be associated with behavioural failures than a lack of technical expertise (Bogner 1994, 2004)

Thankfully, 'bad' behaviour in the operating theatre has improved. Throwing of instruments and temper tantrums are now a thing of the past. However, a recent survey of surgical trainees in Scotland revealed that in some areas as many as 50 per cent of trainees reported experiencing bullying by senior staff which made them feel unable to express their views (National Trainee Survey 2007), and this is clearly liable to influence how likely these trainees are to speak up if they observe problems in the operating theatre. This finding is unlikely to be unique to Scotland.

Streamlining of training has reduced the number of years for specialist training and introduction of the European Working Time Directive (EWTD) and similar limits to working hours in other countries has progressively reduced the number of hours that doctors are permitted to work. While on one hand, reduction in hours of work has been demonstrated to reduce error in clinical environments (Lockley et al. 2004), the increase in shift working increases the number of handovers of complex patient care and highlights the need for good and effective communication. The reduction in hours of training time means that we no longer have the luxury of training redundancy and need to make all parts of the curriculum explicit. While this has been done well for the knowledge and technical-skill-based competencies, there is now an urgent need to define the implicit skills (such as non-technical skills) required to work in the healthcare system and to embed them into the curriculum (Glavin and Maran 2003). The fixed 'firm' team has been replaced by transient teams of individuals who may come together for only short periods and once again this highlights the need for individuals to develop portable team skills, or non-technical skills, which will equip them to work in these situations. This book brings together, for the first time, the leading researchers who are carrying out observational research in the operating theatre. We have been lucky enough to be directly involved in the work of some of these groups and have learned much from the others. It is useful, perhaps to consider how this work can be of relevance to the operating theatre clinician.

Some seminal studies (Brennan et al. 1991, Vincent et al. 2001) and government responses to these (Kohn et al. 1999, Department of Health 2000) have helped us to understand the importance of human factors in adverse events and have driven much of the patient safety agenda. All of the researchers who have contributed to this volume have helped to increase our understanding of how non-technical skills influence the way we work more specifically in the operating theatre. Increasing our understanding of where things are going wrong will help us to develop strategies to deal with these issues or to focus training on improving the situation. Although we like to think that behaviour in the operating theatre has improved over the last ten years, it is sobering to look at the findings in observational work. What is described is exactly what happens – it is just that it is so 'normal' that we don't notice how absurd our behaviour can sometimes be. Many problems in the operating theatre stem from the ineffectiveness or lack of communication (see Lingard et al., Chapter 17 in this volume). Although communication is a major component of undergraduate and postgraduate curricula, the emphasis is almost exclusively on doctor–patient or nurse–patient communication and very little if any consideration given to the importance of doctor–doctor or doctor–nurse communication. This issue is now being addressed in various safety tools which are being introduced including the WHO patient safety briefing tool (World Health Organization) and the use of SBAR (Situation, Background, Assessment, Recommendation) (Leonard et al. 2004) as part of the IHI initiatives in improving handovers.

The non-technical skills taxonomies (Fletcher et al. 2003, Yule et al. 2006) which have been developed not only give us a vocabulary with which to express and discuss non-technical skills ourselves but also a framework which can be used to give feedback to help understand where we are and improve our own non-technical skills. The definition of non-technical skills also helps to allow us to integrate these skills into curricula (Canadian Patient Safety Institute 2005, National Patient Safety Education Framework 2004) and we will increasingly see non-technical skills being incorporated into workplace-based assessment. Using these taxonomies in clinical practice (see Glavin and Patey, Chapter 11 in this volume) will help us to recognize when trainees are failing to develop good NTS early and introduce remediation. Further research is needed to explore whether this can be effective and if not, this clearly has implications for selection in the future.

Many of the research groups included in this volume are working in simulation environments. The fidelity of the training mannequins which are now available means that the simulator is the ideal place to study behaviour in emergency situations without having to wait for these unusual events to happen in real practice

(Flin and Maran 2008). The same situation can be recreated on multiple occasions to allow observation of cohorts of participants. Although human factors training can commence in the classroom, in order to develop skills, individuals need feedback on behaviours and an opportunity to practise these skills. The simulator provides an optimal environment which is safe for both patient and learner to allow observation of self and rehearsal of skills. Simulators will clearly have a role to play in helping individuals to develop the skills required in emergency situations and are also likely to have a role in 'remedial' training. The fidelity of the surgical simulators currently available is still not high enough to allow good intra-operative non-technical skills training for surgeons. However this is likely to be overcome in the next few years as the technology develops and simulators become more widely available. Transfer of skills from the simulator to clinical practice is vital and NTS frameworks such as ANTS and NOTSS are designed to give feedback in both the simulated environment and in the operating theatre.

The development of our understanding of the impact of non-technical skills on patient outcomes should also be reflected in the use of systems to analyse behaviours when errors occur such as during incident reporting and morbidity and mortality meetings. The Australian AIMS study (Webb et al. 1993) analyses critical incidents from a human factors perspective, but this methodology should be more widely used.

Challenges for the future include training trainers to become familiar with assessing and providing feedback on non-technical skill as (see Graham et al., Chapter 12 in this volume) have clearly demonstrated that inter-rater reliability of such systems is not high unless assessors are both experienced in the observation of skills and have been well calibrated. The aviation model of trainer accreditation for both teaching and assessing non-technical skills (Civil Aviation Authority 2003) is one that we can only aspire to in healthcare.

We have come a long way in healthcare over the last ten years and many of those who have contributed to this book have helped to drive this change. In the next ten years, non-technical skills will become an implicit part of the curriculum for doctors, nurses and all other health professionals involved in the delivery of healthcare. As a result, the assessment of non-technical skills will become the norm, and understanding the importance of non-technical skills in certain specialties will drive the need to identify individuals with good NTS early in training for selection to certain specialities. Future generations will find the operating theatre a very different place to work in and, as a result, ultimately a safer place for patients.

References

Bogner M. (ed.) (1994) *Human Error in Medicine.* Hillsdale, NJ: LEA.

Bogner M. (ed.) (2004) *Misadventures in Health Care.* Mahwah, NJ: LEA.

Brennan, T., Leape, L., Laird, N.M., Herbert, L., Localio, A.R., Lawthers, A.G., Newhouse, J.P., Weiler, P.C. and Hiatt, H.H. (1991) Incidence of adverse events and negligence in hospitalised patients: Results of the Harvard Medical Practice Study I. *New England Journal of Medicine* 324, 370–6.

Canadian Patient Safety Institute. (2007) *Safety Competencies Framework – Groundbreaking Project on Interprofessional Education.* Available from: <http://www.patientsafetyinstitute.ca/education/safetycompetencies.html> [last accessed March 2009].

Catchpole, K.R., Giddings, A.E., Wilkinson, M., Hirst, G., Dale T. and de Leval, M.R. (2007) Improving patient safety by identifying latent failures in successful operations. *Surgery* 142(1), 102–10.

Chantler, C. (1999) The role and education of doctors in the delivery of healthcare. *Lancet* 353, 1178–81.

Civil Aviation Authority (2003) *Crew Resource Management (CRM) Training. Guidance for Flight Crew, CRM Instructors (CRMIS) and CRM Instructor-examiners (CRMIES).* CAP 737. London: Civil Aviation Authority.

de Leval, M.R., Carthey, J., Wright D.J. and Reason, J.T. (2000) Human factors and cardiac surgery: A multicenter study. *Journal of Thoracic Cardiovascular Surgery,* 119, 661–72.

Department of Health (2000) *An Organisation with a Memory: Learning from Adverse Events in the NHS.* London: The Stationery Office.

Fletcher, G., Flin, R., McGeorge, P., Glavin, R., Maran, N. and Patey, R. (2003) Anaesthetists' Non-Technical Skills (ANTS): Evaluation of a behavioural marker system. *British Journal of Anaesthesia* 90(5), 580–8.

Flin, R. and Maran, N. (2008) Non-technical skills. In R. Riley (ed.) *Simulation in Medicine.* Oxford: Oxford University Press.

Glavin, R.J. and Maran, N.J. (2003) Integrating human factors into the medical curriculum. *Medical Education* 37(Suppl.1), 59–64.

Kohn, L, Corrigan, J and Donaldson, M. (eds) (1999) *To Err is Human. Building a Safer Healthcare System.* Washington, DC: Institute of Medicine National Academy Press.

Leonard, M., Graham, S. and Bonacum, D. (2004) The human factor: The critical importance of effective teamwork and communication in providing safe care. *Quality and Safety in Health Care* 13(Suppl 1), i85–i90.

Lockley, S., Cronin, J., Evans, E., Cade, B., Lee, C., Landrigan, C., Rothschild, J., Katz, J., Lilly, C., Stone, P., Aeschbach, D., Czeisler, C. and Harvard Work Hours, Health and Safety Group (2004) Effect of reducing interns' weekly work hours on sleep and attentional failures. *The New England Journal of Medicine* 351(18), 1829–37.

National Patient Safety Education Framework (2004) *An Initiative of the Australian Council for Safety and Quality in Health Care.* Available from: <http://www.patientsafety.org.au/framework/index.html> [last accessed 11 March 2009].

National Trainee Survey (2007) *Postgraduate Medical Education and Training Board.* Available from: <www.pmetb.org.uk/reports> [last accessed March 2009].

Safe Surgery Saves Lives (2008) *World Health Organization*. Available from: <www.who.int/patientsafety/safesurgery/> [last accessed March 2009].

Vincent, C., Neale, G. and Woloshynowych, M. (2001) Adverse events in British Hospitals: Preliminary retrospective record review. *British Medical Journa,* 322, 517–19.

Webb, R.K. Currie, M., Morgan, C.A., Williamson, J.A., Mackay, P., Russell, W.J. and Runciman, W.B. (1993) The Australian Incident Monitoring Study: An analysis of 2000 incident reports. *Anaesthesia and Intensive Care* 21(5), 520–8.

Yule, S., Flin, R., Paterson-Brown, S., Maran, N. and Rowley, D. (2006) Development of a rating system for surgeons' non-technical skills. *Medical Education* 40, 1098–104.

Index